AIDS and the
Heterosexual Population

AIDS and the
Heterosexual Population

Edited by

Lorraine Sherr
St Mary's Hospital, London, UK

hoap

harwood academic publishers
Switzerland • Australia • Belgium • France • Germany • Great Britain
India • Japan • Malaysia • Netherlands • Russia • Singapore • USA

Copyright © 1993 by Harwood Academic Publishers GmbH, Poststrasse 22,
7000 Chur, Switzerland. All rights reserved.

Harwood Academic Publishers

Private Bag 8
Camberwell, Victoria 3124
Australia

3-14-9, Okubo
Shinjuku-ku, Tokyo 169
Japan

12 Cour Saint-Eloi
75012 Paris
France

Emmaplein 5
1075 AW Amsterdam
Netherlands

Christburger Strasse II
10405 Berlin
Germany

Post Office Box 90
Reading, Berkshire RG1 8JL
Great Britain

820 Town Center Drive
Langhorne, Pennsylvania 19047
United States of America

Library of Congress Cataloging-in-Publication Data

AIDS and the heterosexual population / edited by Lorraine Sherr.
    p.   cm.
  Includes bibliographical references and index.
  ISBN 3-7186-5459-8. -- ISBN 3-7186-5460-1 (soft)
    1. AIDS (Disease)--Epidemiology.   2. AIDS (Disease)--Transmission.
  3. AIDS (Disease)--Social aspects.   4. AIDS (Disease)--Prevention.
  I. Sherr, Lorraine.
  RA644.A25A3534   1993
  614.5'993--dc20

                                                              93-29061
                                                              CIP

Contents

To
Avrom

Acknowledgements

This book evolved from many discussions and coincided with my maternity leave. Although it had no sixteen hour labour and no emergency caesarean section, it was not without its own birth traumas. Many of the usual suspects were rounded up and contributed fascinating pieces of work in an orchestra of timetabling. Chapters arrived in inverse proportion to their proximity, with those from the room next door never arriving at all! A large group of people put in tremendous effort, for which I am exceedingly grateful. Some worked despite difficult conditions, and I give especial thanks to Lee Strunin.

Academic pursuit is often facilitated by the help and encouragement of many people. I owe a special tribute to inspirational individuals particularly Professor Don Jefferies, Professor Catherine Peckham, Professor Ruben Sher and Dr Peter Exon. Ari Ilan Yonatan and Liora played their part and tiptoed around the scatter during the embryonic period of the book. Ester listened and Jaqui smiled. Yet much of my inspiration, as always, comes from those who teach by example, such as Sue, Karen, Sarah, Rose and David — a few stars in a constellation.

Contributors

KAREN BARLOW
Infectious Diseases Unit, City Hospital, Edinburgh, UK

ROBERT BOR
City Univeristy, London, UK

PETER DAVIS
Project Sigma, Department of Social Sciences, The University of the South Bank, London, UK

CHARLES ERIN
The Centre for Social Ethics and Policy, Manchester University, UK

SAMUEL R FRIEDMAN
Narcotic and Drug Research, National Development & Research Institutes Inc, New York, USA

JOHAN GIESECKE
Huddinge University Hospital, Sweden

ELEANOR GOLDMAN
Katherine Dormandy Haemophilia Centre and Haemostasis Unit, The Royal Free Hampstead NHS Trust, London, UK

MARJORIE GOLDSTEIN
Narcotic and Drug Research, National Development & Research Institutes Inc, New York, USA

CATHERINE HANKINS
Centre for AIDS Studies, Department of Community Health, Montreal General Hospital, Canada

JOHN HARRIS
The Centre for Social Ethics and Policy, Manchester University, UK

RALPH HINGSON
Boston University, School of Public Health Social and Behavioural Science, USA

DON DES JARLAIS
Chemical Dependency Institute, Beth Israel Medical Center, New York, USA

BENNY JOSE
Narcotic and Drug Research, National Development & Research Institutes Inc, New York, USA

DONNA LAMPING
Academic Department of Public Health, Parkside Health Authority, and London School of Hygiene and Tropical Medicine, London, UK

RIVA MILLER
District AIDS/HIV Counselling Service, The Royal Free Hampstead NHS Trust, London, UK

JACQUELINE MOK
Infectious Diseases Unit, City Hospital, Edinburgh, UK

ALAN NEAIGUS
Narcotic and Drug Research, National Development & Research Institutes Inc, New York, USA

NANCY S PADIAN
University of California, San Francisco, Dept of Epidemiology & Biostatistics, USA

MARTIN PLANT
Alcohol Research Group, Department of Psychiatry, University of Edinburgh, UK

SUSAN QUINN
AIDS Unit, Swandean Hospital, Sussex, UK

KRISTINA RAMSTEDT
Department of Dermato-Venereology, Gothenburg University, Sweden

MICHAEL ROSS
Center for Health Education Research and Development, School of Public Health, University of Texas at Houston, USA

ITESH SACHDEV
Department of Applied Linguistics, Birkbeck College, London, UK

LORRAINE SHERR
St Mary's Hospital, London, UK

GERRY STIMSON
Centre for Research on Drugs & Health Behaviour, London, UK

LEE STRUNIN
Boston University, School of Public Health Social and Behavioural Science, USA

PAUL TURNBULL
Centre for Research on Drugs & Health Behaviour, London, UK

THOMAS P WARD
Narcotic and Drug Research, National Development & Research Institutes Inc, New York, USA

PETER WEATHERBURN
Project Sigma, Department of Social Sciences, The University of the South Bank, London, UK

JANNEKE H H M VAN DE WIJGERT
University of California, San Francisco, Dept of Epidemiology & Biostatistics, USA

DAVID WILSON
Department of Psychology, University of Zimbabwe, Zimbabwe

Introduction

Innumerable outstanding achievements have been made in the quest against Human Immunodeficiency Virus (HIV) and the associated Acquired Immune Deficiency Syndrome (AIDS). Yet despite such advances there is still a long way to go. The most spectacular headway has been in the true utilisation of interdisciplinary and multidisciplinary approaches to the many hurdles created by HIV infection and AIDS. As with all progress, the gaps are usually more startling than the progress. In AIDS a skewed focus has often resulted in disproportionate information, attention and understanding for some groups, some approaches and some solutions at the expense of a more comprehensive approach.

It is into this niche that this text on AIDS in the heterosexual community has emerged. In addition this text is an attempt to present a comprehensive examination of the psychological and sociological ramifications of HIV disease for this group. It is surprising that so many years have evolved without direct study of the group given that they comprise the largest numbers, worldwide, of people affected with and by HIV. It may be that they do not fall naturally into a group but are comprised of sub groups, overlapping and interweaving with such specific nuances that a global, general picture is difficult to formulate. On the other hand cynics may note that the group as a whole contains the most disenfranchised, the most powerless, the most disadvantaged and the most needy. Their voices may not be heard in the clamour, their needs may not be foremost in the overwhelming rush and their problems may be so enormous that they anaesthetise the observer.

The individual chapters in this text provide a wide coverage of problems either generally or specifically targeted at one of a number of facets of the heterosexual population. There are issues beyond those covered here, but it should stand as a comprehensive psychosocial text. Each chapter attempts to provide a systematic overview from a psychosocial standpoint, and to examine, where appropriate, theoretical and practical implications for future care and planning.

The book provides an initial overview of the epidemiology of heterosexual transmission of HIV (van de Wijgert and Padian) exploring current knowledge on male-female and female-male transmission rates and a range of possible cofactors in such transmission including sexual practices, contraception and biological factors. Hankins (chapter 2) then gives a thorough account of HIV infection and women, which represents a fast growing sector. Studies of women have suffered from a history of neglect. This chapter outlines epidemiology, transmission, natural history, psychosocial issues and prevention. Drug injectors have been affected by HIV infection both through their drug using and their sexual behaviour. Friedman, Des Jarlais and coworkers (chapter 3) give a comprehensive account of the problems and challenges for this disparate group, both in the west and east. They provide a detailed examination of behavioural factors associated with HIV transmission for drug users worldwide and examine prevention and intervention. Wilson (chapter 4) provides a challenging chapter on the role of prevention within heterosexual prostitution. He examines the varying international roles, life style factors and barriers presented by this group with a critique of prevention initiatives. Sherr (chapter 5) examines the particular circumstances experienced by discordant couples not only in terms of transmission factors and transmission risks, but also in terms of psychological and reproductive problems which may confront those within such dyads, such as disclosure, support and bereavement. Miller and Goldman (chapter 6) provide an overview of similar issues as they apply to those affected by both HIV and haemophilia. As the epidemic progresses, there are a growing number of children both infected and affected by HIV. Given that the majority are infected vertically there are specific issues associated with HIV and children (Barlow and Mok chapter 7). Similarly adolescents, with their emerging adulthood and sexuality, represent the challenge of tomorrow in terms of prevention and education (Strunin and Hingson chapter 8). Bor (chapter 9) explores the growing need to examine HIV infection in terms of the family — however broadly this is defined. This approach allows for an understanding at the systems level in terms of relationships, stress, coping, support, communication and response. Weatherburn and Davies (chapter 10) examine the issues of behavioural bisexuality among men. They provide an examination of the prevalence and implications this may have for HIV disease.

It is important to focus on situational factors as well as individual or group factors as they provide a broader understanding of HIV disease. Turnbull and Stimson (chapter 11) examine the role of prisons as a risk environment for heterosexual spread of HIV infection in terms of risk behaviours and populations within the population and the prison's response which may hinder, encourage or ignore prevention efforts. Sherr and Quinn (chapter 12) critically examine the effects of HIV counselling and testing on behaviour change. This serves not only as an overview of the range of outcome behaviours measured globally, but also as an insight into the uses and limitations of some counselling approaches. The theme of psychological needs and services is carried forward in chapter 13 (Lamping and

Sachdev). Plant (chapter 14) provides an overview of situational use of alcohol and how this may have implications for sexual behaviour and AIDS. This wide array of topics then draws on the chapter by Erin and Harris (Chapter 15) who examine the role of ethics and ethical dilemmas which relate directly to the heterosexual population. They examine the notion of AIDS providing a "gender neutral" threat and how this may interact with justice and individual responsibility. Ross and Kelaher (chapter 16) provide an overview of the vast array of knowledge, attitude and behaviour studies which seems to overwhelm much of the research. Finally Ramstedt and Gieseck (chapter 17) examine the difficult issues of partner management in HIV infection.

This book should hopefully provide a point from which much more in-depth study can evolve. As the world grows weary of the drama of AIDS, overwhelmed by the impact of AIDS and saturated with the messages of AIDS, the time has come to look back critically in order to forge relevant longer term strategy. The way forward must utilise broad based knowledge, lateral approaches and an integration of the psychological, social and medical.

Lorraine Sherr

1

Heterosexual Transmission of HIV

JANNEKE H.H.M. VAN DE WIJGERT AND
NANCY S. PADIAN

DESCRIPTIVE EPIDEMIOLOGY OF HETEROSEXUAL TRANSMISSION OF HIV

Though the actual number of people infected with human immunodeficiency virus (HIV) by heterosexual transmission remains relatively low in Europe and the United States, it is the fastest growing risk group. The percentage of AIDS cases attributed to heterosexual contact with persons known to be HIV infected or at increased risk for HIV infection, excluding persons who were born in pattern II countries, increased steadily from 0.9% in the first quarter of 1983, to 5.2% in the third quarter of 1992 (CDC, 1992). The percentage of new cases attributed to heterosexual contact reported from October 1990 to September 1991 was 6.4%, and from October 1991 to September 1992 was 7.8% (CDC, 1992). Similar patterns are seen in Europe where now 11% of the cases acquired their infection through heterosexual transmission (Downs, Ancelle-Park & Brunet, 1990). In contrast, as much as 80% of HIV infection in Africa is acquired heterosexually (N'Galy & Ryder, 1988; Quinn, Mann, Curran & Piot, 1986).

This chapter discusses the efficiency of male-to-female and female-to-male sexual transmission of HIV and the factors that influence these transmission rates.

HETEROSEXUAL SPREAD OF HIV: THE LIKELIHOOD OF CHOOSING AN INFECTED PARTNER

The likelihood of sexual transmission of HIV depends first on the likelihood of choosing an HIV infected partner (who is infectious) and then on the likelihood of transmission given exposure. The probability of choosing an infected partner depends on the rate of new partner acquisition: the greater number of new partners a susceptible person has per unit time the more likely it is that one partner is infected. In most parts of the world, the prevalence of HIV is higher is certain high risk groups, such as prostitutes, homo- and bisexual men and intravenous drug users, but relatively low in the population at large. Choosing large numbers of partners from the low risk population might then be less significant than choosing few partners from one of these high risk groups (Brunham, 1991; Padian, Shiboski & Hitchcock, 1991). Thus, it also matters who your partners are in addition to how many you have. The potential for spread of HIV into the population at large depends on the sexual interaction between members of high risk groups and persons from the population at large, as well as on the efficiency of sexual transmission from male-to-female and from female-to-male (Anderson & May, 1988).

MALE-TO-FEMALE TRANSMISSION RATES

The first reports of HIV transmission from HIV infected males to their female sex partners were published from 1982 to 1984 (CDC, 1983; Harris *et al.*, 1983; Masur, Michelis & Wormser, 1982; Pitchenik, Fischi and Spira, 1983; Pitchenik, Shafron, Glasser & Spira, 1984; Ratnoff, Lederman & Jenkins, 1984; Redfield *et al.*, 1985a). Several later studies have examined the efficiency of male-to-female transmission (table 1.1). In these studies, the rates of HIV infection among female sexual partners were examined by risk group of the male index case. The rates range from 0 to 21% among the female sex-partners of haemophiliacs, 18 to 25% among the female partners of patients with transfusion-associated AIDS or HIV infection, 19 to 32% among the female partners of bisexual men, and 14 to 42% among the female partners of intravenous drug users (table 1.1). In a Belgian study, the transmission rate among the partners of men who acquired their infection in Central Africa was 53%. Similar transmission rates have been observed in studies among Africans in central Africa (reviewed in N'Galy *et al.*, 1988; Quinn *et al.*, 1986).

The data in table 1.1 suggest that the mode by which the index case acquired HIV infection may influence the likelihood that a person will transmit HIV to a sex partner, although this is not a universal finding. Female partners of intravenous drug users or men who acquired their infection through heterosexual contact in Africa seem more likely to be HIV positive than are female partners of haemophilic men or transfusion recipients. However, these female partners may also be more likely to have multiple routes of exposure to HIV. Additional routes of exposure include exposure to infected needles, and having other high risk partners outside of

Table 1.1:
Partner studies of the sexual transmission of HIV from men to women,
Europe and the United States

Major risk factor in male index case	No. Pos/total	(%)	Place	Reference
Haemophiliac	2/21	(9.5)	U.S.A.	(Kreiss, 1985)
Haemophiliac	2/33	(6)	U.S.A.	(Jason, 1986)
Haemophiliac	10/148	(6.8)	France	(Allain, 1986)
Haemophiliac	4/24	(17)	U.S.A.	(Goedert, 1987)
Haemophiliac	4/19	(21)	U.S.A.	(Padian, 1987)
Haemophiliac	77/772	(10)	U.S.A.	(CDC, 1987)
Haemophiliac	1/14	(7)		(Kim, 1988)
Haemophiliac	0/35	(0)	Netherl.	(Van der Ende, 1988)
Haemophiliac	5/46	(10)	U.S.A.	(Lawrence, 1988)
Haemophiliac	6/45	(13)	U.S.A.	(Ragni, 1989)
Haemophiliac	1/10	(10)	Europe	(ESG, 1992)
Blood transfusion	1/4	(25)	U.S.A.	(Padian, 1987)
Blood transfusion	10/55	(18)	U.S.A.	(Peterman, 1988)
Blood transfusion	3/13	(23)	Europe	(ESG, 1992)
Bisexual	12/55	(22)	U.S.A.	(Padian, *et al.*, 1987)
Bisexual	4/21	(19)	U.K.	(Johnson, 1989)
Bisexual	21/65	(32)	Europe	(ESG, 1992)
IV druguser	5/12	(42)	U.S.A.	(Padian, 1987)
IV druguser	7/50	(14)	U.K.	(Johnson, 1989)
IV druguser	90/325	(27.7)	Italy	(Lazzarin, 1991)
IV druguser	46/250	(18)	Europe	(ESG, 1992)
Mixed	13/22	(59)	Italy	(Luzi, 1985)
Mixed	14/28	(50)	U.S.A.	(Fischl, 1987)
Mixed	22/97	(23)	U.S.A.	(Padian, 1987)
Mixed	15/78	(19)	U.K.	(Johnson, 1989)
Mixed	42/155	(27)	Europe	(ESG, 1989)
Mixed	99/368	(27.7)	Italy	(Lazzarin, 1991)
Mixed	82/404	(20)	Europe	(ESG, 1992)
Mixed, 87% heterosex. contact Africa	34/64	(53)	Belgium	(Laga, 1989)
Heterosexual	40/70	(57)	Kenya	(Moss, 1991)

the studied relationship. Furthermore, the presence of cofactors (discussed below) may be different among the different risk groups and could explain in part the observed transmission rate differences.

The risk of acquiring HIV from a single heterosexual contact with an infected man for a woman is not known, but has been estimated to be between 1 per 1,000 to 1 per 100 sexual contacts (Grant, Wiley & Winkelstein, 1987; Hearst & Hulley, 1988; Holmberg, Horsburgh, Ward & Jaffe, 1989; Padian *et al.*, 1987; Piot *et al.*, 1987a). The probability of transmission is however highly dependent on individual variations in infectivity or susceptibility and the presence of other cofactors, as discussed below.

FEMALE-TO-MALE TRANSMISSION RATES

Female-to-male transmission of HIV was documented in 1985 (Calabrese & Gopalakrishna, 1986; Polk, 1985; Redfield *et al.*, 1985b). Some of these early studies were controversial because they included persons who may not acknowledge other risk factors for acquiring HIV. Redfield's study in military recruits for example, has been heavily criticized because military recruits face the possibility of discharge from military service for homosexuality and/or intravenous drug use and are therefore less likely to report these behaviours (Polk, 1985; Schultz, Milberg, Kristal & Stoneburner, 1986; Wykoff, 1986).

Because relatively few women are infected at this point in the epidemic in the United States and Europe, male partners of infected women (who have no other risk factors for HIV infection such as intravenous drug use) are relatively rare. Thus studies of female-to-male transmission in these countries are based on small numbers, making generalizations uncertain (ESG, 1992; Johnson *et al.*, 1989). Female-to-male transmission has been studied more extensively in Africa, mostly among prostitutes (Kreiss *et al.*, 1986; Mann *et al.*, 1988; Moss *et al.*, 1991; Nzila *et al.*, 1991; Simonsen *et al.*, 1990) and women attending prenatal care clinics (Allen *et al.*, 1991a,b).

Table 2 shows female-to-male transmission rates from several studies that enrolled female index cases and their male sexual partners. Transmission rates vary from 0% to 33% with the exception of two studies that found extraordinarily high transmission rates (61% and 71%) (Fischl *et al.*, 1987; Pape, Stanback & Pamphile, 1987). Although transmission rates may differ depending on the study, the fact that male-to-female transmission is more efficient than female-to-male transmission is an almost universal finding in Europe and the United States (table 1.1 and table 1.2). The risk of acquiring HIV from a single heterosexual contact from an infected

Table 2:
Studies of the heterosexual transmission of HIV from women to men

Major risk factor female index case	No. pos/total	(%)	Place	Reference
Artif. insemin.	0/4	(0)	Australia	(Stewart, 1985)
Blood transfusion	2/25	(8)	U.S.A.	(Peterman, 1988)
Blood transfusion	0/4	(0)	Arabia	(Al-Nozha, 1990)
Blood transfusion	3/9	(33)	Europe	(ESG, 1992)
IV druguser	1/17	(6)	U.K.	(Johnson, 1989)
IV druguser	13/99	(13)	Europe	(ESG, 1992)
Mixed	1/76	(1.3)	U.S.A.	(Padian, 1992)
Mixed	12/17	(71)	U.S.A.	(Fischl, 1987)
Mixed	23/38	(61)	Haiti	(Pape, 1987)
Mixed	1/18	(5.6)	U.K.	(Johnson, 1989)
Mixed	19/159	(12)	Europe	(ESG, 1992)
Mixed, 69% heterosex. contact Africa	2/16	(13)	Belgium	(Laga, 1989)

woman to a man is estimated to be anywhere from twice to twenty time less likely than transmission from men to women (ESG, 1992; Laga *et al.*, 1989; Padian, Shiboski & Jewell, 1991; Rehmet *et al.*, 1992).

THE LIKELIHOOD OF HIV TRANSMISSION GIVEN EXPOSURE: COFACTORS FOR HETEROSEXUAL TRANSMISSION probability.

After choosing an infected partner, the likelihood of sexual transmission depends on the likelihood of transmission given exposure. Although some people become infected after one or just a few sexual encounters, others remain uninfected after hundreds of unprotected sexual contacts (Brown, Siddiqui, Phillips & Ajulu-chukwu, 1992; Johnson *et al.*, 1989; Padian, Shiboski & Jewell, 1989; Padian, Wiley, Glass, Marquis & Winkelstein, 1988; Peterman, Stoneburner, Allen, Jaffe & Curran, 1988; Sion *et al.*, 1992). These observations imply that certain cofactors can affect the likelihood of sexual HIV transmission. The likelihood of HIV transmission given exposure, depends on three factors: infectiousness of the index case, susceptibility of the partner, and cofactors that modify either the infectiousness of the host or the susceptibility of the partner.

The exact biological mechanism of heterosexual transmission, from man to woman and from woman to man, is still unknown. HIV has been cultured from both semen (Ho *et al.*, 1984; Zagury *et al.*, 1984), and vaginal/cervical secretions of symptomatic and asymptomatic subjects (Vogt *et al.*, 1986; Wofsy *et al.*, 1986). It has been hypothesized that for male-to-female transmission, contact between HIV in semen and the target cells present on the mucosa of the vagina, cervix, endometrium, or rectum can result in transmission (Miller & Scofield, 1989). Transmission of HIV by HIV positive semen used for artificial insemination, indicates that the virus can be transmitted without trauma of the mucosa and without other bodily contact (Stewart *et al.*, 1985). It seems likely however, that trauma or inflammation of the mucosa will facilitate viral entry. A study in Rwanda showed that lymphocytes are the major source of HIV in cervicovaginal secretions of infected women (van de Perre *et al.*, 1988). Conditions that increase the lymphocyte population in the female genital tract, such as other sexually transmitted diseases (STDs), chronic inflammation of the cervix, and menstruation may facilitate male-to-female transmission of HIV during sexual intercourse. In addition, conditions that increase the concentration of virus in semen, such as later stages of disease, might increase male-to-female transmission (Simmonds, 1990).

Female-to-male transmission could take place when virus is shed in the vagina and cervix of the infected woman and enters target cells on the penis of the male partner. Conditions that influence viral shedding in the vagina and cervix, such as stage of disease, phase of the menstrual cycle, and inflammation, might influence female-to-male transmission. Conditions that enhance viral entry into the male are less clear. Minor abrasions on the penis due to certain STDs or trauma during sex, might enhance transmission. Direct contact with (menstrual) blood of an HIV infected women, with or without lesions on the penis, might also increase the probability of transmission but this remains uncertain.

Cofactors of sexual HIV transmission that have been studied so far can be divided into three groups (table 1.3): sexual practices, contraceptive practices, and biological factors that influence infectivity as well as susceptibility.

COFACTORS IN TRANSMISSION: SEXUAL PRACTICES

The practice of anal intercourse has shown to increase the risk of male-to-female HIV transmission in a number of studies (ESG, 1989; ESG, 1992; Guimaraes *et al.*, 1992; Lazzarin, Saracco, Musicco & Nicolosi, 1991; Padian *et al.*, 1987). Couples who engaged in anal sex were 2–6 times more likely to be concordant than couples who did not. In studies that did not find an increased risk with anal intercourse, the number of couples who engaged in anal intercourse was too small to reach adequate statistical power to detect associations (Fischl *et al.*, 1987; Johnson *et al.*, 1989; Peterman *et al.*, 1988). There is no evidence for an increased risk of

Table 1.3:
Factors associated with heterosexual transmission of HIV

Factor	Male-to-female	Female-to-male
SEXUAL PRACTICES		
anal intercourse	yes	no
oral intercourse	no	no
sex during menses	no	yes
bleeding from trauma	possibly	possibly
number of sexual contacts	yes	yes
number of exposures	yes	yes
CONTRACEPTIVE PRACTICES		
lack of condoms	yes	yes
oral contraceptives	possibly	unknown
IUD use	possibly	unknown
spermicides	possibly	possibly
BIOLOGICAL FACTORS		
lack of male circumcision	possibly	yes
advanced disease state	yes	yes
variations in viral strain	possibly	possibly
host immunological profile	possibily	unknown
genital sores, infections		
or inflammations	yes	yes
cervical ectopy	yes	unknnown
smoking	possibly	unknown
AZT	yes	unknown

female-to-male transmission with the practice of anal intercourse (ESG, 1992; Simonsen *et al.*, 1988). Several biological mechanisms have been proposed to explain why HIV is transmitted more efficiently during anal intercourse than during vaginal intercourse. One of these proposed mechanisms is that anal intercourse often causes mucosal lesions in the rectum of the woman which may facilitate entry of the virus.

In contrast, the majority of studies in heterosexual populations failed to find any association between oral sex and transmission of HIV (ESG, 1989; ESG, 1992; Johnson *et al.*, 1989; Mann *et al.*, 1988; Nzila *et al.*, 1991; Padian *et al.*, 1987; Peterman *et al.*, 1988; Ragni, Kingsley, Nimorwicz, Gupta and Rinaldo, 1989). The practice of oral sex however, is likely to be confounded by the practices of anal and vaginal sex and should therefore be studied in couples who exclusively engage in oral sex. These couples are extremely difficult to find.

It has been hypothesized that sexual intercourse during menses might put women and their partners at increased risk for HIV infection. The vaginal secretion of a healthy non-menstruating reproductive-aged woman is acidic and presents a hostile environment for HIV particles and infected lymphocytes. Vaginal pH is higher (less acidic) in postpartum, postmenopausal, and menstruating women, which could cause these women to be more susceptible and more infectious to their sexual partners (Guinee, 1992). Mucosal alterations and alterations in local immunity in the female genital tract during menses might also influence a woman's susceptibility and infectiousness. However, no associations have been found between sex during menses and male-to-female transmission (Allen *et al.*, 1991a; Castelli *et al.*, 1992; ESG, 1989; Johnson *et al.*, 1989; Lazzarin *et al.*, 1991; Mann *et al.*, 1988; Moss *et al.*, 1991; Nzila *et al.*, 1991; Ragni *et al.*, 1989; Siraprapasiri *et al.*, 1991). In contrast, the European Study Group on heterosexual transmission of HIV found that female-to-male transmission was 3.4 times more likely in couples who engaged in sex during menses (ESG, 1992).

Bleeding during sex from trauma has been reported as a risk factor for heterosexual transmission (Allen *et al.*, 1991a; ESG, 1989; Padian and Shiboski, 1992) but has not been studied extensively. Pain during intercourse (ESG, 1992) and defloration by an HIV infected partner (Bouvet, De Vicenzi, Ancelle & Vachon, 1989) could facilitate transmission via similar mechanisms.

COFACTORS IN TRANSMISSION: CONTRACEPTIVE PRACTICES

Most epidemiological studies have shown that consistent and correct condom use is protective (ESG, 1989; Fischl, Lai, Strickman-Stein and Resnick, 1992; Fischl *et al.*, 1987; Guimaraes *et al.*, 1992; Lazzarin *et al.*, 1991; Mann *et al.* 1988; Moss *et al.*, 1991; Nzila *et al.*, 1991; Padian *et al.*, 1992; Siraprapasiri *et al.*, 1991). Laboratory tests (van de Perre, Jacobs & Sprecher-Goldberger, 1987) and human studies (ESG, 1989; Mann, Quinn & Piot, 1987; Peterman *et al.*, 1988; Roumeliotou, Papautsakis, Kallinikos & Papeyanegelou, 1988; Smith & Smith, 1986) have shown that condoms can prevent exposure to the virus during sexual intercourse and reduce the risk of transmission. Alcohol and drug use decrease the likelihood that couples will use condoms and can therefore indirectly increase the likelihood of HIV infection (Allen *et al.*, 1991a).

The role of oral contraceptive use in heterosexual HIV transmission remains controversial. Some studies have detected an increased risk of acquiring HIV infection (Allen, *et al.*, 1991a; Boschi *et al.*, 1992; Chao *et al.*, 1992; Guimaraes, *et al.*, 1992; Hitti *et al.*, 1992; Kapiga *et al.*, 1992; Moss *et al.*, 1991; Simonsen *et al.*, 1990), others have found no association (Boulos *et al.*, 1990; ESG, 1989; Latif *et al.*, 1989; Moss *et al.*, 1991; Nzila *et al.*, 1991; Siraprapasiri *et al.*, 1991) and one study has actually found a protective effect (Lazzarin *et al.*, 1991). Because the use of oral contraceptives could simply be a marker for lack of condom use, all these studies were controlled for condom use. In a study among Nairobi prostitutes, there appeared to be a dose-response relationship: of 85 women who never used oral contraceptives 60% seroconverted, compared with 76% of 21 women who used intermittently and 89% of 18 women who used throughout the study period (Moss *et al.*, 1991).

Oral contraceptives might alter the thickness of the cervical mucus and the cell mediated immunity in the female genital tract. Women who use oral contraceptives are also known to be at higher risk for acquisition of chlamydia and candida infections (Tait, Rees, Hobson, Byng & Tweedie, 1980), and the same phenomenon could hold true for HIV. A third possibility is a direct immunosuppressive effect of oral contraception, making women more susceptible to HIV (Grossman, 1985).

Another hypothesis has to do with the association between oral contraceptives and cervical ectopy. A study in Kenya showed that cervical ectopy (defined as at least 10% of the ectocervix upon pelvic examination) was a strong risk factor of acquiring HIV infection in wives of HIV positive men (Moss *et al.*, 1991). It has been hypothesized that oestrogen-containing oral contraceptives can increase the frequency and the size of the area of ectopy. Cervical ectopy was present in 88% of the women who used oral contraceptives (7/8), compared with 51% of the women who did not use oral contraceptives (30/59). The possibility that HIV infection caused the ectopy could not be excluded. Prospective studies are needed to determine the independent associations of oral contraceptive use, chlamydia infection and cervical ectopy on HIV transmission.

Use of intrauterine devices might increase the risk of HIV infection (Lazzarin *et al.*, 1991) but more studies are needed to confirm this finding. The possible biological mechanism is that intrauterine devices provoke a stable local inflammatory state of the uterine mucosa which could predispose to infections. Chronic inflammation of the uterus subsequently increases the lymphocyte population in the female genital tract, and therefore the number of target cells for HIV as proposed earlier.

A study in Zaire showed that prostitutes who inserted products for douching, lubrication, pregnancy prevention, or menstrual care into the vagina, were significantly more likely to be seropositive than prostitutes who did not. No single practice was associated with HIV seropositivity (Mann *et al.*, 1988). The prostitutes also reported inserting substances to 'tighten' the vagina. Additional reports show that women from certain ethnic groups in Africa insert substances into the vagina, such as certain leaves, to enhance sexual stimulation for themselves and their partners (Brown, Brown & Ayowa, 1992; Jingu *et al.*, 1992). These substances could provoke inflammatory reactions and epithelial damage and could therefore facilitate HIV transmission.

Similarly, douching and tampon use might cause damage to the vaginal or cervical mucosa. These practices are very common in Europe and the United States, but have yet not been studied in detail.

COFACTORS IN TRANSMISSION: BIOLOGICAL FACTORS

Sexually Transmitted Diseases (STDs)

The relationship between HIV infection and other STDs is very complex. STDs could facilitate HIV transmission and accelerate HIV disease progression. HIV infection could increase susceptibility to other STDS and alter their natural history and response to therapy (Wasserheit, 1992). In this chapter, the influence of STDs on the transmission of HIV will be reviewed.

The conclusion of a recently published review of 163 studies on the interrelationships between HIV infection and other STDs (Wasserheit, 1992) was that both ulcerative and non-ulcerative STDs increase the risk of HIV transmission 3- to 5-fold after adjustment for sexual behaviour. This relative risk was based on the review of 8 prospective or nested case-control studies and 17 cross-sectional case-control studies that adjusted for sexual behaviour in a multivariate analysis.

Several methodologic issues were discussed in these studies. First of all, the presence of a STD could be a marker for the practice of high risk behaviours, such as lack of condom use and having large numbers of sexual partners. As mentioned above, the association persists when adjusted for these behaviours. The often very strong associations between STDs and HIV infection in Africa, where many of the studies were performed, could be confounded by exposure to unsterilized needles for the treatment of STDs. However, after adjustment for injections and other cofactors of HIV transmission in Africa, the association persists.

From retrospective and cross-sectional studies it is hard to determine whether the presence of a STD enhanced HIV transmission or whether HIV infection rendered someone more susceptible to infection with STDs. Genital warts, vaginitis, cervicitis and candidiasis could all be early signs of immunologic impairment induced by HIV infection (Fischl *et al.*, 1987; Lazzarin *et al.*, 1991). Evidence for the causal relationship between increased risk of HIV transmission and ulcerative STDs comes from prospective studies. Two prospective studies in the United States have shown that genital herpes preceded seroconversion for HIV antibody in homosexual men (Holmberg, *et al.*, 1988; Stamm *et al.*, 1988), and a prospective cohort study in prostitutes in Nairobi showed that genital ulcers were independently associated with an increased risk for HIV seroconversion (Plummer *et al.*, 1990). These studies suggest that genital ulcers increase susceptibility to HIV infection. Another study in

Kenya suggests that people with HIV who also have genital ulceration are more infectious than people with HIV but without genital ulceration. Four hundred and twenty two men who had acquired a STD from a group of prostitutes in Nairobi with a prevalence of HIV infection of 85%, were followed prospectively (Cameron *et al.*, 1989). Twenty four of 293 initially HIV negative men seroconverted and all of them had also acquired genital ulcers. The association between HIV seroconversion and acquisition of a genital ulcer was significant with a relative risk of 4.7. According to the authors, these men had been exposed to genital ulcer disease and HIV simultaneously, suggesting that prostitutes with genital ulcers were more infectious.

Data on the association between non-ulcerative STDs, such as gonorrhoea, chlamydia and trichomoniasis, and HIV infection are far more limited. The prevalence of non-ulcerative STDs is much higher than the prevalence of ulcerative STDs. If non-ulcerative STDs facilitate HIV infection, many HIV infections will be attributable to them. Two prospective studies in African prostitutes did find an increased risk of HIV seroconversion with chlamydia cervicitis (Laga, Nzila & Manoka, 1990; Moss *et al.*, 1991) but two case-control studies did not (Hayes, Manaloto & Basaca-Sevilla, 1990; Simonsen *et al.*, 1990). Similarly, the association between gonorrhoea and HIV seroconversion (Figueroa *et al.*, 1992; Kreiss *et al.*, 1986; Laga *et al.*, 1990; Piot *et al.*, 1987b) and trichomoniasis and HIV seroconversion (Hayes *et al.*, 1990; Laga *et al.*, 1990) remains controversial because of inconsistent results.

STDs in the woman may increase male-to-female transmission rates by damaging the mucosal epithelium of the female genital tract or increasing the number of target cells for HIV on the mucosa. STDs in the man may increase male-to-female transmission by increased viral shedding from the lesions caused by the STD (Latif *et al.*, 1989), although men who have severe lesions are less likely to have sexual intercourse (Cameron *et al.*, 1989). Analogous biological mechanisms have been postulated to explain female-to-male transmission in the presence of STDs. HIV has been isolated from the surface of genital ulcers in HIV infected women, which suggests that women might be more infectious when ulcers are present (Cameron *et al.*, 1989; Kreiss *et al.*, 1989).

Genital ulcers in the man might provide a direct portal of entry for the virus. Furthermore, repeated STD-related activation of T-lymphocytes could increase the susceptibility to HIV infection for both men and women (Quinn *et al.*, 1987). If STDs facilitate the transmission of HIV and if HIV infection prolongs the infectiousness of persons with STDs, these infections may greatly amplify each other.

Circumcision

Lack of circumcision as a risk factor was first observed in a study of Nairobi prostitutes and their clients (Cameron *et al.*, 1989) and among men attending a STD clinic in Nairobi, Kenya (Greenblatt *et al.*, 1988). However, lack of circumcision was not an independent risk factor: it was highly associated with a history of genital ulceration. Another study among men attending a STD clinic in

Nairobi showed an interesting relationship between circumcision, genital ulcers and HIV. In uncircumcised men the increased risk of HIV infection was independent of the occurrence of genital ulcer disease. Among circumcised men, a history of genital ulcer disease was strongly associated with HIV seropositivity (Simonsen *et al.*, 1988).

Lack of circumcision could be a risk factor for both male-to-female and female-to-male transmission. Evidence for the association with female-to-male transmission comes from studies in clients of prostitutes and men attending a STD clinic in Nairobi (Cameron *et al.*, 1989; Greenblatt *et al.*, 1988; Hellmann *et al.*, 1992; Simonsen *et al.*, 1988; Tyndall *et al.*, 1992). The association with male-to-female transmission is more controversial. Several studies among African women have failed to show an association (Allen *et al.*, 1991a; Carael *et al.*, 1988; Moss *et al.*, 1991) but data are limited. An ecological study compared the prevalence of circumcision with the prevalence of HIV infection in different regions in Africa and found a high correlation (Bongaarts, Reining, Way & Conant, 1989).

How the foreskin increases susceptibility to HIV is uncertain. Several mechanisms have been proposed. The prepuce could trap infected vaginal secretions and provide an environment in which the virus can survive. The intact foreskin provides a larger surface area of contact with infected secretions and may be more susceptible to trauma during sexual intercourse (Stone, Grimes, Magder *et al.*, 1986). Also, minor inflammatory conditions, that attract HIV target cells to the epithelium or can act as a portal of virus entry, are more common in uncircumcised men (Parker, Stewart, Wren *et al.*, 1983; Piot, Duncan, van Dyck *et al.*, 1986).

Viral Load

Laboratory studies show that virus load (the proportion of provirus bearing and virus expressing peripheral blood mononuclear cells and levels of circulating free virus) is usually higher in persons with AIDS related complex or AIDS than for asymptomatic persons. But it is also clear that there are considerable interindividual differences in virus load at similar stages of disease (reviewed in Simmonds, 1990).

The relationship between virus load and the efficiency of sexual transmission remains unclear. In several studies, transmission probabilities increase with progression to disease where individuals, who are sicker as measured by low CD4 counts, presence of P24 antigen, or AIDS diagnoses are more likely to transmit than individuals who are asymptomatic (Castelli *et al.*, 1992; ESG, 1989; ESG, 1992; Goedert, Eyster, Biggar & Blattner, 1987; Jingu *et al.*, 1992; Laga *et al.*, 1989; Latif, *et al.*, 1989; Lazzarini *et al.*, 1991; Musicco *et al.*, 1992; Perroni Alberoni & Soscia, 1992; Rehmet *et al.*, 1992). This finding however, is not confirmed by all partner studies (Guimaraes *et al.*, 1992; Johnson *et al.*, 1989; Moss, *et al.*, 1991; Ragni *et al.*, 1989). One problem is that low CD4 count could just be a marker for longer duration of infection in the man and consequently, of longer virus exposure for the woman. Most studies therefore adjust for the (average) number of exposures or the duration of the relationship. A lack of an association, even after these adjustments, may simply mirror the lack of a clear relationship between virus load and symptomatology, especially in studies with relatively small numbers of study subjects. Another problem with most of these studies is that the disease stage of the index case is determined after heterosexual transmission already has occurred. A study in haemophiliacs, who all seroconverted in 1982–1983, showed that, at the time of the study in 1989, six of the 45 spouses had seroconverted (Ragni *et al.*, 1989). Transmissions occurred within one year of the time of first exposure (on the average), when all the men in the study were asymptomatic. More studies are needed to address this problem.

A recent study showed that zidovudine therapy may decrease the virus load in semen (Anderson, May, Ng & Rowley, 1992). Early treatment with zidovudine could therefore decrease the probability of sexual transmission, in addition to slowing down disease progression. An Italian heterosexual partner study found that partners of untreated men were 2.6 times more likely to seroconvert than partners of treated men (95% confidence interval: 1.1, 6.6) (Musicco *et al.*, 1992).

Immune Competence

As discussed above, susceptibility clearly depends on cofactors that determine the integrity of the vaginal or rectal mucosa. Susceptibility could also depend on human genetic variation, and factors that determine host immunity, such as nutritional status, general health, stress and drug use. These factors have been studied in much less detail. An association between smoking and HIV seroconversion was shown in two studies (Boulos *et al.*, 1990; Chao *et al.*, 1992) and deserves further attention. More research is needed to determine whether different variants of HIV differ in their ability to infect a new host.

It has been hypothesized that the immune systems of African heterosexuals, similar to those of U.S. homosexual men, are in a chronically activated state associated with chronic viral and parasitic antigenic exposure, which may cause them to be particularly susceptible to HIV infection or disease progression. A study that compared African and U.S. AIDS patients, African and U.S. heterosexual men and women, and U.S. homosexual men, found that all groups, except for the U.S. heterosexual men and women, had high prevalence of antibodies to various microbial pathogens (Quinn *et al.*, 1987). Studies in Rwanda however, did not confirm these findings (Allen *et al.*, 1991b). These studies did not find any correlation between HIV seropositivity and raised antibody levels to various parasites, including malaria.

CONCLUSION

Some of the cofactors discussed in this chapter are subject to intervention. Early education to increase condom use, decrease high risk sexual and contraceptive practices and teach people to choose their sexual partners carefully remains necessary. However, even without the presence of any known cofactors, transmission can take place. The intensification of STD control programmes may limit the spread of HIV in certain populations (Nkowane & Lwanga, 1990; Padian, Hitchcock, Fullilove, Kohlstadt & Brunham, 1990). Biological cofactors are not always subject to intervention but increasing epidemiological knowledge in this area might be helpful in the search for prophylactic and curative therapies.

REFERENCES

Al-Nozha, M., Ramia, S., Al-Frayh, A., Arif, M. (1990). Letters to the Editor: Female-to-Male: An Inefficient Model of Transmission of Human Immunodeficiency Virus (HIV). *Journal of Acquired Immune Deficiency Syndromes*, 3(2), 193–194.

Allain, J.P. (1986). Prevalence of HTLV-III/LAV Antibodies in Patients with Haemophilia and in Their Sexual Partners in France. *New England Journal of Medicine*, 315(8), 517–518.

Allen, S., Lindan, C., Serufilira, A., van de Perre, P., Rundle, A.C., Nsengumuremyi, F., Carael, M., Schwalbe, J., Hulley, S. (1991a). Human Immunodeficiency Virus Infection in Urban Rwanda: Demographic and Behavioural Correlates in a Representative Sample of Childbearing Women. *Journal of the American Medical Association*, 266(12), 1657–1663.

Allen, S., van de Perre, P., Serufilira, A., Lepage, P., Carael, M., DeClercq, A., Tice, J., Black, D., Nsengumuremyi, F., Ziegler, J., Levy, J., Hulley, S. (1991b). Human Immunodeficiency Virus and Malaria in a Representative Sample of Childbearing Women in Kigali, Rwanda. *Journal of Infectious Diseases*. 164, 64–71.

Anderson, R.M., May, R.M. (1988). Epidemiological Parameters of HIV Transmission. *Nature*, 333, 514–518.

Anderson, R.M., May, R.M., Ng, T.W., Rowley, J.T. (1992). Age-Dependent Choice of Sexual Partners and the Transmission Dynamics of HIV in Sub-Saharan Africa. *Philosophical Transactions of the Royal Society of London. Series B: Biological Sciences*, 336(1277), 135–155.

Bongaarts, J., Reining, P., Way, P., Conant, F. (1989). The Relationship between Male Circumcision and HIV Infection in African Populations. *AIDS*, 3(6), 373–377.

Boschi, C., Castilho, E., Guimaraes, M.D.C., Morgado, M., Cavalcante, S., Sereno, A., Lima, L.A., Berbara, V., Hart, D. (1992). Association Between Oral Contraceptive Use and HIV-1 Infection. *VIII International Conference on AIDS/III STD World Congress, Amsterdam, 1992* (PoC 4355).

Boulos, R., Halsy, N.A., Holt, E., Ruff, A., Brutus, J.-R., Quinn, T.C., Adrien, M., Boulos, C. (1990). HIV-1 in Haitian Women, 1982–1988. *Journal of Acquired Immunodeficiency Syndromes*, 3(7), 721–728.

Bouvet, E., De Vicenzi, I., Ancelle, R., Vachon, F. (1989). Defloration as Risk Factor for Heterosexual HIV Transmission. *Lancet*, 1, 615.

Brown, L., Siddiqui, N., Phillips, R., Ajuluchukwu, D. (1992). No Seroconversions Among Steady Sex Partners of HIV-1 Seropositive Injecting Drug Users in New York City. *VIII International Conference on AIDS/III STD World Congress, Amsterdam, 1992* (PoC 4168).

Brown, R.C., Brown, J.E., Ayowa, O.B. (1992). Vaginal Inflammation in Africa. *New England Journal of Medicine*, 324(16), 572.

Brunham, R.C. (1991). The Concept of Core and its Relevance to the Epidemiology and Control of Sexually Transmitted Diseases. *Sexually Transmitted Diseases*, 19, 67–68.

Calabrese, L.H., Gopalakrishna, K.V. (1986). Correspondence: Transmission of HTLV-III Infection From Man to Woman to Man. *New England Journal of Medicine*, 314(15), 987.

Cameron, W., D'Costa, L.J., Maitha, G.M., Cheang, M., Piot, P., Simonsen, J.N., Ronald, A.R., Gakinya, M.N., Ndinya-Achola, J.O., Brunham, R.C., Plummer, F.A. (1989). Female to Male Transmission of Human Immunodeficiency Virus Type 1: Risk Factors for Seroconversion in Men. *Lancet*, 2, 403–407.

Carael, M., van de Perre, P.H., Lepage, P.H., Allen, S., Nsengumuremyi, F., van Goethem, C., Ntahorutaba, N., Nzaramba, D., Clumeck, N. (1988). Human Immunodeficiency Virus Transmission among Heterosexual Couples in Central Africa. *AIDS*, 2, 201–205.

Castelli, F., Casari, Donisi, A., Tomasoni, L., Rodella, A., Carosi, G. (1992). Risk Factors for Heterosexual HIV Transmission. *VIII International Conference on AIDS/III STD World Congress, Amsterdam, 1992* (PoC 4152).

Centers for Disease Control, Atlanta, USA (1983). Immunodeficiency among Female Sexual Partners of Males with Acquired Immune Deficiency Syndrome (AIDS) — New York. *Morbidity and Mortality Weekly Report*, 31(52), 697–698.

Centers for Disease Control, Atlanta, USA (1992). *HIV/AIDS Surveillance, Third Quarter Edition: US AIDS Cases Reported Through September 1992.*

Centers for Disease Control, Atlanta, USA (1987). HIV Infection and Pregnancies in Sexual Partners of HIV-Seropositive Haemophiliac Men — United States. *Morbidity and Mortality Weekly Report*, 36(35), 593–595.

Chao, A., Habimana, P., Bulterys, M., Bulterys, K., Mukafaranswa, B., Dushimimana, A., Nawrocki, P., Hill, T., Saah, A. (1992). Oral Contraceptive Use, Cigarette Smoking, Age at First Sexual Intercourse, and HIV-1 Infection among Rwandan Women. *VIII International Conference on AIDS/III STD World Congress, Amsterdam, 1992* (PoC 4338).

Downs, A.M., Ancelle-Park, R.A., Brunet, J.-B. (1990). Surveillance of AIDS in the European Community: Recent Trends and Predictions to 1991. *AIDS*, 4(11), 1117–1124.

European Study Group on Heterosexual Transmission of HIV (1989). Risk Factors for Male to Female Transmission of HIV. *British Medical Journal*, 298, 411–414.

European Study Group on Heterosexual Transmission of HIV (1992). Comparison of Female to Male and Male to Female Transmission of HIV in 563 Stable Couples. *British Medical Journal*, 304, 809–813.

Figueroa, J.P., Brathwaite, A., Morris, J., Ward, E., Peruga, A., Blattner, W., Vermund, S., Hayes, R. (1992). Risk Factors for HIV in Heterosexual STD Patients in Jamaica. *VIII International Conference on AIDS/III STD World Congress, Amsterdam, 1992* (PoC 4322).

Fischl, M.A., Lai, S., Strickman-Stein, N., Resnick, L. (1992). Seroprevalence and Risk Factors Associated with the Heterosexual Transmission of HIV in a Sexually Active Non-Drug Abusing Population. *VIII International Conference on AIDS/III STD World Congress, Amsterdam, 1992 (PoC 4161).*

Fischl, M.A., Dickinson, G.M., Scott, G.B., Klimas, N., Fletcher, M.A., Parks, W. (1987). Evaluation of Heterosexual Partners, Children, and Household contacts of Adults with AIDS. *Journal of the American Medical Association*, 257(5), 640–644.

Goedert, J.J., Eyster, M.E., Biggar R.J., Blattner, W.A. (1987). Heterosexual Transmission of Human Immunodeficiency Virus: Association with Severe Depletion of T-Helper Lymphocytes in Men with Haemophilia. *AIDS Research and Human Retroviruses*, 3(4), 355–360.

Grant, R.M., Wiley, J.A., Winkelstein, W. (1987). Infectivity of the Human Immunodeficiency Virus: Estimates from a Prospective Study of Homosexual Men. *Journal of Infectious Diseases*, 156(1), 189–192.

Greenblatt, R.M., Lukehart, S.A., Plummer, F.A., Quinn, T.C., Critchlow, C.W., Ashley, R.L., D'Costa, L.J., Ndinya-Achola, J.O., Corey, L., Ronald, A.R., Holmes, K.K. (1988). Genital Ulceration as a Risk Factor for Human Immunodeficiency Virus Infection. *AIDS*, 2, 47–50.

Grossman, C.J. (1985). Interactions Between Gonadal Steroids and the Immune System. *Science*, 227, 257–261.

Guimaraes, M.D.C., Castilho, E., Sereno, A., Cavalcante, S., Lima, L.A., Gomes, V., Berbara, V., Hart, D., Boschi, C. (1992). Heterosexual Transmission of HIV-1: A Multicenter Study in Rio de Janeiro. *VIII International Conference on AIDS/III STD World Congress, Amsterdam, 1992* (PoC 4156).

Guinee, V.F. (1992). Heterosexual Transmission of HIV. *Journal of the American Medical Association*, **267**(14), 1918.

Harris, C., Small, C.B., Klein, R.S., Friedland, H., Moll, B., Emeson, E.E., Spigland, I., Steigbigel, N.H. (1983). Immunodeficiency in Female Sexual Partners of Men with the Acquired Immunodeficiency Syndrome. *New England Journal of Medicine*, **308**(20), 1181–1184.

Hayes, C.G., Manaloto, C.R., Basaca-Sevilla, V. (1990). Epidemiology of HIV Infection among Prostitutes in the Philipinnes. *Journal of Acquired Immunodeficiency Syndromes*, **3**, 913–920.

Hearst, N., Hulley, S.B. (1988). Preventing the Heterosexual Spread of AIDS. *Journal of the American Medical Association*, **259**(16), 2428–2430.

Hellmann, N.S., Grant, R.M., Nsubuga, P.S., Walker, C.K., Kamya, M., Tager, I.B., Jacobs, B., Mbidde, E.K. (1992). Modifiers of the Protective Effect of Circumcision. *VIII International Conference on AIDS/III STD World Congress, Amsterdam, 1992* (PoC 4299).

Hitti, J., Walker, C.K., Nsubuga, P.S.J., Grant, R.M., Tager, I.B., Mdibbe, E.K. (1992). Oral Contraceptive Use and HIV Infection. *VIII International Conference on AIDS/IIII STD World Congress, Amsterdam, 1992* (PoC 4309).

Ho, D.D., Schooley, R.T., Rota, T.R., Kaplan, J.L., Flynn, T., Syed, Z., Salahuddin, S.Z., Gonda, M.A., Hirsch, M.S. (1984). HTLV III in the Semen and Blood of a Healthy Homosexual Men. *Science*, **226**, 452–453.

Holmberg, S.D., Horsburgh, C.R., Ward, J.W., Jaffe, H.W. (1989). Biologic Factors in the Sexual Transmission of Human Immunodeficiency Virus. *Journal of Infectious Diseases*, **160**(1), 116–125.

Holmberg, S.D., Stewart, J.A., Gerber, A.R., Byers, R.H., Lee, F.K., O'Malley, P.M., Nahmias, A.J. (1988). Prior Herpes Simplex Virus Type 2 Infection as a Risk Factor for HIV Infection. *Journal of the American Medical Association*, **259**(7), 1048–1050.

Jason, J.M., McDougal, S., Dixon, G., Lawrence, D.N., Kennedy, M.S., Hillgartner, M., L., A., Evatt, B.L. (1986). HTLV-III/LAV Antibody and Immune Status of Household Contacts and Sexual Partners of Persons With Haemophilia. *Journal of the American Medical Association*, **255**(2), 212–215.

Jingu, M., St. Louis, M.E., Mbuyi, K., Mbu, L., Ndilu, M., Kaseka, N., Assina, Y., Kolo, M., Kazadi, C., Ryder, R.W. (1992). Risk Factors for HIV Transmission: A Case-Control Study among Married Couples Concordant and Discordant for HIV-1 Infection. *VIII International Conference on AIDS/III STD World Congress, Amsterdam, 1992* (PoC 4176).

Johnson, A.M., Petherick, A., Davidson, S.J., Brettle, R., Hooker, M., Howard, L., McLean, K.A., Osborne, L.E.M., Robertson, R., Sonnex, C., Tchamouroff, S., Shergold, C., Adler, M.W. (1989). Transmission of HIV to Heterosexual Partners of Infected Men and Women. *AIDS*, **3**(6), 367–372.

Kapiga, S., Hunter, D.J., Shao, J.F., Lwihula, G., Mtui, J., Mbena, E. (1992). Contraceptive Practice and HIV-1 Infection among Family Planning Clients in Dar Es Salaam, Tanzania. *VIII International Conference on AIDS/III STD World Congress, Amsterdam, 1992* (PoC 4343).

Kim, H.C., Raska, K., Clemow, L., Eisele, J., Matts, L., Saidi, P., & Raska, K.J. (1988). Human Immunodeficiency Virus Infection in Sexually Active Wives of Infected Hempohilic Men. *American Journal of Medicine*, **85**, 472–476.

Kreiss, J.K., Coombs, R., Plummer, F.A., Holmes, K.K., Nikora, B., Cameron, W., Ngugi, E., Ndinya Achola, J.O., Corey, L. (1989). Isolation of Human Immunodeficiency Virus from Genital Ulcers in Nairobi Prostitutes. *Journal of Infectious Diseases*, **160**(3), 380–384.

Kreiss, J.K., Kitchen, L.W., Prince, H.E., Kasper, C.K., Essex, M. (1985). Antibody to Human T-Lymphotropic Virus Type III in Wives of Haemophiliacs; Evidence for Heterosexual Transmission. *Annals of Internal Medicine*, **102**, 623–626.

Kreiss, J.K., Koech, D., Plummer, F.A., Holmes, K.K., Lightfoote, M., Piot, P., Ronald, A.R., Ndinya-Achola, J.O., D'Costa, L.J., Roberts, P., Ngugi, E.N., Quinn, T.C. (1986). AIDS Virus Infection in Nairobi Prostitutes. *New England Journal of Medicine*, 314(7), 414–418.

Laga, M., Nzila, N., Manoka, A.T. (1990). Non Ulcerative Sexually Transmitted Diseases (STD) as Risk Factors for HIV Transmission. *Sixth International Conference on AIDS, San Francisco, 1990* (Th.C. 97)

Laga, M., Taelman, H., van der Stuyft, P., Bonneux, L., Vercauteren, G., Piot, P. (1989). Advanced Immunodeficiency as a Risk Factor for Heterosexual Transmission of HIV. *AIDS*, 3(6), 361–366.

Latif, A.S., Katzenstein, D.A., Bassett, M.T., Houston, S., Emmanuel, J.C., Marowa, E. (1989). Genital Ulcers and Transmission of HIV Among Couples in Zimbabwe. *AIDS*, 3, 519–523.

Lawrence, D.N., Jason, J.M., Holman, R.C., Heine, P., Evatt, B.L. (1988). Sex Practice Correlates of Human Immunodeficiency Virus Transmission and Acquired Immuno Deficiency Syndrome Incidence in Heterosexual Partners and Offspring of U.S. Hemophilic Men. *American Journal of Hematology*, 30, 68–76.

Lazzarin, A., Saracco, A., Musicco, M., Nicolosi, A. (1991). Man-to-Woman Sexual Transmission of the Human Immunodeficiency Virus. *Archives of International Medicine*, 151(12), 2411–2416.

Luzi, G., Ensoli, B., Turbessi, G., Scarpati, B., Aiuti, F. (1985). Transmission of HTLV-III Infection by Heterosexual Contact. *Lancet*, 2, 1018.

Mann, J., Quinn, T.C., Piot, P. (1987). Condom Use and HIV Infection among Prostitutes in Zaire. *New England Journal of Medicine*, 316–345.

Mann, J.M., Nzilambi, N., Piot, P., Bosenge, N., Kalala, M., Francis, H., Colebunders, R.C., Azila, P.K., Curran, J.W., Quinn, T.C. (1988). HIV Infection and Associated Risk Factors in Female Prostitutes in Kinshasa, Zaire. *AIDS*, 2, 249–254.

Masur, H., Michelis, M.A., Wormser, G.P. (1982). Opportunistic Infection in Previously Healthy Women: Initial Manifestations of a Community Acquired Cellular Immunodeficiency. *Annals of Internal Medicine*, 97, 533–539.

Miller, V.E., Scofield, V.L. (1989). Transfer of HIV by Semen. In: Alexander. Gabelnick & Spieler (Ed.), *Heterosexual Transmission of AIDS* (pp. 147–154).

Moss, G.B., Clemetson, D., D'Costa, L., Plummer, F.A., Ndinya-Achola, J.O., Reilly, M., Holmes, K.K., Piot, P., Maitha, G.M., Hillier, L., Kiviat, N.C., Cameron, C.W., Wamola, I.A., Kreiss, J.K. (1991). Association of Cervical Ectopy with Heterosexual Transmission of Human Immunodeficiency Virus: Results of a Study of Couples in Nairobi, Kenya. *Journal of Infectious Diseases*, 164(3), 588–591.

Musicco, M., Angarano, G., Saracco, A., Nicolosi, A., Gasparini, M., Arici, C., Ricchi, E., Lazzarin, A. (1992). Antiretroviral Therapy Reduces the Rate of Sexual Transmission of HIV-1 from Man to Woman. *VIII International Conference on AIDS/III STD World Congress, Amsterdam, 1992* (WeC 1088).

N'Galy, B., Ryder, R.W. (1988). Epidemiology of HIV Infection in Africa. *Journal of Acquired Immunodeficiency Syndromes*, 1, 551–558.

Nkowane, B.M., Lwanga, S.K. (1990). HIV and Design of Intervention Studies for Control of Sexually Transmitted Diseases. *AIDS*, 4(suppl 1), S123–S126.

Nzila, N., Laga, M., Thiam, M.A., Mayimona, K., Edidi, B., van Dyck, E., Behets, F., Hassig, S., Nelson, A., Mokwa, K., Ashley, R.L., Piot, P., Ryder, R.W. (1991). HIV and Other Sexually Transmitted Diseases among Female Prostitutes in Kinshasa. *AIDS*, 5, 715–721.

Padian, N.S., Hitchcock, P.J., Fullilove, R.E., Kohlstadt, V., Brunham, R. (1990). Report of the NIAID Study Group on Integrated Behavioural Research for Prevention and Control of Sexually Transmitted Diseases; Part I: Issues in Defining Behavioural Risk Factors and their Distribution. *Sexually Transmitted Diseases*, 17(4), 200–210.

Padian, N.S., Marquis, L., Francis, D.P., Anderson, R.E., Rutherford, G.W., O'Malley, P.M., Winkelstein, W. (1987). Male-to-Female Transmission of Human Immunodeficiency Virus. *Journal of the American Medical Association*, **258**(6), 788–790.

Padian, N.S., Shiboski, S.C. (1992). Partner Studies in the Heterosexual Transmission of HIV (submitted).

Padian, N.S., Shiboski, S.C., Hitchcock, P.J. (1991). Risk Factors for Acquisition of Sexually Transmitted Diseases and Development of Complications. In J.N. Wasserheit et al. (Ed.), *Research Issues in Human Behaviour and Sexually Transmitted Diseases in the AIDS Era* (pp. 83–96). Washington, DC 20005: American Society for Microbiology.

Padian, N.S., Shiboski, S.C., Jewell, N.P. (1989). The Effect of Number of Exposures on the Risk of Heterosexual HIV Transmission. *Journal of Infectious Diseases*, **161**(5), 883–887.

Padian, N.S., Shiboski, S.C., Jewell, N.P. (1991). Female-to-Male Transmission of Human Immunodeficiency Virus. *Journal of the American Medical Association*, **266**(12), 1664–1667.

Padian, N.S., Wiley, J., Glass, S., Marquis, L., Winkelstein, W. (1988). Anomalies of Infectivity in the Heterosexual Transmission of HIV. *IV International Conference on AIDS, Stockholm, 1989* (4062).

Pape, J.W., Stanback, M., Pamphile, M. (1987). Seroepidemiology of HIV in Haiti. *Clinical Research*, **35**, 486.

Parker, S.W., Stewart, A.J., Wren, M.N., (1983). Circumcision and Sexually Transmitted Diseases. *Medical Journal of Australia ii*, 288–290,

Perroni, L., Alberoni, F., Sogcia, F. (1992). Transmission of HIV Infection in Heterosexual Partners of HIV + Subjects. *VIII International Conference on AIDS/III STD World Congress, Amsterdam 1992)* (PoC 4164).

Peterman T.A., Stoneburner, R.L., Allen, R., Jaffe, H.W., Curran, J.W. (1988). Risks of Human Immunodeficiency Virus Transmission from Heterosexual Adults with Transfusion-Associated Infections. *Journal of the American Medical Association*, 259(1), 55–58.

Piot, P., Duncan, M., van Dyck, E. (1986). Ulcerative Balanoprosthitis Associated with non-Syphilic Spirochaetal Infection. *Genitourinary Medicine*, **62**, 44–46.

Piot, P., Kreiss, J.K., Ndinya-Achola, J.O., Ngugi, E.N., Simonsen, N., Cameron, D.W., Taelman, H., Plummer, F.A. (1987a). Editorial Review: Heterosexual Transmission of HIV. *AIDS*, 1(4), 199–206.

Piot, P., Plummer, F.A., Rey, M.-A., Ngugi, E.N., Rouzioux, C., Ndinya-Achola, J.O., Vercauteren, G., D'Costa, L.J., Laga, M., Nsanze, H., Fransen, L., Haase, D., Brunham, R.C., Ronald, A.R., Brun-Vezinet, F. (1987b). Retrospective Seroepidemiology of AIDS Virus Infection in Nairobi Populations. *Journal of Infectious Diseases*, 155(6), 1108–1112.

Pitchenik, A.E., Fischl, M.A., Spira, T.J. (1983). Acquired Immunodeficiency Syndrome in Low Risk Patients: Evidence for Possible Transmission by an Asymptomatic Carrier. *Journal of the American Medical Association*, 250, 1310–1312.

Pitchenik, A.E., Shafron, R.D., Glasser, R.M., Spira, T.J. (1984). The Acquired Immunodeficiency Syndrome in the Wife of a Haemophiliac. *Annals of Internal Medicine*, 100, 62–65.

Plummer, F.A., Simonsen, J.N., Cameron, D.W., Ndinya-Achola, J.O., Kreiss, J.K., Gakinya, M.N., Waiyaki, P., Cheang, M., Piot, P., Ronald, A.R., Ngugi, E.N. (1990). Cofactors in Male-Female Sexual Transmission of Human Immunodeficiency Virus Type 1. *Journal of Infectious Diseases*, 163(2), 233–239.

Polk, B.F. (1985). Female-to-Male Transmission of AIDS. *Journal of the American Medical Association*, **254**(22), 3177–3178.

Quinn, T., Piot, P., McCormick, J.B., Feinsod, F.M., Taelman, H., Kapita, B., Stevens, W., Fauci, A.S. (1987). Serologic and Immunologic Studies in Patients with AIDS in North America and Africa. *Journal of the American Medical Association*, 257(19), 2617–2621.

Quinn, T.C., Mann, M., Curran, J.W., Piot, P. (1986). AIDS in Africa: An Epidemiologic Paradigm. *Science*, **234**, 955–963.

Ragni, M.V., Kingsley, L.A., Nimorwicz, P., Gupta, P., Rinaldo, C.R. (1989). HIV Heterosexual Transmission in Haemophilia Couples: Lack of Relation to T4 Number, Clinical Diagnosis, or Duration of HIV Exposure. *Journal of the Acquired Immunodeficiency Syndromes*, **2**(6), 557–563.

Ratnoff, O.D., Lederman, M.M., Jenkins, J.J. (1984). Lymphadenopathy in a Haemophiliac Patient and his Sexual Partner. *Annals of Internal Medicine,* **100**, 915.

Redfield, R.R., Markham, P.D., Salahuddin, S.Z., Sarngadharan, M.G., Bodner, A.J., Folks, T .M., Ballou, W.R., Wright, D.C., Gallo, R.C. (1985a). Frequent Transmission of HTLV-III Among Spouses of Patients with AIDS-Related Complex and AIDS. *Journal of the American Medical Association*, **253**(11), 1571–1573.

Redfield, R.R., Markham, P.D., Salahuddin, S.Z., Wright, D.C., Sarngadharan, M.G., Gallo, R.C. (1985b). Heterosexually Acquired HTLV-III/LAV Disease (AIDS-Related Complex and AIDS): Epidemiologic Evidence for Female-to-Male Transmission. *Journal of the American Medical Association*, **254**(15), 2094–2096.

Rehmet, S., Staszewski, S., Muller, R., Doerr, H.W., Bergmann, L., von Wangenheim, G., Helm, E.B., Stille, W. (1992). Transmission Rates and Co-Factors of Heterosexual HIV Transmission. *VIII International Conference on AIDS/III STD World Congress, Amsterdam, 1992* (PoC 4165).

Roumeliotou, A., Papautsakis, G., Kallinikos, G., Papeyanegelou, G. (1988). Effectiveness of Condom Use in Preventing HIV Infection in Prostitutes. *Lancet*, **2**, 1249.

Schultz, S., Milberg, J.A., Kristal, A.R., Stoneburner, R.L. (1986). Female-to-Male Transmision of HTLV-III. *Journal of the American Medical Association*, **255**(13), 1703–1704.

Simmonds, P. (1990). Variation in HIV Virus Load of Individuals at Different Stages in Infection: Possible Relationship with Risk of Transmission. *AIDS*, **4**(suppl 1), S77–S83.

Simonsen, J.N., Cameron, D.W., Gakinya, M.N., Ndinya-Achola, J.O., D'Costa, L.J., Karasira, P., Cheang, M., Ronald, A.R., Piot, P., Plummer, F.A. (1988). Human Immunodeficiency Virus Infection among Men with Sexually Transmitted Diseases. *New England Journal of Medicine,* **319**(5), 274–278.

Simonsen, J.N., Plummer, F.A., Ngugi, E.N., Black, C., Kreiss, J.K., Gakinya, M.N., Waiyaki, P., D'Costa, L.J., Ndinya-Achola, J.O., Piot, P., Ronald, A. (1990). HIV Infection among Lower Socioeconomic Strata Prostitutes in Nairobi. *AIDS*, **4**(2), 139–144.

Sion, F.S., Signorini, D.J.H.P., Santos, E.A., Merces, R.N., Cassalta, N., Morals de Sa, C.A., Passman, L.J., van der Borghth, B.O.H., Rubini, N.P.H., Rachid de Lacerda, M.C., Ismael, C. (1992). Absence of Female-to-Male Transmission of HIV in Stable Couples in Rio de Janeiro, Brazil, *VIII International Conference on AIDS/III STD World Congress, Amsterdam, 1992* (PoC 4169).

Siraprapasiri, T., Thanprasertsuk, S., Rodklay, A., Srivanichakorn, S., Sawanpanyalert, P., Temtanarak, J. (1991). Risk Factors for HIV among Prostitutes in Chiangmai, Thailand. *AIDS*, **5**, 579–582.

Smith, G.L., Smith, K.F. (1986). Lack of HIV Infection and Condom Use in Licensed Prostitutes *Lancet*, **1**, 1392.

Stamm, W.E., Handsfield, H.H., Rompalo, A.M., Ashley, R.L., Roberts, P.L., Corey, L. (1988). The Association between Genital Ulcer Disease and Acquisition of HIV Infection in Homosexual Men. *Journal of the American Medical Association,* **260**, 1429–1433.

Stewart, G.J., Tyler, J.P.P., Cunningham, A.L., Barr, J.A., Driscoll, G.L., Gold, J., Lamont, B .J. (1985). Transmission of Human T-Cell Lymphotropic Virus Type III (HTLV-III) by Artificial Insemination by Donor. *Lancet*, **2**, 581–584.

Stone, K.M., Grimes, D.A., Magder, L.S. (1986). Primary Prevention of Sexually Transmitted Diseases-State-of-the-Art Review. *Journal of the American Medical Association*, 255, 1763–1765.

Tait, I.A., Rees, E., Hobson, D., Byng, R.E., Tweedie, M.C.K. (1980). Chlamydia Infection of the Cervix in Contacts of Men with Non-Gonococcal Urethritis. *British Journal of Venereal Diseases*, 56, 37–45.

Tyndall, M., Agoki, E., Malisa, W., Ronald, A.R., Ndinya-Achola, J.O., Plummer, F.A. (1992). HIV-1 Prevalence and Risk of Seroconversion among Uncircumcised Men in Kenya. *VIII International Conference on AIDS/III STD World Congress, Amsterdam, 1992* (Poc 4308).

van de Perre, P., DeClerq, A., Cogniaux-LeClerc, J., Nzaramba, D., Butzler, J.-P., Sprecher-Goldberger, S. (1988). Detection of HIV p17 Antigen in Lymphocytes but not Epithelial Cells from Cervicovaginal Secretions of Women Seropositive for HIV: Implications for Heterosexual Transmission of the Virus. *Genitourinary Medicine*, 64, 30–33.

van de Perre, P., Jacobs, D., Sprecher-Goldberger, S. (1987). The Latex Condom, an Efficient Barrier Against Sexual Transmission of AIDS-Related Viruses. *AIDS*, 1, 49–52.

van der Ende, M.E., Rothbarth, P., Stibbe, J. (1988). Heterosexual Transmission of HIV by Haemophiliacs. *British Medical Journal*, 297, 1102–1103.

Vogt, M.W., Witt, D.J., Craven, D.E., Byington, R., Crawford, D.F., Schooley, R.T., Hirsch, M.S. (1986). Isolation of HTLV-III/LAV from Cervical Secretions of Women at Risk for AIDS. *Lancet*, 1, 525–527.

Wasserheit, J.N. (1992). Epidemiological Synergy Interrelationships between Human Immunodeficiency Virus Infection and Other Sexually Transmitted Diseases. *Sexually Transmitted Diseases*, 19(2), 61–77.

Wofsy, C.B., Cohen, B., Hauer, L.B., Padian, N.S., Michaelis, B.A., Evans, L.A., Levy, J.A. (1986). Isolation of AIDS-Associated Retrovirus from Genital Secretions of Women with Antibodies to the Virus. *Lancet*, 1, 527–529.

Wykoff, R.F. (1986). Female-to-Male Transmission of HTLV-III. *Journal of the American Medical Association*, 255(13), 1704–1705.

Zagury, D., Bernard, J., Liebowitch, J., Safai, B., Groopman, J.E., Feldman, M., Sam-Gadharan, M.G., Gallo, R.C. (1984). HTLV III in Cells Cultured from Semen of Two Patients with AIDS. *Science*, 226, 449–451.

2

Women and HIV Infection

CATHERINE HANKINS

INTRODUCTION

In many respects, the epidemic of acquired immune deficiency syndrome (AIDS) of the 1990s, which follows on the heels of the epidemic of human immunodeficiency virus (HIV) infection of the 1980s, is only in its infancy. The World Health Organization (WHO) predicts that, by the year 2000, 90% of all new AIDS cases in the world will have been acquired through heterosexual activity and that more women than men will be infected, even in many developed countries (Merson, 1992). These estimates for the future contrast with current figures suggesting that 75% of cumulative infections in adults have been acquired via heterosexual transmission and that the male to female ratio for HIV infection is now five to four (World Health Organization, 1992a). By the beginning of 1992 more than 4.7 million women had become infected by HIV and of the one million persons newly infected in the first half of 1992 the Global Programme on AIDS estimates that nearly one-half have been women (World Health Organization, 1992b).

Only now is increased attention beginning to be paid to the unique features of HIV in women after years of scientific neglect. A significant body of work does exist already concerning pregnancy and maternal-foetal HIV transmission, a subject of significant interest to women but one which also tends to conceptualize women as transmitters of HIV infection. Among the reasons for the delay in addressing the subject of HIV and women has been the preponderance of AIDS cases among gay and bisexual men during the first decade of the AIDS epidemic in many industrialized countries. Recent discourse concerning a syndrome in medicine entitled "The Yentl syndrome" suggests, however, that underemphasis on women in the context of HIV/AIDS may not be unique (Healy, 1991). The Yentl syndrome refers to an increasingly recognized phenomenon of gender bias in medicine creating disparate, unequal chances of having symptoms taken seriously, appropriate diagnostic testing ordered, and correct diagnoses made. This bias has been clearly documented to occur in women with cardiovascular disease (Ayanian & Epstein, 1991; Steingart *et al.*, 1991).

In this chapter, a brief overview of current knowledge concerning women and HIV is presented addressing epidemiology and transmission, clinical manifestations, psychosocial aspects, and prevention dilemmas. Several other chapters in this book include complementary information enlarging in more detail on many of the issues presented here.

EPIDEMIOLOGY AND TRANSMISSION

Epidemiology

Heterosexual activity in the context of marriage may well be the predominant risk factor for HIV infection in women worldwide with estimates that as many as 1500 women who have only their own husband as a sexual partner are becoming infected on a daily basis (Reid, 1990). This risk factor may have played a less important role in earlier phases of the epidemic when heterosexual men and a core group of women were those primarily affected in some countries (Cameron & Padian, 1990). Increased heterosexual transmission to women in general is now becoming increasingly evident in AIDS case surveillance, a lag time discrepancy that reflects the long incubation period from HIV infection to AIDS. Based on current estimates as many as 40% of individuals have not developed AIDS by 12 to 13 years after initial infection (World Health Organization, 1992a). The overall result is a dynamically evolving epidemiological picture with current HIV transmission to women expected to be evident in changing male-to-female case ratios for years to come.

Prevalence

In the absence of information concerning HIV incidence among women, the prevalence of HIV infection throughout many parts of the world has been estimated using mandatory testing, unlinked anonymous studies, and surveys of women attending reproductive health services, working as prostitutes or entering drug treatment programmes. In Africa, HIV prevalence rates vary dramatically with estimates ranging from 1.4% of women in a population-based study in Southeastern Gabon (Schrijvers, Delaporte, Peeters, Dupont, & Meheus, 1991), 9.0% of women having delivered a low birth weight baby or stillbirth in Nairobi (Temmerman *et al.*, 1990), 28.6% of women residents in Kagera, Tanzania (Killewo *et al.*, 1990), to 62% of women working as prostitutes in Nairobi (Simonsen *et al.*, 1990).

In the United States HIV prevalence in women has been estimated to be 0.032% in female military recruits (Burke *et al.*, 1990), 0.15% in childbearing women

(Gwinn *et al.*, 1991), 0.22% in women seeking reproductive health services (Sweeney, Onorato, Allen, Byers, & the Field Services Branch, 1992), 3% among women receiving publicly funded HIV testing and counselling services (Centers for Disease Control, 1991), and 2.5–14.7% among incarcerated women (Vlahov *et al.*, 1991). In inner London, England, HIV-1 prevalence has been estimated to be 0.10% among childbearing women over the period 1988–1991 (Ades *et al.*, 1991) in comparison with 0.18% for Montreal, Canada in 1989 (Hankins *et al.*, 1990). Estimates of HIV-1 infection for women in Salvador, Brazil include 0.9% of childbearing women and 0.8% of pregnant women from lower socioeconomic classes attending a sexually transmitted disease clinic (Ivo-dos-Santos *et al.*, 1991). In Chiangmai, Thailand reported estimates of HIV-1 infection among women working as prostitutes are as high as 36.5% with seropositivity associated with lower pay for sexual service (Siraprapasiri *et al.*, 1991).

HIV and Sexually Transmitted Disease

An epidemiological synergy is hypothesized to exist between sexually transmitted diseases (STD) and HIV infection with three different groups of STD postulated to have distinct interactions with HIV infection (Wasserheit, 1992). This synergy is of particular importance to women since the risk of heterosexual transmission of HIV may be substantially reduced by efficacious treatment and control programmes which are accessible to women with both symptomatic and asymptomatic sexually transmitted diseases.

Genital ulcer diseases, such as chancroid, genital herpes, and syphilis, interact with HIV infection to reinforce both the prevalence and incidence of each other. Genital herpes, for example, may facilitate HIV transmission while HIV infection itself may simultaneously prolong or augment the infectiousness of individuals with genital herpes. This interaction of HIV and ulcerative STD would help explain not only the dramatic levels of heterosexual HIV transmission in parts of Africa in which risk of HIV seroconversion is clearly associated with genital ulcer disease (Plummer *et al.*, 1991) but also the interaction between syphilis and HIV in North America among heterosexuals (Castro *et al.*, 1988; Cannon *et al.*, 1989) and between primary genital herpes and HIV in gay men (Holmberg *et al.*, 1988).

The discharge syndromes such as gonorrhoea, chlamydial infection, and trich-omonas probably interact with HIV infection in a unidirectional fashion by promoting HIV transmission without a synergistic increase in their own prevalence or incidence. Although gonorrhoea rates have declined in many industrialized countries and gonorrhoea appears to be restricted somewhat to a core group, gonorrhoea outbreaks continue to occur and chlamydial infection is widespread. Estimates from industrialized countries indicate that between 10 and 30 percent of sexually active girls under 20 years of age have chlamydial infection (Judson, 1985; Mårdh, Helin, Bobeck, Laurin & Nilsson, 1986). A greater emphasis should be placed on the diagnosis and treatment of both symptomatic and asymptomatic discharge STD, which act in a similar fashion to the ulcerative STD to increase the risk of HIV transmission from 3- to 5-fold (Wasserheit, 1992). These strategies would reduce the risk of HIV acquisition as well as the risk of infertility, both of which constitute major concerns for women.

Human papilloma virus (HPV) infection may participate in a third type of HIV-STD interaction with HPV appearing to represent a traditional opportunistic infection, the expression and progression of which are augmented by HIV. In addition to causing anogenital warts, human papilloma virus infection is the agent which increasingly has an established role in the aetiology of disease of the uterine cervix (Franco, 1991; Vermund & Kelley, 1991). Geographical variation in HPV prevalence is marked with recent studies conducted in family planning, university health services, and general clinics suggesting HPV prevalence rates in North America and Britain in the range of 20 to 46%, based on sensitive polymerase chain reaction detection methods and large sample sizes (Bauer *et al.*, 1991; Bavin *et al.*, 1992; Burmer, Parker, Bates, East, & Kulander, 1990). Evidence is accumulating to suggest that HIV-induced immunodeficiency facilitates the expression of HPV as a causal agent in the development of cervical lesions and cancer.

Other Risk Factors for Sexual Transmission

Younger women may be at increased risk of acquiring infection if they are exposed to HIV because of a higher prevalence of cervical ectopy, a biological vulnerability which has been demonstrated for chlamydial infection (Saltz, Linnemann, Brookman, and Rauh, 1981); (Oriel *et al.*, 1978); (Rees *et al.*, 1977). The possibility that immaturity of the genital tract may influence risk underscores the importance of assisting young women to prolong first coitus and to negotiate consistent partner condom use (Guinan, 1992).

Factors which increase the risk of sexual transmission of HIV for women include the clinical stage of the male partner with increased infectivity postulated to occur in the early viraemic stages of HIV infection and late in the clinical course when CD4$^+$ cell counts decline (Goedert, Eyster, & Biggar, 1987). Use of oral contraceptives may increase risk for HIV perhaps by increasing the area of cervical ectopy (Moss *et al.*, 1991) or through the indirect mechanism of increased prevalence of chlamydial infection (Tait, Rees, Hobson, Byng, & Tweedie, 1980). Further investigation is required to better characterize the association between oral contraceptive use and the risk of HIV acquisition, suggested by some studies (Plourde *et al.*, 1992; Plummer *et al.*, 1991) but not by others (Pepin *et al.*, 1991; European Study Group, 1989; Allen *et al.*, 1991). The practice of anal intercourse, which is reported to range from 20–25% for total lifetime experience (King *et al.*, 1989; Colon, Robles, Aponte, & Matos, 1990) and from 8–10% as a regular activity (Bolling, 1977; Hankins *et al.*, 1989) in studies of non-prostitute women, appears to double the risk of HIV acquisition over vaginal intercourse (Padian, 1987). Sexual activity during menstruation has also been postulated to increase risk of HIV acquisition for women although firm evidence to support this association is lacking. To the extent that lack of male circumcision may increase risk of HIV in the male partner (Piot *et al.*, 1987; Bongaarts, Reining, Way, & Conant, 1989; Simonsen, Cameron, & Gajinya, 1988), sexual activity with a non-circumcised man may increase the risk for women depending on the sexual history of the male partner.

Mother-to-Child Transmission

Based on prospective studies and accounting for loss to follow-up, the likelihood that mothers who have HIV infection during pregnancy ("Report of a Consensus Workshop," 1992) may transmit HIV infection to offspring appears to be closer to 20% to 30% in the industrialized world and to 30% to 40% in the developing world. A recent meta-analysis by Dunn, Newell, Ades & Peckham (1992) of studies examining the risk of transmission from a mother who becomes infected while breastfeeding, either via blood transfusion or sexual activity, suggests a rate of 29% (95% CI 16–42%). This has clear implications for the prevention of HIV acquisition in women who are breastfeeding. Dunn *et al*. (1992) also calculate the incremental risk of transmission attributable to breastfeeding by a mother who was already infected during pregnancy to be 14% (95% CI 7–22%). Studies by Kennedy *et al*. (1990) and Heymann (1990) have modelled the survival outcomes of children born to HIV-infected women in relation to whether they are breastfed or bottle-fed in countries where the infant mortality reaches 10%, as it does in many non-industrialized countries. Even when HIV prevalence is as high as 40% among mothers, the WHO recommendation to maintain breastfeeding as protection against infectious diseases still holds as long as HIV transmission does not surpass 30%, a rate which is situated well outside the confidence limits of the meta-analysis estimate of Dunn *et al*. (1992). Breastfeeding should therefore continue to be promoted for women with HIV infection wherever no safe alternative for infant feeding exists.

NATURAL HISTORY

Although the natural history of HIV disease in women has not been well studied to date, and little is known concerning co-factors for progression, some information is now available concerning both the comparative survival of women with HIV infection and specific gynaecological manifestations.

HIV Disease Progression

The presence and the severity of symptoms in men at the time of seroconversion may be associated with an increased risk of development of AIDS (Schechter *et al*., 1990; Tindall & Cooper, 1991). No studies to date have examined whether an acute symptom complex in women predicts HIV disease progression. In men, older age at the time of infection, repeated sexually transmitted diseases, smoking, continued injection drug use, and genetic HLA type are among the co-factors which appear to play a role in HIV disease progression (Moss & Bacchetti, 1989; Lifson, Rutherford, & Jaffe, 1988). These potential co-factors have yet to be examined in women.

Several studies have attempted to define a role for pregnancy in HIV disease progression separate from the effects of the passage of time. Pregnancy does not appear to accelerate the onset of symptoms associated with HIV in women who are asymptomatic at the time of conception (Berrebi *et al*., 1991). Those who are already ill prior to pregnancy, however, are more likely to experience clinical deterioration, with Pneumocystis carinii pneumonia (PCP) constituting a significant cause of maternal mortality in women with AIDS (Koonin *et al.*, 1989). Pregnant women with a CD4$^+$ cell count of less than 200 cells/μL, or having clinical signs predictive of a low CD4$^+$ count when immunological parameters are not available, should receive prophylaxis for PCP in addition to other preventive measures (Sperling *et al.*, 1992).

Studies comparing the immune responses of women with and without HIV infection during pregnancy suggest that the normal rebound in the immediate post-partum period to pre-pregnancy levels of immune function does not occur in women with HIV infection (Biggar *et al.*, 1989; Lapointe, Boucher, Samson, & Charest, 1991). Studies comparing women who become pregnant with those who do not are needed to clarify whether these findings provide support for the unconfirmed hypothesis that pregnancy may accelerate HIV-induced depletion of CD4$^+$ cells increasing the risk of AIDS.

AIDS-Defining Illnesses

The diagnosis of AIDS in women in industrialized countries generally features opportunistic infections, with Pneumocystis carinii pneumonia predominating either with or without other illnesses. Cryptococcal meningitis, cytomegalovirus disease, toxoplasmosis, and lymphoma are reported in women, however, wasting syndrome, Candida oesophagitis, and Herpes simplex disease appear to be more frequently associated with an AIDS diagnosis in women than in men (Nahlen, Nwanyanwa, Chu, & Berkelman, 1991; Fleming, Clesielski, & Berkelman, 1991). Women rarely develop Kaposi's sarcoma (KS), a disease which appears to be more common in women infected through sexual intercourse with a bisexual man (Beral, Peterman, Berkelman, & Jaffe, 1990; Chu, Buehler, Fleming, & Berkelman, 1990). A comparative study in Uganda has suggested more aggressive disease manifestations and shorter survival times in women with KS than in men (Desmond-Hellmann, Mbidde, Kizito, & Hellman, 1990).

Although early reports and uncontrolled studies did suggest a differential survival in women with AIDS compared with men, it is now clear that when age at diagnosis, AIDS-defining illness, and zidovudine treatment are taken into account in comparative studies, gender differences in survival disappear (Hankins & Handley, 1992). In the United States, the differences which have been observed appear to be related to the unequal access to treatment experienced by women (Moore, Hidalgo, Sugland, & Chaisson, 1991). In countries where this barrier theoretically does not exist, delays in diagnosis and misdiagnosis (Chu, Buehler, & Berkelman, 1990) due to either patient or physician factors may create a similar effect on the potential for survival in women.

Gynaecological Manifestations

Various gynaecological disorders have been described in women at all stages of HIV disease, with studies reporting that as many as three out of four women with HIV infection may experience one or more manifestations such as vaginal candidiasis, persistent vulvo vaginitis, abnormal cervicovaginal cytology, human papilloma virus (HPV) infection, trichomonas, Chlamydia, bacterial vaginosis, pelvic inflammatory disease, Herpes simplex virus infection, and genital tract cancers (Carpenter *et al.*, 1991; Iman *et al.*, 1990; Buehler, Farizo, & Berkelman, 1991; Anastos, Denenberg, Solomon, & Rein, 1992).

Women with HIV infection may complain of changes in the nature or frequency of their menstrual periods. These may include dysmenorrhoea, increased or decreased menstrual flow, and irregular periods (Shah *et al.*, 1992). Premenstrual symptoms may become more evident with increased breast tenderness, oedema, anxiety, and depression. More research is warranted to further document these changes and to elucidate their pathogenesis. They may be the result of direct HIV viral effects, may be secondary to medications such as zidovudine, may be influenced by cocaine or crack use, or may be secondary to weight loss. It is suspected that premature menopause may be more common in women with immunosuppression.

The importance of regular gynaecological evaluation has not been well recognized by physicians and by their women patients who have HIV infection. Among HIV-positive women referred to an AIDS out-patient clinic in New York City, two thirds did not complain of gynaecological symptoms, but more than half had detectable clinical abnormalities upon examination (Stein *et al.*, 1991).

The extent to which women who present with cervical dysplasia and other gynaecological conditions may have undetected HIV infection is not known. Recurrent vaginal candidiasis may be a common initial clinical manifestation of HIV infection (Carpenter *et al.*, 1991) with one study reporting that almost half of the women with previous vaginal Candida infections observed an increase in the frequency and severity of symptoms six months to three years prior to testing positive for HIV antibodies (Iman *et al.*, 1990). Chronic vaginal candidiasis refractory to treatment has been observed among women with advanced HIV infection (Rhoads, Wright, Redfield, & Burke, 1987), however, vaginal candidiasis can be recurrent and often severe in the absence of either indicators or symptoms of immune suppression (Iman *et al.*, 1990).

HIV and Genital Cancers

An association between HIV infection and cancers of the cervix, vulva, and perianal region has been reported (Vermund *et al.*, 1991; Feingold *et al.*, 1990; Maiman *et al.*, 1990, 1991). This association appears to be strongest in the presence of human papilloma virus (HPV) infection with the clinical severity of co-infection demonstrated by reports of HPV disease recurrence, lack of HPV disease regression, and shortened survival time among women with HIV infection and detectable HPV disease (Maiman *et al.*, 1990; Agarossi *et al.*, 1991; Conti *et al.*, 1992).

Human papilloma virus infection is more likely to be detected in symptomatic HIV-positive women than in either asymptomatic HIV-positive or HIV-negative women (Feingold *et al.*, 1989; Vermund *et al.*, 1990) with HPV prevalence estimates among symptomatic women reported to be above 70% using various techniques. For asymptomatic women and for women without HIV infection, the comparative prevalence of HPV infection does not differ, with estimates ranging between 20% and 27% (Burk, Fleming, Ho, & Klein, 1991; Miotti *et al.*, 1992). This suggests a positive association between immunosuppression and the detection of HPV, as has been found with renal transplant patients (Vermund and Kelley, 1991).

The hypothesis that HIV-induced immunosuppression mediates the expression of a sexually transmitted causal agent, such as HPV, is supported by previous studies reporting increased occurrence of cervical cancer among women with immunosuppression unrelated to HIV infection (Vermund & Kelley, 1991). Maiman *et al.* (1991) reported mean CD4$^+$ counts of <500 cells/μL for women with abnormal Papanicolaou smears of all grades. More research is required to determine the interactions of HPV prevalence, cervical disease, and HIV infection in the presence of immunosuppression.

In the absence of sentinel surveillance studies and with genital tract neoplasia not included in the AIDS case definition, it has been impossible to assess the true extent of underestimation of HIV-related disease and death in women with cervical cancer. The Centers for Disease Control in Atlanta, Georgia has recently proposed that invasive cancer of the cervix be added to the list of AIDS-defining illnesses as of January 1993. If invasive cervical cancer becomes subject to AIDS reporting a better understanding of the prevalence and severity of this disease in the presence of HIV infection may be possible.

Clinical Management

Some studies have suggested that standard cervicovaginal cytology as assessed via Pap smear may underdiagnose dysplasia which is subsequently detected by colposcopy or biopsy, particularly in the presence of vaginal infections (Minkoff *et al.*, 1992). Other studies have shown good correspondence between cervicovaginal cytology and colposcopic findings (Kell, Shah, & Barton, 1992), with one study indicating no difference in the proportion of false negative cytological results found in women with HIV infection compared with those without (Kell *et al.*, 1992). Pending further evidence, the standard Pap smear screening procedure, with colposcopy as indicated, should be performed at least once a year after two negative Pap smears six months apart, as long as CD4$^+$ cell counts are high. As evidence of immune suppression appears, the frequency of gynaecological examinations with cervicovaginal cytology should increase to at least semi-annually. Women with CD4$^+$ counts below 500 cells/μL should be considered for baseline colposcopy.

Therapeutic interventions for gynaecological problems and STD should be accompanied by standard evaluation and treatment for HIV disease. Antiretroviral agents such as zidovudine or ddI should be offered as CD4$^+$ counts fall below 500 cells/μL and prophylaxis for Pneumocystis carinii pneumonia using trimethoprim-sulfamethoxazole or pentamidine should be offered at CD4$^+$ counts below 200 cells/μL. A course of prophylactic isoniazid (INH) is recommended for women with a positive PPD tuberculin test on baseline evaluation.

More information is required concerning gynaecological manifestations of HIV disease and, in particular, of the presentation and clinical course of dysplasia in relation to immune status and response to treatment in women with HIV infection.

PSYCHOSOCIAL ISSUES

Unequal Burden

Jonathan Mann, former director of the Global Programme on AIDS, speaks of three epidemics: the epidemic of HIV, the epidemic of AIDS, and the epidemic of discrimination (Mann, 1992). Women's unequal status in most societies renders them vulnerable to the social and psychological effects that form part of the third epidemic of discrimination. As HIV infection has spread increasingly to women in the Western world and as women in developing countries have been shown to be as equally affected as men by the virus, there have been significant delays in developing a focus on the unique needs of women in the HIV pandemic.

The vast majority of women with HIV infection worldwide are from the most disadvantaged, poorest sectors of society and are therefore often least able to advocate for themselves. Mays and Cochran (1988) highlighted the dual set of psychosocial problems arising from the combination of gender and minority group status in industrialized countries. De Bruyn (1992) points to the greater psychological and social burdens born by women in the HIV epidemic both as lay persons and as professionals. The increasing role being played by heterosexual transmission in industrialized countries, in which until now injection drug use has constituted the major risk for women, is creating psychosocial dilemmas that present different facets from pre-existing ones. The chapter on the psychological impact of HIV explores several aspects particular to heterosexual transmission.

The delayed recognition of the special needs of women in much of the industrialized world occurred in part because women have lacked a natural community to speak for them such as is shared by many gay men. This lack of social support is revealed in the extreme isolation and marginalization that women experience as they strive to keep their infection and the status of their children rigorously secret (Wofsy, 1987). They may fear stigmatization of their families as well as loss of employment, in particular if they are sole providers for the family. Fear of abandonment by the male partner may lead to secrecy regarding their infection status within their own sexual units. Many women are dependent for material and social resources on their male partners and cannot risk the possible effects of disclosure on themselves and their children. Women who develop AIDS-related symptoms before their partners do, are more likely than men to be abandoned by their spouse (Ankrah, 1991). If they are not abandoned and family members become aware of the woman's infection, they may isolate her within the family and find themselves, as a family, isolated within their own neighbourhood or subculture.

Sexuality

With respect to her basic need for intimacy and sexual expression the woman with HIV infection may encounter negative attitudes among professionals rather than a discussion of positive constructive alternatives. Guilt-induction and deprivation reinforce already potent feelings inside that say *"I am unlovable, dirty, unwanted and undesirable"*. The decline in physical attractiveness due to weight loss, hair loss, and other physical manifestations in young previously healthy women can be devastating.

Preliminary results of a Montreal study of sexual activity and satisfaction among women with HIV infection indicate that over half of the women in reasonably good health report being sexually active (Hankins *et al.*, 1993). Many women appear to pass through a period of reduced sexual functioning and loss of libido, however, around the time that they learn that they have HIV infection. They may be afraid of infecting sexual partners and may fear being reinfected by them with HIV or another sexually transmitted disease. Knowledge of safer sex techniques and support from non-judgemental professionals to address sexual issues are important if women with HIV infection are to find ways of achieving safe sexual satisfaction.

Fertility

The direct association between HIV infection in women and the epidemiology of pediatric AIDS creates psychosocial issues concerning the acceptability of contraception and abortion as well as the personal and societal implications of childbearing for the woman with HIV infection. Many women have deep-seated concerns over fertility and the regulation of the time and number of pregnancies. Regardless of the cultural context, anxiety about future childbearing potential may be paramount (Wofsy, 1987) and grief for the perceived loss of reproductive choice may be profound. In societies where self-esteem and societal acceptance may be based on the number of healthy children that they produce, women with HIV infection may express the desire to increase the number of pregnancies that they will have in order to ensure that at least some of their offspring are not HIV infected (Temmerman *et al.*, 1990).

Women who are already pregnant may wish to terminate the pregnancy, however, in many countries legal and safe abortions are not available. It is estimated that 40 per cent of all maternal mortality worldwide is related to illegal abortion (Blum, 1990). Even if therapeutic abortion is legal, available services may not accept women with known HIV infection (Franke, 1989).

Factors which may influence women to take a pregnancy to term include a desire for a child to fulfil needs related to motherhood, a gender self-image which requires childbearing, an acceptable odds risk evaluation, personal morality opposed to therapeutic abortion, unavailability of therapeutic abortion, personal optimism, increasing age, religious faith, and prior experience with an antibody-positive child who sero-reverted (Kurth & Hutchinson, 1990). On the other hand, factors influencing reproductive decisions to terminate or avoid pregnancy may include lack of adoption options for the child, prior experience with HIV and the stress of waiting for children to sero-revert, prior experience with infant death, desire to avoid physical illness in their child, fear of inability to care for the child, and desire to avoid HIV stigma for the child (Levasseur, Pineault, & Hankins, 1991).

The decision to bear a child for women with HIV infection presents a personal dilemma framed by the uncertain risks of transmission, the essential human desire to reproduce, and gender-role and societal expectations (Levine & Dubler, 1990). Women with HIV infection require the latest available scientific information and culturally sensitive professional assistance in exploring the consequences of proceeding with or renouncing pregnancy in order to arrive at a decision with which they themselves can live.

PREVENTION OF HETEROSEXUAL TRANSMISSION OF HIV TO WOMEN

Status of Women

Serious efforts have been devoted to characterize and better understand the conditions which foster the sexual transmission of HIV to women since the recognition that prevention programmes aimed at empowering women to initiate behaviour change and to maintain healthy sexual behaviours could not succeed without the political and economic empowerment of women (Hankins, 1990; Ulin, 1992; de Bruyn, 1992). The interrelationships between the status of women and risk of HIV infection have been explored (Toolanen, 1990), with clear concerns expressed not only about the cultural, social, and economic constraints which increase the risk of HIV in all countries but also with regard to the potential for the AIDS epidemic to undermine gains that have been achieved in improving the status of women (United Nations Division for the Advancement of Women, 1990). This is an important area for scientific endeavour and for ongoing surveillance in light of the major sociodemographic and economic effects of the HIV/AIDS epidemic (United Nations Development Program, 1991).

Mechanical and Chemical Barriers

Prevention messages have promoted abstinence, reducing the number of sexual partners and knowing one's sexual partner, endogamy, which is the choice of a sexual partner of one's own age, and the condom. The latter is the primary method of protection advocated to date in many countries. Since partner condom use depends on the full cooperation of the male partner, a call has been made for greater emphasis on preventive methods that women can use in a clandestine fashion. Stein (1990) argues that a vaginally inserted barrier or virucide would fill the need if it was not only efficacious but also convenient to use, non-irritant, non-toxic, and low-priced. Although *in vitro* studies of the properties of the spermicide nonoxynol-9 are promising (Cates & Stone, 1992) and spermicidal gels and sponges have shown protection against gonorrhoea and chlamydia (Louv, Austin, Alexander, Stagno, & Cheeks, 1988) a recently published *in vivo* study by Kreiss *et al*. (1992) shows no protective effect. On the contrary, frequent nonoxynol-9 sponge use appeared to be associated with HIV infection, a result which may be attributable to inflammation secondary to chemical irritation from the relatively high dose of spermicide contained in the sponge. As Stone and Peterson (1992) have declared, new vaginal products are urgently needed to act as mechanical or chemical barriers to expand the armamentarium available to women for HIV prevention.

Gender Relations

Dilemmas are posed to HIV prevention efforts by paradigms, such as the ethos of male superiority and the conception of all sexual intercourse in terms of the schema of penetration (Foucault, 1985), and by patriarchal ideologies which influence the identities, expectations, and practices of young men (Holland, Ramazanoglu, Scott, Sharpe, & Thomson, 1992). As a result, gender and power relations as well as socialized concepts of masculinity and femininity limit the capacity of young women to negotiate the boundaries of sexual encounters so as to ensure both their safety and their satisfaction.

Holland *et al*. (1992) call for a gendered dimension in prevention which would nurture and develop in young women a sense of self-worth and self-esteem as well as awareness of their own needs for experiencing and requiring sexual pleasure. For young men the legitimation of alternatives to stereotypical gender notions and increased sensitivity to the sexual and social needs of young women would be encouraged. St. Lawrence *et al*. (1992) recommend skill building interventions for young women which would assist in self-expression, assertion, and partner negotiation as well as interventions for young men which would help them to develop greater self-control, increased perceptions of vulnerability, and a more internal locus of control.

With respect to commercial sex work more research is required to determine how differences in the organisation of work and working conditions for various types of prostitutes can influence risk practices while working (Jackson, Highcrest, & Coates, 1992). A better understanding is needed of the mechanisms by which economic recession and increased police enforcement create financial hardships rendering women more vulnerable to demands for unsafe sexual services.

Short-term solutions to these prevention dilemmas lie in the development of clandestine, woman-controlled, methods of HIV prevention, however, in the medium- to long-term only the empowerment of women to achieve economic autonomy and equal social and sexual status will protect them from exposure to HIV infection through heterosexual activity.

CONCLUSION

Increased attention is now beginning to be paid to the unique features of HIV in women after years of scientific neglect. An estimated 4.7 million women had become infected with the human immunodeficiency virus by the beginning of 1992. Women living with HIV experience many of the same clinical manifestations as do men and have comparative survival when important clinical, demographic, and treatment variables are taken into consideration. It has only recently become apparent, however, that there are important gynaecological manifestations in women which require aggressive investigation and intervention. Psychosocial and sexual issues play a large role in the lives of women with HIV infection. Worldwide, women who are most at risk of HIV infection are disadvantaged and disenfranchised. Prevention of HIV infection in women requires a critical examination of societal forces and gender-based power inequalities that put women at risk.

ACKNOWLEDGEMENTS

The assistance of Margaret Handley and Sylvie Gauthier in the preparation of this manuscript is gratefully acknowledged.

REFERENCES

Ades, A.E., Parker, S., Berry, T., Holland, F.J., Davison, C.F., Cubitt, D., Hjelm, M., Wilcox, A. H., Hudson, C.N., Briggs, M., Tedder, R.S., Peckham, C.S. (1991). Prevalence of maternal HIV-1 infection in Thames Regions: results from anonymous unlinked neonatal testing. *The Lancet*, **337**, 1562-1565.

Agarossi, A., Casolati, E., Muggiasca, L., Ravasi, L., Brambilla, T., Conti, M. (1991). Natural history of cervical HPVi and CIN in HIV positive women [Abstract M.B.2425]. *VII International Conference on AIDS*, 1, 288.

Allen, S., Lindan, C., Serufilira, A., Van de Perre, P., Chen Rundle, A., Nsengumuremyi, F., Carael, M., Schwalbe, J., Hulley, S. (1991). Human immunodeficiency virus infection in urban Rwanda. *Journal of the American Medical Association*, **266**, 1657–1663.

Anastos, K., Denenberg, R., Solomon, L., Rein, S. (1992). Relationship of CD4 cell counts to cervical cytologic abnormalities and gynecologic infections in 150 HIV-infected women [Abstract TuB0532]. *VIII International Conference on AIDS/III STD World Congress, Final Program & Oral Abstracts*, Tu32.

Ankrah, M. (1991). AIDS and the social side of health. *Social Science and Medicine*, **32**(9), 967–980.

Ayanian, J.Z., Epstein, A.M. (1991). Differences in the use of procedures between women and men hospitalized for coronary heart disease. *New England Journal of Medicine*, **325**, 221–225.

Bauer, H.M., Ting, Y., Greer, C.E., Chambers, J.C., Tashiro, C.J., Chimera, J., Reingold, A., Manos, M. (1991). Genital human papillomavirus infection in female university students as determined by a PCR-based method. *Journal of the American Medical Association*, **265**, 472–477.

Bavin, P.J., Giles, J.A., Hudson, E., Williams, D., Crow, J., Griffiths, P.D., Emery, V.C., Walker, P.G. (1992). Comparison of cervical cytology and the polymerase chain reaction for HPV16 to identify women with cervical disease in a general practice population. *Journal of Medical Virology*, **37**, 8–12.

Beral, V., Peterman, T.A., Berkelman, R.L., Jaffe, H.W. (1990). Kaposi's sarcoma among persons with AIDS: a sexually transmitted infection? *Lancet*, **335**, 123–128.

Berrebi, A., Chraibi, J., Kobuch, W.E., Puel, J., Grandjean, H., Fournie, A. (1991). Influence of pregnancy on HIV disease [Abstract W.B.2046]. *VII International Conference on AIDS*, 2, 193.

Biggar, R.J., Pahwa, S., Minkoff, H., Mendes, H., Willoughby, A., Landesman, S., Goedert, J.J. (1989). Immunosuppression in pregnant women infected with human immunodeficiency virus. *American Journal of Obstetrics and Gynecology*, **161**, 1239–1244.

Blum, R.W. Global trends in adolescent health. (1990). *Journal of the American Medical Association*. **265**, 2711–2719.

Bolling, D.R. (1977). Prevalence, goals and complications of heterosexual anal intercourse in a gynecologic population. *The Journal of Reproductive Medicine*, **19**(3), 120–124.

Bongaarts, J., Reining, P., Way, P., Conant, F. (1989). The relationship between male circumcision and HIV infection in African populations. *AIDS*, **3**, 373–377.

Buehler, J., Farizo, K., Berkelman, R. (1991). The spectrum of HIV disease in women [Abstract M.D.4253]. *VII International Conference on AIDS*, **1**, 453.

Burk, R.D., Fleming, I., Ho, G.Y.F., Klein, R.S. (1991). Cervical squamous intraepithelial lesions (SIL) in women with HIV: relationship to persistent human papilloma virus (HPV) infection of the cervix [M.A.1246]. *VII International Conference on AIDS*, **1**, 153.

Burke, D.S., Brundage, J.F., Goldenbaum, M., Gardner, L.I., Peterson, M., Visintine, R., Redfield, R.R., & the Walter Reed Retrovirus Research Group. (1990). Human immunodeficiency virus infection in teenagers — Seroprevalence among applicants for U.S. Military Service. *Journal of the American Medical Association*, **263**(15), 2074–2077.

Burmer, G.C., Parker, J.D., Bates, J., East, K., Kulander, B.G. (1990). Comparative analysis of human papillomavirus detection by polymerase chain reaction and virapap/viratype kits. *American Journal of Clinicial Pathology*, **94**, 554–560.

Cameron, D.W., Padian, N.S. (1990). Sexual transmission of HIV and the epidemiology of other sexually transmitted diseases. *AIDS*, **4**(suppl. 1), S99-S103.

Cannon, R.O., Quinn, T., Rompalo, A., Glasser, D., Groseclose, S., Hook, E. (1989). Syphilis is strongly associated with HIV infection in Baltimore STD clinic patients independent of risk group [Abstract Th.A.O.18]. *V International Conference on AIDS, Abstracts*, 74.

Carpenter, C.C.J., Mayer, K.H., Stein, M.D., Leibman, B.D., Fisher, A., Fiore, T.C. (1991). Human immunodeficiency virus infection in North American women: Experience with 200 cases and a review of the literature. *Medicine*. **70**, 307–325.

Castro, K.G., Lieb, S., Jaffe, H.W., Narkunas, J.P., Calisher, C.H., Bush, T.J., Witte, J.J. & the Belle Glade Field-Study Group. (1988). Transmission of HIV in Belle Glade, Florida: Lessons for other communities in the United States. *Science*, **239**, 193-197.

Cates, W., Stone, K.M. (1992). Family planning, sexually transmitted diseases, and contraceptive choice: a literature update—part 1. *Family Planning Perspective*, **24**, 75–84.

Centers for Disease Control. (1991). Characteristics of, and HIV infection among, women served by publicly funded HIV counselling and testing services—United States, 1989–1990. *Morbidity and Mortality Weekly Report*, **40**, 195–203.

Chu, S.Y., Buehler, J.W., Berkelman, R.L. (1990). Impact of the human immunodeficiency virus epidemic on mortality in women of reproductive age, United States. *Journal of the American Medical Association*, **264**(2), 225–229.

Chu, S.Y., Buehler, J.W., Fleming, P.L., Berkelman, R.L. (1990). Epidemiology of reported cases of AIDS in Lesbians, United States 1980–1989. *American Journal of Public Health*, **80**, 1380–1381.

Colon, H., Robles, R., Aponte, L., Matos, T. (1990). HIV status and risk behaviours among women sexual partners of IVDUs in Puerto Rico [Abstract 3008]. *VI International Conference on AIDS, Final Program and Abstracts*, **2**, 404.

Conti, M., Agarossi, A., Muggiasca, M., Ravasi, L., Ghetti, E., Carlini, N., Boldorini, R. (1992). High progression rate of HPV and CIN in HIV [Poster PoB3050]. *VIII International Conference on AIDS/III STD World Congress, Poster Abstracts*, B95.

de Bruyn, M. (1992). Women and AIDS in developing countries. *Social Science and Medicine*, **34**(3), 249-262.

Desmond-Hellmann, S., Mbidde, E.K., Kizito, A., Hellman, N.S. (1990). The epidemiology and clinical features of Kaposi's sarcoma in African women with HIV infection [Abstract S.B.508]. *VI International Conference on AIDS, Final Program and Abstracts*, **3**, 213.

Dunn, D.T., Newell, M.L., Ades, A.E., Peckham, C.S. (1992). Risk of human immunodeficiency virus type 1 transmission through breastfeeding. *The Lancet*, **340**, 585–588.

European Study Group. (1989). Risk factors for male to female transmission of HIV. *British Medical Journal*, **298**, 411–415.

Feingold, A.R., Vermund, S.H., Burk, R.D., Kelley, K.F., Schrager, L.K., Klein, R.S., *et al.* (1989). HIV infection increases frequency and severity of papillomavirus induced cervical cytolic abnormalities [Poster presentation]. *V International Conference on AIDS, Abstracts*, 158.

Feingold, A.R., Vermund, S.H., Burk, R.D., Kelley, K.F., Schrager L.K., Munk, G., Friedland, G.H., Klein, R.S. (1990). Cervical cytologic abnormalities and papillomavirus in women infected with human immunodeficiency virus. *Journal of Acquired Immune Deficiency Syndromes*, **3**, 896–903.

Fleming, P.L., Clesielski, C.A., Berkelman, R.L. (1991). Sex-specific differences in theprevalence of reported AIDS-indictive diagnoses, United States, 1988–1990 [Abstract M.C.3210]. *VII International Conference on AIDS*, **1**, 350.

Foucault, M. (1985). History of Sexuality, Vol. 2. *The Use of Pleasure*. Harmondsworth, Viking.

Franco, E.L. (1991). Viral etiology of cervical cancer: A critique of the evidence. *Review of Infectious Diseases*, **13**, 1195–1206.

Franke, K.M. (1989). Discrimination against HIV positive women by abortion clinics in New York City [Abstract]. *V International Conference on AIDS*, 855.

Goedert, J.J., Eyster, M.E., Biggar, R.J. (1987). Heterosexual transmission of human immunodeficiency virus (HIV): Association with severe T4-cell depletion in male haemophiliacs [Abstract 2.6]. *III International Conference on AIDS*.

Guinan, M.E. (1992). HIV, heterosexual transmission, and women. *Journal of the American Medical Association*, **268**(4), 520–521.

Gwinn, M., Pappaioanou, M., George, J.R., Hannon, H., Wasser, S.C., Redus, M.A., Hoff, R. Grady, G.F., Willoughby, A., Novello, A.C., Petersen, L.R., Dondero, T.J. Curran, J.W. (1991). Prevalence of HIV infection in childbearing women in the United States. *Journal of the American Medical Association*, **265**, 1704–1708.

Hankins, C., Corobow, G., Gendron, S., Elmslie, K. (1989). Une étude séro-épidémiologique portant sur la clientèle féminine de quatre cliniques de MTS à Montréal [Abstract]. *Annales de l'Association canadienne-française pour l'avancement des sciences*. **57**, 328.

Hankins C. (1990). Issues involving women, children and AIDS primarily in the developed world. *Journal of AIDS*, **3**, 443–448.

Hankins, C.A., Laberge, C., Lapointe, N., Lai Tung, M.T., Racine, L., O'Shaughnessy, M. (1990). HIV infection among Quebec women giving birth to live infants. *Canadian Medical Association Journal*, **143**(9), 885–893.

Hankins, C.A., Handley, M.A. (1992) HIV disease and AIDS in women: Current knowledge and a research agenda. *Journal of Acquired Immune Deficiency Syndromes*, **5**, 957–971.

Healy, B. (1991). The Yentl syndrome. *New England Journal of Medicine*, **325**, 274–276.

Heymann, S.J. (1990). Modeling the impact of breast-feeding by HIV-infected women on child survival. *American Journal of Public Health*, **80**, 1305–1309.

Holland, J., Ramazanoglu, C., Scott, S., Sharpe, S., Thomson, R. (1992). Risk, power and the possibility of pleasure: young women and safer sex. *AIDS Care*, **4**(3), 273–283.

Holmberg, S.D., Stewart, J.A., Gerber, A.R., Byers, R.H., Lee, F.K., O'Malley, P.M., Nahmias, A.J. (1988). Prior herpes simplex virus type 2 infection as a risk factor for HIV infection. *Journal of the American Medical Association*, **259**, 1048–1050.

Iman, N., Carpenter, C.J., Mayer, K.H., Fisher, A., Stein, M., Danforth, S.B. (1990). Hierarchical pattern of mucosal Candida infections in HIV-seropositive women. *American Journal of Medicine*, **89**, 142–146.

Ivo-dos-Santos, J., Couto-Fernandez, J.C., Santana, A. J., Luna, T.M.S., Cunha, G.C.M., Moreira, L., Lemos, A.C., Dutra, M., Miranda, C., Galvo-Castro, B. (1991). Prevalence of HIV-1 antibodies in selected groups of a Brazilian city with African sociodemographic characteristics [Letter to the editor]. *Journal of Acquired Immune Deficiency Syndromes*, **4**(4), 448–449.

Jackson, L., Highcrest, A., Coates, R.A. (1992). Varied potential risks of HIV infection among prostitutes. *Social Science Medicine*, **35**(3), 281-286.

Judson, F.N. (1985). Assessing the number of genital chlamydial infections in the United States. *Journal of Reproductive Medicine*, **30**, 269–272.

Kell, P.D., Shah, P.N., Barton, S.E. (1992). Colposcopic screening of HIV seropositive women - help or hindrance? [Poster PoB3055]. *VIII International Conference on AIDS/III STD World Congress, Poster Abstracts*, B96.

Kennedy, K.I., Fortney, J.A., Bonhomme, M.G., Potts, M., Lamptey, P., Carswell, W. (1990). Do the benefits of breast-feeding outweigh the risk of postnatal transmission of HIV via breastmilk? *Tropical Doctor*, **20**, 25–29.

Killewo, J., Nyamuryekunge, K., Sandström, A., Bredberg-Rådén, U., Wall, S., Mhalu F., Biberfeld, G. (1990). Prevalence of HIV-1 infection in the Kagera region of Tanzania: a population-based study. *AIDS*, **4**, 1081–1085.

King, A.J.C., Beazley, R.P., Warren, W.K., Hankins, C.A., Robertson, A.S., Radford, J.L. (1989). Highlights from the Canada Youth and AIDS Study. *Journal of School Health*, **59**, 139–145.

Koonin, L.M., Ellerbrock, T.V., Atrash, H.K., Rogers, M.F., Smith, J.C., Hogue, C.J.R., Harris, M.A., Chavkin, W., Parker, A.L., Halpin, G.J. (1989). Pregnancy-associated deaths due to AIDS in the United States. *Journal of the American Medical Association*, **261**, 1306–1309.

Kreiss, J., Ngugi, E., Holmes, K., Ndinya-Achola, J., Waiyaki, P., Roberts, P.L., Ruminjo, I., Sajabi, R., Kimata, J., Fleming, T.R., Anzala, A., Holton, D., Plummer, F. (1992). Efficacy of nonoxynol 9 contraceptive sponge use in preventing heterosexual acquisition of HIV in Nairobi prostitutes. *Journal of the American Medical Association*, **268**, 477–482.

Kurth A., Hutchinson, M. (1990). Reproductive health policy and HIV: Where do women fit in? *Pediatric AIDS and HIV Infection: Fetus to Adolescent*, **1**, 121-133.

Lapointe, N., Boucher, M., Samson, J., Charest, J. (1991). Significant markers in the modulation of immunity during pregnancy and post-partum in a paired HIV positive and HIV negative population [Abstract W.B.2054]. *VII International Conference on AIDS*, **2**, 195.

Levasseur, C., Pineault, R., Hankins, C. (1992). Facteurs psychosociaux influençant l'intention de femmes infectées par le VIH d'avoir un enfant : étude de cas. *Santé mentale au Québec*, **XVII**(1), 177-194.

Levine, C., Dubler, N.N. (1990). HIV and childbearing: 1. Uncertain risks and bitter realities: The reproductive choices of HIV-infected women. *The Milbank Quarterly*, **68**, 321–351.

Lifson, A.R., Rutherford, G.W., Jaffe, H.W. (1988). The natural history of human immunodeficiency virus infection. *Journal of Infectious Diseases*, **158**, 1360–1366.

Louv, W.C., Austin, H., Alexander, W.J., Stagno, S., Cheeks, J. (1988). A clinical trial of nonoxynol-9 for preventing gonococcal and chlamydial infections. *Journal of Infectious Diseases*, **158**, 518–523.

Maiman, M., Fruchter, R.G., Serur, E., Remy, J.C., Feuer, G., Boyce, J. (1990). Human immunodeficiency virus infection and cervical neoplasia. *Gynecology and Oncology*, **38**, 377–382.

Maiman, M., Tarricone, N., Vieira, J., Suarez, J., Serur, E., Boyce, J. (1991). Colposcopic evaluation of human immunodeficiency virus-seropositive women. *Obstetrics & Gynecology*, **78**, 84-88.

Mann, J. (1992). The Conference and the pandemic. [Plenary address]. *VIII International Conference on AIDS/III STD World Congress*.

Mårdh, P-A., Helin, I., Bobeck, S., Laurin, J., Nilsson T. (1986). Colonization of pregnant and puerperal women and neonates with Chlamydia trachomatis. *British Journal of Venereal Diseases*, **56**, 96–100.

Mays, V.M., Cochran, S.D. (1988). Issues in the perception of AIDS risk and risk reduction activities by Black and Hispanic/Latina women. *American Psychologist*, **43**, 949–957.

Merson, M. (1992). Epidemiological trends in the epidemic [Plenary address]. *VIII International Conference on AIDS/III STD World Congress*.

Minkoff, H.L., Kelly, P., Maiman, M., Fruchter, R., Fink, M.J., Clarke, L., DeHovitz, J.A. (1992). The relationship of cytology, colposcopy histology, and vaginal cultures among HIV infected women [Poster PoB3059]. *VIII International Conference on AIDS/III STD World Congress, Poster Abstracts*, B96.

Miotti, R., Dallabetta, G., Liomba, G., Wangel, A., Daniel, R., Saah, A., Shah, K., Chiphangwi, J. (1992). Cervical abnormalities in Malawian women co-infected with human papilloma virus (HPV) and HIV-1 [Abstract TuB0529]. *VIII International Conference on AIDS/III STD World Congress, Final Program & Oral Abstracts*. Tu32.

Moore, R.D., Hidalgo, J., Sugland, B.W., Chaisson, R.E. (1991). Zidovudine and the natural history of acquired immunodeficiency syndrome. *New England Journal of Medicine*, **324**, 1412–1416.

Moss, A.R., Bacchetti, P. (1989). Natural history of HIV infection. *AIDS*, **3**, 55–61.

Moss, G.B., Clemetson, D., D'Costa, L., Plummer, F.A., Ndinya-Achola, J.O., Reilly, M., Holmes, K.K., Piot, P., Maitha, G.M., Hillier, S.L., Kiviat, N.C., Cameron, C.W., Wamola, I.A., Kreiss, J.K. (1991). Association of cervical ectopy with heterosexual transmission of human immunodeficiency virus: results of a study of couples in Nairobi, Kenya. *Journal of Infectious Diseases*, **164**, 588–591.

Nahlen, B., Nwanyanwa, O., Chu, S., Berkelman, R. (1991). HIV wasting syndrome in the U.S. [Abstract M.C.47]. *VII International Conference on AIDS*, **1**, 34.

Oriel, J.D., Johnson, A.L., Barlow, D., Thomas, B. J., Mayyar, K., Reeve, P. (1978). Infection of the uterine cervix with Chlamydial trachomatis. *Journal of Infectious Diseases*, **137**(4), 443–451.

Padian, N., Marquis, L., Francis, D.P., Anderson, R.E., Rutherford, G.W., O'Malley, P.M., Winkelstein, W., Jr. (1987). Male-to-female transmission of immunodeficiency virus. *Journal of the American Medical Association*, **258**, 788–790.

Pepin, J., Dunn, D., Gaye, I., Alonso, P., Egboga, A., Tedder, R., Piot, P., Berry, N., Schellenberg, D., Whittle, H., Wilkins, A. (1991). HIV-2 infection among prostitutes working in The Gambia: association with serological evidence of genital ulcer diseases and with generalized lymphadenopathy. *AIDS*, **5**, 69-75.

Piot, P., Plummer, F.A., Rey, M.A., Ngugi, E.N., Rouzioux, C., Ndinya-Achola, J.O., Veracauteren, G., D'Costa, L.H., Laga, M., Nsanze, H., Fransen, L., Haase, D., van der Groen, G., Brunham, R.C., Ronald, A.R., Brun-Vézinet, F. (1987). Retrospective seroepidemiology of AIDS virus infection in Nairobi populations. *Journal of Infectious Diseases*, **155**, 1108–1112.

Plourde, P.J., Plummer, F.A., Pepin, J., Agoki, E., Moss, G., Ombette, J., Ronald, A.R., Cheang, M., D'Costa, L., Ndinya-Achola, J.O. (1992) Human immunodeficiency virus type 1 infection in women attending a sexually transmitted disease clinic in Kenya. *Journal of Infectious Diseases*, 166, 86–92.

Plummer, F.A., Simonsen, J.N., Cameron, D.W., Ndinya-Achola, J.O., Kreiss, J.K., Gakinya, M.N., Waiyaki, P., Cheang, M., Piot, P., Ronald, A.R., Ngugi, E.N. (1991). Cofactors in male-female sexual transmission of human immunodeficiency virus type 1. *Journal of Infectious Diseases*, 163, 233–239.

Rees, E., Tait, I.A., Hobson, D. Johnson, F.W. (1977). Chlamydia in relation to cervical infection and pelvic inflammatory disease. In D. Hobson, K. K. Holmes (Eds.), *Nongonoccocal Urethritis and Related Infections* (pp. 67–76). Washington, DC: American Society for Microbiology.

Reid, E. (1990). Placing women at the centre of the analysis. In *Panel Discussion Proceedings, CIDA World AIDS Day Series, Women in Development with the Health and Population Directorates* (pp. 24–31). Hull, Quebec, Canada.

Report of a Consensus Workshop, Siena, Italy, January 17–18, 1992: Maternal factors involved in mother-to-child transmission of HIV-1. (1992). *Journal of Acquired Immune Deficiency Syndromes*, 5, 1019–1029.

Rhoads, J.L., Wright, D.C., Redfield, R.R., Burke, D.S. (1987). Chronic vaginal candidiasis in women with human immunodeficiency virus infection. *Journal of the American Medical Association*, 257, 3105–3107.

Saltz, G.R., Linnemann, C.C., Brookman, R.R., Rauh, J.L. (1981). Chlamydia trachomatis cervical infections in female adolescents. *Journal of Pediatrics*, 98, 981–985.

Schechter, M.T., Craib, K.J.P., Le, T.H., Montaner, J.S., Douglas, B., Sestak, P., Willoughby, B., O'Shaughnessy, M.V. (1990). Susceptibility to AIDS progression appears early in HIV infection. *AIDS*, 4, 185–190.

Schrijvers, D., Delaporte, E., Peeters, M., Dupont, A., Meheus, A. (1991). Seroprevalence of retroviral infection in women with different fertility status in Gabon, western equatorial Africa. *Journal of Acquired Immune Deficiency Syndromes*, 4, 468-470.

Shah, P., Smith, R., Kitchen, V., Wells, C., Barton, S., Steer, P. (1992). Menstrual abnormalities in HIV seropositive women [Poster PoB3062]. *VIII International Conference on AIDS/III STD World Congress, Poster Abstracts*, B97.

Simonsen, J., Cameron, D., Gajinya, M. (1988). Human immunodeficiency virus infection among men with sexually transmitted diseases. *New England Journal of Medicine*, 319, 274–278.

Simonsen, J.N., Plummer, F.A., Ngugi, E.N., Black, C., Kreiss, J.K., Gakinya, M.N., Waiyaki, P., D'Costa, L.H., Ndinya-Achola, J.O., Piot, P., Ronald, A. (1990). HIV infection among lower socioeconomic strata prostitutes in Nairobi. *AIDS*, 4, 139–144.

Siraprapasiri, T., Thanprasertsuk, S., Rodklay, A., Srivanichakorn, S., Sawanpanyalert, P., Temtanarak, J. (1991). Risk factors for HIV among prostitutes in Chiangmai, Thailand. *AIDS*, 5(5), 579–582.

Sperling, R.S., Stratton, P., & the Members of the Obstetric-Gynecologic Working Group of the AIDS Clinical Trials Group of the National Institute of Allergy and Infectious Diseases. (1992). Treatment options for human immunodeficiency virus-infected pregnant women. *Obstetrics & Gynecology*, 79(3), 443-448.

St. Lawrence, J.S., Davis, J., Brasfield, T., Alleyne, E., Jefferson, K., Banks, P., Jones, M., Simms, S., Shirley, A., Moore, D. (1992). Gender differences relevant to AIDS prevention with African-American adolescents. [Poster PoD5449]. *VIII International Conference on AIDS/III STD World Congress, Poster Abstracts*, D461.

Stein, Z.A. (1990). HIV prevention: the need for methods women can use. *American Journal of Public Health*, 80, 460–462.

Stein, J., Roche, N., Mathur-Wagh, U., Wilets, E., Weber, J., Middleton, S., Gomez, R. (1991). Gynecologic findings in an HIV-positive out-patient population [Abstract M.B.2427]. *VII International Conference on AIDS*, 1, 288.

Steingart, M.S., Packer, M., Hamm, P., Coglianese, M.E., Gersh, B., Geltman, E.M., Sollano, J., Katz, S., Moyé, L., Basta, L.L., Lewis, S.J., Gottlieb, S. S., Bernstein, V., McEwan, P., Jacobson, K., Brown, E.J., Kukin, M.L., Kantrowitz, N.E., Pfeffer, M.A. (1991). Sex differences in the management of coronary artery disease. *New England Journal of Medicine*, 325, 226–230.

Stone, K., Peterson, H.B. (1992). Spermicides, HIV, and the vaginal sponge [Editorial]. *Journal of the American Medical Association*, 268, 521–523.

Sweeney, P.A., Onorato, I.M., Allen, D.M., Byers, R.H., & the Field Services Branch. (1992). Sentinel surveillance of human immunodeficiency virus infection in women seeking reproductive health services in the United States, 1988–1989. *Obstetrics & Gynecology*, 79(4), 503–510.

Tait, I.A., Rees, E., Hobson, D., Byng, R.E., Tweedie, M.C.K. (1980). Chlamydia infection of the cervix in contacts of men with nongonococcal cervicitis. *British Journal of Venereal Diseases*, 56, 37–45.

Temmerman, M., Moses, S., Kiragu, D., Fusallah, S., Wamola, I.A., Piot, P. (1990). Impact of single session post-partum counselling of HIV infected women on their subsequent reproductive behaviour. *AIDS Care*, 2(3), 247–252.

Tindall, B., Cooper, D.A. (1991). Primary HIV infection: host responses and intervention strategies. *AIDS*, 5, 1–14.

Toolanen, D. (1990). *Interrelationships between the status of women and HIV epidemic: A review of published literature* (EGM/AIDS/1990/BP.2). Vienna, Austria.

Ulin, P.R. (1992). African women and AIDS: Negotiating behavioural change. *Social Science and Medicine*, 34, 63–75.

United Nations Development Program. (1991). *Annual Report: HIV and Development*.

United Nations Division for the Advancement of Women. (1990). *Interrelationships between the status of women and the AIDS epidemic: A conceptual approach for intervention* (EGM/AIDS/1990/BP.1). Vienna, Austria.

Vermund, S.H., Kelley, K.F., Burk, R.D., Feingold, A.R., Schreiber, K., Munk, G., Schrager, L.K., Klein, R.S. (1990). Risk of human papillomavirus and cervical squamous intraepithelial lesions highest among women with advanced HIV disease [Abstract S.B.517]. *VI International Conference on AIDS, Final Program and Abstracts*, 3, 215.

Vermund, S.H., Kelley, K.F. (1991). Human papillomavirus in women: Methodologic issues and role of immunosuppression. In Michele Kiely (Ed.), *Reproductive and Perinatal Epidemiology* (pp. 143-168). Boca Raton: CRC Press.

Vermund, S.H., Kelley, K.F., Klein, R.S., Feingold, A.R., Schreiber, K., Munk, G., Burk, R.D. (1991). High risk of human papillomavirus infection and cervical squamous intraepithelial lesions highest among women with symtomatic human immunodeficiency virus infection. *American Journal of Obstetrics and Gynecology*, 165, 392–400.

Vlahov, D., Brewer, T.F., Castro, K.G., Narkunas, J.P., Salive, M.E., Ullrich, J., Muñoz, A. (1991). Prevalence of antibody to HIV-1 among entrants to US correctional facilities. *Journal of the American Medical Association*, 265, 1129–1132.

Wasserheit, J.N. (1992). Epidemiology synergy: Interrelationships between human immunodeficiency virus infection and other sexually transmitted diseases. *Sexually Transmitted Diseases*, 19, 61–77.

Wofsy, C.B. (1987). Human immunodeficiency virus infection in women. *Journal of the American Medical Association*, 257, 2074–2076.

World Health Organization Global Programme on AIDS. (1992a). *Current and Future Dimensions of the HIV/AIDS Pandemic: A Capsule Summary.*

World Health Organization Global Programme on AIDS. (1992b). *The Current Global Situation of the HIV/AIDS Pandemic.*

3

Drug Injectors and Heterosexual AIDS

SAMUEL R. FRIEDMAN, DON C. DES JARLAIS,
THOMAS P. WARD, BENNY JOSE, ALAN NEAIGUS
AND MARJORIE GOLDSTEIN

In developed countries with high rates of HIV infection among injecting drug users (IDUs), such as the United States, Scotland, Italy and Spain, drug injectors are the predominant source of heterosexual transmission of HIV (WHO Collaborating Centre, 1991; Friedman & Des Jarlais, 1991). Substantial HIV infection among IDUs has also been observed in many developing countries, including Thailand (Vanichseni & Sakuntanaga, 1990; Choopanya et al., 1991), India (Naik et al., 1991), Brazil (Lima et al., 1991; Mesquita et al., 1991) and Argentina (Boxaca et al., 1990; Calello et al., 1991; Fay et al., 1991). The possible linkages between HIV infection among IDUs and heterosexual transmission have not yet been determined in these developing countries. The situation in Thailand is particularly worrisome, however, because rapid spread of HIV among IDUs was followed several years later by rapid spread among heterosexuals who do not inject illicit drugs (Choopanya, 1991). If rapid bridging from IDUs to non-injecting heterosexuals should occur in other South Asian and South American countries, then controlling HIV in those areas will be particularly difficult.

Despite its epidemiologic importance, heterosexual HIV transmission from injecting drug users to non-injectors is probably the mode of transmission for which there is the least scientific data upon which to base interventions. As will be discussed below, changing the drug injection behaviour of IDUs is easier than changing their sexual behaviour (Becker & Joseph, 1988; Des Jarlais & Friedman, 1988a; Stimson, 1990). This suggests that the most effective method of preventing heterosexual and perinatal transmission from IDUs to others may be to keep the

We would like to acknowledge support from US National Institute on Drug Abuse grants DA06723 and DA03574, and from the World Health Organization Global Programme on AIDS.

IDUs from initially becoming infected through the sharing of injection equipment. However, in areas where there are already large numbers of HIV-infected IDUs, changes in sexual behaviour—which have been difficult to change and maintain among all heterosexuals, and not just among drug injectors—will still be required to prevent further heterosexual and perinatal transmission.

This paper explores several aspects of heterosexual HIV transmission involving drug injectors. First, epidemiologic evidence showing the magnitude of this problem is presented. Then, data about the extent of high-risk sexual behaviours among drug injectors are examined, as are various studies of how these behaviours are affected by IDUs' social relationships. Finally, behavioural change by IDUs to reduce the risk of transmitting HIV to others is examined, along with a review of research about the efficacy of interventions designed to reduce the risk of HIV transmission from IDUs to their heterosexual partners.

CASES OF AIDS AMONG HETEROSEXUAL PARTNERS OF IDUS

One way to study heterosexual transmission of HIV from IDUs to others is to compare the number of AIDS cases among heterosexual drug injectors and heterosexual non-drug injectors in areas where drug injectors are known to be the primary source of heterosexual transmission. Since it takes years for HIV infection to develop into active AIDS after the initial HIV exposure, AIDS case data reflect transmission and its associated behaviours that occurred years previously. Nonetheless, such data minimize many of the sampling problems involved in most other methods of studying drug injectors and their non-injecting sexual partners. Of course, AIDS case data are not completely unbiased, and there may well be distortions in the reporting of risk behaviours when persons with AIDS are interviewed—but most persons with AIDS do seek medical attention, and their condition is likely to be reported to public health authorities. Thus, a relatively complete sampling frame can be constructed.

The relative magnitudes of AIDS cases among heterosexual IDUs and among heterosexuals who do not inject drugs are shown in table 3.1 for three geographical locations where drug injectors are the predominant source of heterosexual transmis-

TABLE 3.1

Cumulative Number of AIDS Cases among Heterosexual IDUs and Heterosexual Non-IDUs in Italy, Spain, and New York City (as of 30 June 1991)

	IDUs	Non-IDUs	Ratio of IDUs to non-IDUs
Italy	6435	628	10.2 to 1
Spain	5809	414	14.0 to 1
New York City	13,193	1245	10.6 to 1

sion and where there are enough cases to facilitate interpretation. Despite the many cultural differences between New York City, Spain, and Italy, and despite the differences in the history of the HIV epidemics in the areas, the ratios of heterosexual IDU cases to heterosexual transmission cases range only from 10:1 to 14:1. This may suggest that such areas may have similar risk behaviours, social networks and patterns of epidemiologic transmission; alternatively, if there are differences in regard to these factors, they may cancel each other out—at least when viewed at the level of entire populations of drug injectors.

SEROPREVALENCE AND SEROCONVERSION STUDIES OF HIV AMONG THE NON-DRUG-INJECTING HETEROSEXUAL PARTNERS OF DRUG INJECTORS

The efficiency and extent of HIV transmission during sex between infected IDUs and their partners is, of course, a matter of considerable importance. It is not, however, the focus of this paper. Although numerous seroprevalence studies have been conducted among the non-drug-injecting sex partners of IDUs, serious sample bias issues threaten their generalizability.

In some studies, for example, couples have been recruited in which the IDU member is known to be seropositive or to have HIV-related disease (e.g., Tor *et al.*, 1991; Johnson *et al.*, 1989). These studies require cooperation both from the index IDU and from his or her sexual partner. Although systematic research into the reasons for agreeing or refusing to take part in such studies has not been conducted, it seems reasonable that powerful feelings such as guilt about having infected a partner with HIV, fear of relationship disruption, anger about possibly having become infected, or conflicts over the IDU's drug use would negatively affect both the willingness to participate and the quality of data obtained about risk behaviours.

Other seroprevalence studies have recruited heterosexual partners of IDUs directly rather than together with an index IDU (e.g., Smith *et al.*, 1991; Garcia *et al.*, 1988; Sogolow *et al.*, 1991; Chiasson *et al.*, 1991a). This strategy also leads to methodological problems (Sterk *et al.*, 1989). No specific, readily available sampling frame exists from which to select such heterosexual partners. Some potential subjects might not identify themselves as heterosexual partners of IDUs because they do not know their partners are IDUs, they are uncertain about how their partner would react to their participation, or due to the stigma of being the partner of an IDU. If they do take part, many subjects would not know the HIV status of their IDU sexual partner.

Moreover, based on a review of a number of relatively large studies of non-drug injecting heterosexual partners of injecting drug users, there is considerable variation in seroprevalence rates (Chiasson *et al.*, 1991; De Vincenzi & Ancelle Park, 1991; Falciano *et al.*, 1991; France *et al.*, 1988; Garcia *et al.*, 1988; Johnson *et al.*, Moore *et al.*, 1990; Smith *et al.*, 1991; Tor *et al.*, 1991). Seroprevalence rates in the couples studies vary from 12% to 48%, and in convenience samples from 7% to 38%. These studies also indicate that condom use may be protective.

Another approach to studying HIV transmission from IDUs to non-IDU sex partners is to conduct longitudinal studies of seroconversion among couples in which the IDU is seropositive and the partner seronegative. Recruitment for such studies, however, is biased by all the aforementioned factors involved in studying seroprevalence among couples; indeed, since participation requires remaining in the project for long periods of time, sample biases are probably even stronger. Furthermore, since researchers counsel subjects in seroconversion studies about how to avoid high-risk behaviour, study participation may itself lead many couples to reduce their behavioural risks and thus their probability of seroconversion. Thus, the rates found in seroconversion studies cannot be generalized to other IDUs and their sexual partners. In addition, these studies vary widely in the seroconversion rates they have found (De Vincenzi & Ancelle Park, 1991; Falciano *et al.*, 1991; Papetti *et al.*, 1991; Tor *et al.*, 1991). Nonetheless, seroconversion data, like seroprevalence studies, indicate that consistent condom use reduces risk of HIV infection.

In summary, then, methodological problems and, perhaps, actual variations in transmission rates or dynamics in different locations, have prevented studies of HIV among the partners of IDUs from yielding a clear picture either of the extent of such transmission or of the behavioural risk factors that facilitate transmission. Hence, even though considerable evidence exists that consistent condom use may be effective, further research is clearly warranted.

"BASELINE" RATES OF HETEROSEXUAL BEHAVIOUR AMONG INJECTING DRUG USERS

Since there were few detailed studies of heterosexual behaviour among injecting drug users prior to AIDS, there is a lack of good baseline data from which to assess AIDS-related changes in their sexual behaviour. (There is also a lack of good baseline data for heterosexuals in general.) Studies conducted in the early part of the HIV/AIDS epidemic in a given city must therefore be used to estimate pre-AIDS baseline behaviour, even though some degree of AIDS-related behaviour change might already have occurred prior to the study.

Selected studies of 'baseline' sexual behaviour are presented in table 3.2. Across these different studies, the great majority of injecting drug users reported that they had sexual partners. In the studies that asked about 'regular partner,' the majority of subjects reported that they had a 'regular' heterosexual partner, and a substantial number reported that they had 'casual' heterosexual partners. Taking the studies as a whole, it would appear that there is a potential for large-scale heterosexual transmission.

Although these studies indicate similarities in the heterosexual behaviour of drug injectors from different geographic areas, there are also some important differences. These differences can be seen most clearly in large-scale, multi-site studies that used similar data collection methods across sites.

One of the largest studies of drug injectors and their sexual partners is the National AIDS Demonstration Research (NADR) project, which is being conducted in 63 cities in the United States and Puerto Rico. Studies of sexual risk

TABLE 3.2

Selected Studies of Baseline HIV Sexual Risk Behaviour Among Drug Injectors and/or Their Heterosexual Partners

Author	Sample	Results
Lewis et al. *AJPH* 1990	San Francisco: 149 male IDUs (70 white, 79 black) with stable heterosexual partners interviewed in early 1987.	During the previous year, 63% had more than one female partner, while 31% had 4 or more female partners. During previous five years, 83.2% had more than one partner, while 59.5% had more than 5, and 38.9% more than ten. Heterosexual anal intercourse was reported by 56 (37.6%) of the men. 108 (72.9%) reported never using condoms. Estimated time condoms were used averaged 9.5%. 51 subjects reported having steady non-IDU partners.
Darke et al. *Br J Addict* 1990	Sydney, Australia: Structured interview of 100 IDUs recruited both from treatment sites (59) and from syringe exchanges (41).	*During the one month previous to the interview:* 30% of subjects had more than one sex partner; 10% had engaged in prostitution during month; 42/63 with regular partners had never used condoms; only 10 of those 63 (15.9%) had always used condoms; nearly one third of subjects had sex with casual partner— of these, 20.7% never, 48.3% always used a condom. 14% of subjects had engaged in anal sex.
Corby et al. AIDS Education & Prevention 1991	Long Beach, CA: Mostly street-recruited sample of 137 non-IDU (within prior 6 months) female sex partners of male IDUs. 56.9% were black, 23.4% Latina, 19.7% white. AIDS Initial Assessment interview was administered.	123 were HIV tested, 4 were HIV+ (none of the 4 had used condoms). *During the previous six months:* 67.2% reported having only one sex partner; 20.4% had engaged in prostitution; 94.9% had vaginal sex without condom; 6.6% had anal sex without condom; 44.5% performed fellatio without condom.

Table 3.2 (cont.) — Selected Studies of Baseline HIV Sexual Risk Behaviour Among Drug Injectors and/or Their Heterosexual Partners

Author	Sample	Results
Feucht et al. *J. Drug Issues* 1990	Cleveland, OH: 662 IDUs (520 male, 142 female) interviewed over 12-month period: 189 from MMTP, 473 street-recruited. 62.7% Black, 28.5% white, 6.8% Hispanic.	*During twelve months prior to interview:* 55.6% of male IDUs, 41.5% of female IDUs had 2 or more heterosexual partners; 37.9% of male IDUs, 66.2% of female IDUs had one or more IDU heterosexual partners; 81.9% of males with one partner never used condoms; 81.4% of females with one partner never used condoms; 59.5% of males with > 1 partner never used condoms; 44.1% of females with > 1 partner never used condoms.
McCusker et al. *AJPH* 1990	Worceser, MA: Survey of 926 recent IDUs (678 males, 248 females) enrolled at treatment centres, clinical sites, and a men's jail.	Number of sex partners: None—15% of males, 17% of females; One—48% of males, 44% of females; 2 or more—37% of males, 39% of females. Risk behaviour within previous three months of subset with multiple partners: Used condoms—only 19% of males, 55% of females; 27% of males had sex with prostitute; 73% of females engaged in prostitution.
Centers for Disease Control *MMWR* 4/27/90	U.S. nationwide (63 sites, 45 cities): 16,998 IDUs not in drug treatment (12,678 male, 4,320 female) recruited through National AIDS Demonstration Research projects.	Condom use during previous six months. Vaginal sex, 10,270 males: 70% never, 20% sometimes; Vaginal sex, 3,635 females: 57% never, 29% sometimes; Anal sex, 2,065 males: 78% never, 11% sometimes; Anal sex, 566 females: 68% never, 16% sometimes.

behaviours (during the 6 months prior to study entry) by over 10,000 IDUs in 19 of these cities (which vary widely in HIV seroprevalence among IDUs) have been conducted by Friedman and his colleagues (Friedman *et al.*, in press). In this sample, subjects report a mean of approximately 20 episodes of vaginal intercourse without a condom per month. Condoms were used 21% of the time when these IDUs have vaginal sex. Anal sex without a condom was also fairly widespread; it was reported by 14% of black male subjects, 18% of white male subjects, 23% of Puerto Rican-origin male subjects, and 22% of Mexican-origin male subjects. Among female subjects, the percentages reporting unprotected anal sex were 9% (blacks), 16% (whites), 17% (Puerto Rican-origin), and 14% (Mexican-origin). Between 40% and 64% of each race/ethnicity-gender combination reported having one or more opposite-sex partners who was not a drug injector. In sum, then, this study indicates that IDUs are engaging in considerable high-risk behaviour, including unprotected anal sex; that condom use is limited; and that social characteristics such as race/ethnicity and sex affect the extent of risk behaviours.

Weissman *et al.* (Centers for Disease Control, 1991) studied NADR data on 6,104 sexual partners (70% of whom were women) of drug injectors. None of these sexual partners had themselves injected drugs within 6 months prior to intake, although over half had used non-injected cocaine during this period. Among men, 5% had had sex only with men during the previous 6 months; 4% with both men and women; and 91% only with women. Among women, 2% had had sex only with women during the previous 6 months; 3% with both men and women; and 95% only with men. 35% of the men, and 22% of the women, reported having had sex with 2 or more IDUs during the previous 6 months. Condom use by these sexual partners of IDUs was rare: approximately 60% of both men and women reported never using condoms (during this 6-month period) while having vaginal sex. Subjects with multiple sex partners report more condom use than those with only one. Finally, among these non-injecting sex partners of IDUs, 15% of the men and 24% of the women report trading sex for money in the preceding 6 months.

The World Health Organization multi-site study of injecting drug users also standardizes methods across different locations and thus permits further comparison of the heterosexual behaviour of injecting drug users. There are important differences among sites in the ratio of male to female drug injectors. In most developed country sites, e.g., New York City, the ratio of male drug injectors to female drug injectors is approximately 2:1. The male-to-female ratio in Bangkok, however, is 19:1 (Des Jarlais *et al.*, 1992). Sex ratios greater than 1:1 are likely to lead to male drug injectors developing heterosexual relationships with women who do not inject drugs; this tends to spread HIV to persons who do not inject drugs. Whether the exceptionally high sex ratio among IDUs in Bangkok was in part responsible for the aforementioned rapid spread of HIV among non-drug injecting heterosexuals in Bangkok has not yet been determined. The extent of such spread would be a function of many factors, including the extent to which male drug injectors in Bangkok have sexual relationships with women who do not inject and the extent to which these women, in turn, have unprotected sex with additional partners.

NETWORKS AND SEXUAL BEHAVIOURS AMONG DRUG INJECTORS AND THEIR HETEROSEXUAL PARTNERS IN BROOKLYN, NEW YORK CITY

These general patterns can be exemplified more concretely by presenting data recently collected from street-recruited drug injectors in a study that Friedman *et al.* have been conducting in Brooklyn. All the subjects who were interviewed are drug injectors who had injected drugs within the previous year. Of 591 subjects, 436 (74%) were men, and 155 (26%) women (table 3.3). This 3-to-1 ratio is not greatly dissimilar to what has been found in other studies of drug injectors in New York City and many other cities. The average subject first had sex at age 14 (13.9 for men, 15.4 for women), and first injected drugs at age 20 (19.6 for men, 22.3 for women). The earliest age of sexual initiation (and, in these cases, abuse) was 5 for male and 6 for female subjects.

Data were collected about the sexual behaviour and sexual partners of these subjects during the two years prior to their participation in the study. Most of the subjects had had partners during this period. Many of the partners of both the men and women were themselves drug injectors, and of course these partners were at risk for both injection-related and sexual transmission of HIV and other infectious agents such as hepatitis B, hepatitis C, and human T-cell lymphotropic viruses types I and II. In addition, more than half of the subjects had partners who had never injected drugs. For these partners, sexual transmission from their drug-injecting partners is probably their primary potential risk for HIV infection. Of the male drug injectors in the study, 69% had had at least one female sexual partner during this time period who had never injected drugs; 31% had had only one such partner, but 37% had had 2 or more. Only 3% had had more than ten non-IDU partners. Among the women, 44% had had at least one male sexual partner during this time period who had never injected drugs; 16% had had only one such partner, but 28% had had 2 or more. About 10% had had more than ten non-IDU male partners.

Sexual frequency varied by gender. Men were more likely to have had sex at least once during the prior two years. Among the subjects who did have sex, women had

TABLE 3.3
Number of sex partners of the opposite sex in the last two years:

	Number of partners					
	0	1	2	3–5	6–10	11 +
Male drug injectors (N = 436)						
All partners	14%	34%	18%	21%	8%	5%
Partners who have injected drugs	55%	30%	7%	6%	2%	0%
Partners who have not injected drugs	31%	31%	15%	14%	5%	3%
Female drug injectors (N = 155):						
All partners	22%	40%	10%	10%	7%	10%
Partners who have injected drugs	47%	43%	6%	2%	1%	1%
Partners who have not injected drugs	56%	16%	5%	7%	6%	10%

sex more often. Thus, 22% of women who had sex did so at an average frequency of once per day, as opposed to only 10% of the men.

Subjects who had sex during the previous two years were asked about the proportion of sex acts in which they used condoms (table 3.4). Only about half of these subjects had used condoms at all, and most of the condom-users did so only part of the time they had sex. Only 16% of men, and 19% of women, reported having always used condoms. Women drug injectors were significantly more likely to use condoms more often than the men; this probably reflects their greater involvement in prostitution. (Only 7 men reported any prostitution in the month before the interview, as opposed to at least 35 of the much smaller number of women subjects. Among the women who engaged in prostitution, 50% report always using condoms with customers during oral sex, and 65% during vaginal sex. Among 85 women who had vaginal sex with a spouse or steady lover during the preceding 30 days, only 27% always used condoms with them; and only 20% of 60 women who had oral sex with a spouse or steady lover during this time period always used condoms.)

Data were also collected about the social network members of the drug injectors in this study. Specifically, subjects were asked to provide data about the persons with whom they had had more than casual contact during the past 30 days. They were particularly asked to describe persons with whom they had used drugs or had sex. Detailed questions were then asked of the subjects about their relationships with, and the characteristics and behaviours of, up to ten of these network members. Here, data are presented on the characteristics of the sex partners who were discussed by subjects in response to this stimulus—and, particularly, of those sex partners who were described as never having injected drugs.

Several characteristics of these data should be understood. First, the unit of analysis is the sex partner as named and described by the drug-injecting study participant. Thus, if one subject named four such partners, and another named one, the data being presented include four times as many partners of one IDU as of the other. Furthermore, it is possible that some persons may be named and described by more than one subject as having been their sex partner in the past 30 days; any such person will appear in the data more than once. Finally, the data are the subject's (one-sided) descriptions of the relationship, of their behaviours with their partner, and of the attributes of their partner. In addition to the normal inaccuracies of

TABLE 3.4

Proportion of times drug injectors used condoms during sex in last two years

	Male (N = 378)	Female (N = 134)
Never	52%	43%
Less than half the time	19	14
About half the time	6	7
More than half the time	7	16
Always	16	19
	Chi-square = 12.819	p < .012

self-report data, then, these data may also be inaccurate due to being one-sided descriptions of an interpersonal relationship or due to the respondent's ignorance of the partner's behaviours.

There were 185 such non-IDU heterosexual partners named by the drug injectors in the study. Ten percent of the sexual relationships had started extremely recently (within the past 2 months or less), another 29% had lasted for 3 to 12 months; 28% for more than a year but no more than 5 years; and 34% of the sexual relationships were more than five years old.

During sex between the IDU subject and the non-IDU partner in the last 30 days, condoms were used always by 47% of the couples. Condom use was a function of the nature of the relationship: condoms were used always by 37% of the couples in which the IDU subject said the relationship was 'very close,' 47% of 'close' relationships, 57% of 'somewhat close' relationships, and 61% of 'distant' and 'very distant' relationships (p < .02 by Mantel-Haenszel chi-square). Similarly, condoms were always used by 32% of spouses, 38% of lovers/boyfriends/girlfriends, 55% of friends, and 85% of acquaintances (p < .004 by chi-square).

Another determinant of condom use during sex between IDU subjects and their non-IDU partners was the HIV serostatus of the IDU subject. Among 100 couples where the IDU subject was seronegative, condoms were always used with 32% of their non-IDU heterosexual partners; whereas among 69 couples where the IDU subject was seropositive, condoms were always used with 72% of the non-IDU partners (p < .001 by chi-square). Of some note, the extent of condom use by seropositive IDU subjects with these non-injecting partners did not differ by whether the relationship was 'very close', 'close,' 'somewhat close,' or 'distant.' These data indicate that many couples in which the IDU partner is infected are deliberately engaging in safer sex.

IDU subjects report a lower level of condom use with their drug-injecting sex partners. Among couples in which the partner was a drug injector, condoms were always used by only 22% (as compared to by 49% where the partner was not an IDU; p < .001 by chi-square). There was a statistical tendency towards more consistent condom use by couples in which the partner did not inject drugs even where the IDU subject was seronegative (32% versus 21%; chi-square = 3.17, p < .10). The extent of consistent condom use with IDU partners was similar regardless of the serostatus of the IDU subject: condoms were always used by 21% of the 113 couples where the IDU subject was seronegative and by 22% of 68 couples where the IDU subject was seropositive. The lower level of condom use with partners who inject drugs suggests that IDU couples probably perceive that they have a considerably greater probability of becoming infected with HIV through their drug injecting (including with each other) than through sex with each other.

BEHAVIOUR CHANGE, WITH EMPHASIS ON RESPONSE TO SPECIFIC PROGRAMMES

Table 3.5 describes a number of studies of heterosexual behaviour change among IDUs and the sexual partners of IDUs. Clearly a variety of intervention pro-

Table 3.5

Selected Studies of Sexual Behaviour Change for AIDS Risk Reduction among Injecting Drug Users and/or Their Heterosexual Partners

Author	Sample	Mechanism of Change	Results
Donoghoe et al. AIDS Care 1989	UK multisite: Questionnaire survey, with re-interview after 2 to 4 months, of 142 clients (120 male, 20 female) of syringe exchanges.	Syringe exchange AIDS education	Changes from intake to follow-up: Number of sexual partners: No partner—23% to 31%; Multiple partners—26% to 21%; Regular partner—49% to 52%. Any condom use: 38% to 30%. Non-IDU partner: 36% to 39%; 46% to 55% for sexually active subset.
Klee et al. AIDS Care 1991	North-West of England: 169 IDUs (46 female, 123 male) re-contacted for structured questionnaire 6 to 9 months after previous interview as part of larger (n = 303) sample.	Unspecified, although overall AIDS awareness was high, and many subjects had already sought HIV testing on their own initiative.	Changes from intake to follow-up: Number of sexual partners: No partner—14% to 18%; Multiple partners—30% to 23%; Regular partner—56% to 59%. Condom use among sexually active subset: 54 (36%) out of 148 report any condom use, while only 22 (15%) always use condoms.
Wyld et al. (Florence '91: W.C.3106)	Edinburgh, Scotland: 115 HIV + IDUs and their heterosexual partners—30 of the couples both HIV +, 85 couples serologically discordant—were interviewed every six months over a 3-year period about their sexual histories since 1983.	HIV testing and repeated counseling.	Report any condom use: 2% in 1983, 48% in 1989; Couples reporting a pregnancy: 23/89 (26%) in 1987, 9/78 (11.5%) in 1989.

Table 5 (cont.) — Selected Studies of Sexual Behaviour Change for AIDS Risk Reduction among Injecting Drug Users and/or Their Heterosexual Partners

Author	Sample	Mechanism of Change	Results
Hart *et al.* AIDS 1989	London, UK: 133 clients of the syringe-exchange scheme of Middlesex Hospital interviewed one month after entry, with 76 contacted for 3-month follow-up.	Syringe exchange with AIDS education.	At 3-month follow-up (n = 76): 20 (26%) had no sexual partner, 41 (54%) had one sexual partner—of these, 27% reported using condoms; 15 (20%) had multiple sex partners—of these, 60% reported using condoms.
Neaigus *et al.* AIDS Education & Prevention 1990	New York City: 121 street-recruited IDUs (65% male, 35% female) re-interviewed at a mean of 4.5 months after intake.	Outreach intervention including AIDS information, condom distribution, and referral to HIV testing.	Changes from intake to follow-up: Proportion engaged in high-risk sexual behaviour: 97 (80%) at intake; 71 (59%) at follow-up. From 10 to 6 instances per month of sex without condom (mean monthly frequency); Among sexually active subset (from 109 to 97): Mean % of sex acts with condom—25% to 42%; % who sometimes use condoms—38% to 55%.

Table 5 (cont.) — Selected Studies of Sexual Behaviour Change for AIDS Risk Reduction among Injecting Drug Users and/or Their Heterosexual Partners

Author	Sample	Mechanism of Change	Results
Friedman et al. (Florence '91: W.D.54)	Brooklyn, NY: 243 IDUs (158 males, 85 females) who were sexually active during 6 months before intake and mean 7.8 months before follow-up. 43% Black, 41% Latino, 16% white–also, 26% prostitutes.	Peer pressure for risk reduction mobilized through group meetings, one-on-one counselling, and while distributing condoms, bleach, etc.	Changes from intake to follow-up: Percent always using condoms–24% to 33%; Mean proportion of sex acts in which condom was used–39% to 48%; Of 185 not always using condoms at intake, 39 (21%) were always using condoms at follow-up. Group attendance in re: always using condoms: 51% of attenders vs. 25% of non-attenders always used condoms; Among prostitutes, 61% of attenders vs. 32% of non-attenders always used condoms; Among non-prostitutes, 42% of attenders vs. 26% of non-attenders always used condoms.
Abdul-Quader et al. AIDS 1990	New York City: 568 IDUs (393 male, 175 female) recruited by ex-user outreach workers and given structured interviews on risk behaviour/reduction during the previous year.	No specific intervention, but overall AIDS awareness was already widespread in the city by the time of interview.	Reported risk reduction during average month in the previous year: 37% reported use of condoms; 44% practiced safer sex, mostly condoms; 10% stopped having sex; 8% reduced number of partners.

Table 5 (cont.) — Selected Studies of Sexual Behaviour Change for AIDS Risk Reduction among Injecting Drug Users and/or Their Heterosexual Partners

Author	Sample	Mechanism of Change	Results
Deren, Davis & Tortu (NADR Conf. presentation, 1990)	New York City: 886 subjects— 707 IDUs (457 male, 250 female) and 179 sex partners (41 male, 138 female)—recruited through street outreach and at Harlem Hospital. Results based on first 500 clients with 6-month follow-up interview.	Social learning model, with "standard" intervention involving basic AIDS information, plus two "enhanced" group sessions involving demonstration and practice of skills in needle cleaning and negotiating condom use.	Changes from intake to follow-up: Subjects with one sex partner: Never use condoms–76% to 47%; Always use condoms–10% to 27%. Subjects with multiple sex partners: Never use condoms–41% to 19%; Always use condoms–10% to 40%.
Schoenbaum et al. (Montreal '89: Th.D.P.59)	Bronx, NY: Out of 661 MMTP patients enrolled in 1985–6, 425 (262 HIV–, 163 HIV+) were followed up for a mean of 30 months. 52% male, 48% female.	HIV testing and counselling, methadone maintenance treatment programme.	Heterosexual contact with IDU partners. decreased 53% among HIV–, 51% among HIV+; Prostitution declined 80% among HIV–, 40% among HIV+.
Sogolow et al. (Florence '91: Th.D.58)	Brooklyn, NY: 146 sexually active, non-IV-drug using females in a high IV-drug use/HIV-endemic area: 88% Black, 11% Hispanic, 1% white.	Overall awareness and change in behaviour since hearing of AIDS.	91/146 (62%) reported some sexual behaviour change: 40% of those reported greater condom use (though only 14% of those use consistently); 24% of those report having fewer partners; 24% report both greater condom use and having fewer partners.

Table 5 (cont.) — Selected Studies of Sexual Behaviour Change for AIDS Risk Reduction among Injecting Drug Users and/or Their Heterosexual Partners

Author	Sample	Mechanism of Change	Results
Bellis, DJ, *J of Alcohol & Drug Educ* 1990	Southern California, 5 cities: Standardized questionnaire given to 72 heroin-addicted female street prostitutes: 47% white, 43% Hispanic, 10% Black.	Overall AIDS awareness.	37 (51%) ''suggested'' but did not require that customers use condoms; 10 (14%) require customers to use condoms.
Jain *et al.* (Montreal '89: W.D.P.79)	Sacramento, CA: 671 IDUs recruited from treatment programmes, hospital and jail, 150 of these returned for follow-up.	Intensive education/prevention programme targeted to IDUs and their sexual partners, including HIV testing.	Changes from intake to follow-up: % never using condoms–from 68% to 62%; % often or always using condoms– from 22% to 26%; Average number of sex partners, last 6 mos: from 11 to 5.6.
Poole *et al.* (Montreal '89: W.D.P.53)	San Francisco, CA: Project AWARE followed up 40 HIV+ females at 6- and 12-month intervals. 16 were IDUs. 16 had an HIV+ sex partner, 4 had a high-risk partner, 3 had no identified risk.	Social influence through peer group organization.	Changes from intake to follow-up: Average number of sex partners– from 5.2 to 2.1 (6 mo.) to 4.0 (12 mo.); Percent with fewer partners– 40% (6 mo.), 50% (12 mo.); Percent abstinent–35% (6 mo.), 8% (12 mo.) Percent having vaginal sex without condom– from 75% (6 mo.) to 37% (12 mo.).

Table 5 (cont.) — Selected Studies of Sexual Behaviour Change for AIDS Risk Reduction among Injecting Drug Users and/or Their Heterosexual Partners

Author	Sample	Mechanism of Change	Results
Roggenburg et al. (NADR Conf. presentation, 1989)	Portland, OR: 157 out-of-treatment IDUs (62% male, 38% female). 105 had been tested for HIV, a control group of 52 had not. A subset of 32 subjects who had sought testing of their own volition was also identified.	HIV testing and counselling.	Condom use among the 73/105 (69.5%) HIV-tested subjects with multiple sex partners–41% never; 34% sometimes; 25% always. Condom use among the 36/52 (69.2%) untested subjects with multiple sex partners–42% never; 44% sometimes; 14% always. Condom use among the 24/32 (75%) who sought testing on their own volition and who have multiple sex partners–50% never; 42% sometimes; 8% always.
Vanichseni et al. J AIDS 1992	Bangkok, Thailand: 601 in-treatment IDUs: 336 with no previous HIV test (NPT), 73 who had tested positive (PT+), 148 who had tested negative (PT−).	HIV testing and counselling.	Frequency of condom use w/ primary partner: Always–PT+ 29%; PT− 11%; NPT 9%; Sometimes–PT+ 43%; PT− 17%; NPT 20%; Never–PT+ 29%; PT− 71%; NPT 72%. Any contraception in past 6 months: PT+ 89%; PT− 73%; NPT 60%. Frequency of condom use w/ casual partner: Always–PT+ 57%; PT− 30%; NPT 33%; Sometimes–PT+ 14%; PT− 22%; NPT 22%; Never–PT+ 29%; PT− 48%; NPT 46%.

grammes have been followed by some changes in the sexual behaviour of injecting drug users. Our ability to compare the specific effectiveness of each different intervention is somewhat limited for a number of reasons, including the following: (1) the interventions aimed at changing drug-related risk as well as sexual risk; (2) the variables used to describe sexual risk behaviours vary across studies; and (3) subject characteristics vary across studies, but are not reported in sufficient detail to allow statistical controls to adjust for them. Furthermore, since interventions succeed largely by establishing personal rapport with subjects, the validity of follow-up questionnaires may be even more subject to response bias than is the case in cross-sectional studies (Friedman, in press).

Nevertheless, there are several generalizations that can be made at this point. First, sexual behaviour change has occurred among both injecting drug users and their heterosexual partners even in the absence of formal intervention programmes. Successive studies of IDUs in one area of New York City show progressive increases in the percentage who report that they have made some change in their sexual behaviour because of AIDS, with 61% reporting by 1987–89 that they had changed their sexual behaviour (Friedman *et al.*, 1987; Abdul-Quader, 1990). The most frequently reported sexual behaviour changes among these drug injectors were reductions in the number of sexual partners and an increase in the use of condoms.

Sexual behaviour change has also occurred among current and/or potential partners of IDUs in the absence of participation in formal AIDS prevention programmes. Sogolow and colleagues (1991) studied non-drug-injecting sexually active women who had more than a single partner in the previous 12 months from central Brooklyn (a high injecting-drug-use/AIDS-incidence area in New York City). They found that 62% of the subjects reported already having changed their sexual behaviour because of AIDS. Reducing the number of partners and increasing the use of condoms were the most frequently reported forms of behaviour change.

Comparing changes in drug-injection and sexual AIDS risk behaviours is conceptually and methodologically difficult for many reasons. There is no single common metric for comparing these two types of risk and there are different baseline levels of risk behaviour. Nevertheless, in all studies that we know of in which the authors made such a specific comparison, the change in drug-injection behaviour was considered greater (e.g., Des Jarlais & Friedman, 1988; Fazey, 1990; Jain *et al.*, 1989). The reasons for this discrepancy have yet to be determined. It has been suggested by a number of authors (Cohen, 1991; Sotheran *et al.*, 1989; Sotheran, 1991; Worth, 1989) that the fact that sex usually involves interpersonal social relationships, and often involves important social and emotional concerns, may make sexual behaviour more difficult to change than drug behaviour.

Of particular importance is evidence from New York that the two types of risk reduction are associated with each other. Subjects who reported changing their drug-injection behaviour because of AIDS were also much more likely to report that they had changed their sexual behaviour for this reason (Abdul-Quader *et al.*, 1990). This study needs to be replicated across drug injectors from other cultures and localities, but it does suggest that the goals of drug-injection risk reduction and sexual risk reduction among IDUs are complementary rather than conflicting.

The studies also agree that an increase in the use of condoms by drug injectors is more likely with 'casual' partners than with 'regular' partners. This parallels our finding in the Brooklyn network study that consistent condom use was greater in more distant relationships with non-IDU partners. A study of syringe exchange clients in the United Kingdom shows how the closeness of relationships affects sexual risk reduction due to an intervention (Donoghoe *et al.*, 1989). The participants in the exchange changed their sexual behaviour by reducing the numbers of casual partners, with whom condoms were likely to be used, and forming more regular sexual partnerships, within which condoms were less likely to be used. Thus, ironically, the overall extent of condom use actually declined. The specific reasons for this finding have not been determined, but it is important to note that reported condom use with casual partners was also higher than with regular partners in the "baseline" pre-AIDS studies.

This finding is also consistent with studies of AIDS-related behaviour change among homosexual men, where condom use is also more frequent with casual partners (National Research Council, 1989), and among female prostitutes, who likewise show much higher rates of condom use with customers or clients than with 'boyfriends' (J. Cohen, personal communication). Given the consistency of this finding across different groups, it is likely that there are several reasons why condom use is less likely with 'regular' sexual partners. Casual partners may be seen as more likely to be carrying HIV, and thus more of a risk to persons who presume that they themselves are seronegative. Also, there may be greater uncertainty about the likelihood that casual partners are infected, and condoms may be used to avoid subjective uncertainty. Regular partners may know or believe that they have the same serostatus, so that transmission is less likely to be perceived as a concern. Not using a condom also may be symbolic of the emotional closeness of a 'regular' or 'primary' relationship.[1] The expression of a desire to use a condom may also pose a threat to the relationship since it may imply one has 'cheated' on one's partner. Finally, among regular heterosexual partners, not using condoms may be connected to a desire to have children.

Providing the physical means for behaviour change, e.g. condoms, is an important part of many different intervention programmes. The studies of female prostitutes in particular suggest that the ready availability of condoms is important for their use (Bellis, 1990; Jose *et al.*, in press). This finding parallels findings that the ready availability of sterile syringes and bleach is important in getting injecting drug users to practice 'safer' injection (Des Jarlais & Friedman, 1992).

However, it is not just the physical availability of condoms that is needed. IDUs and their partners also need to know both how to use condoms properly and also how to discuss condom use with sexual partners ('negotiating safer sex'). Condom use can be taught with the use of any phallic-shaped object, and negotiating skills can be taught through role-playing. Negotiating skills are particularly important

---

[1] Interestingly, the "boyfriends" of female prostitutes expect the prostitutes to use condoms with their customers (Cohen, personal communication). Similarly, females from central Brooklyn who suspect that their "primary" male partners are not faithful expect that the male partner will use condoms with his "secondary" partners (Strug *et al.*, 1991) Pimps have on some occasions expressed their appreciation for projects that provide condoms to prostitutes (Jose *et al.*, in press).

because suggesting that condoms should be used may be taken as a sign that the person making the suggestion has been unfaithful. Skills-building exercises are not only useful in themselves, but can also provide opportunities for humorous release of tensions provoked by talking about taboo topics such as sex and death. Moreover, creating a social context in which condom use is perceived as legitimate may be as important as teaching negotiating skills, or even more so (Friedman *et al.* 1991; Friedman & Lipton, 1991; Jose *et al.*, in press).

While cognitive beliefs and the provision of physical means for behaviour change both appear to contribute to reducing sexual risk behaviour among IDUs, they do not explain all of the change that has been reported. Peer influence and group processes have been important factors in AIDS risk reduction among gay men (Turner, Miller & Moses, 1989) and in drug-use risk reduction among IDUs (Friedman *et al.*, 1987; Huang, Watters & Lorvick, 1989; Neaigus *et al.*, 1991). Peer influence and group processes also seem to be important in changing the sexual behaviour of IDUs and their sexual partners. Studies of IDUs (Abdul-Quader *et al.*, 1990; Neaigus *et al.*, 1991) and of women who are at risk for heterosexual transmission of HIV (Sogolow *et al.*, 1991) have both shown strong positive associations between the subjects' own sexual behaviour risk reduction and their friends' sexual behaviour risk reduction. Tross *et al.* (1992) report that drug injectors who say their friends have tried to reduce their sexual risks are themselves more likely to use condoms.

Social influence to initiate behaviour change and social support to maintain behaviour change both require that persons be able to discuss the relevant behaviour within peer groups. Indeed, at least one study has found that discussing AIDS with those with whom one feels close social ties is associated with both drug and sexual risk reduction (Neaigus *et al.*, 1991). Unfortunately, in many cultures, and among many drug injectors, sexual activity is considered to be highly private and not an appropriate topic for public discussion (see, for example, McKeganey & Barnard, 1992). Social norms about inappropriate behaviour may also greatly inhibit discussion of sexual behaviour in many cultures.

Despite the problems involved in mobilizing social influence for AIDS-related behaviour change, several intervention studies have deliberately built upon these social-influence processes by incorporating group organization into the behaviour change processes. In both the Community AIDS Prevention Outreach Demonstration (CAPOD) project in New York City and the AWARE (AIDS Women's Awareness, Research and Education) project in San Francisco, the participants were encouraged to form self-help groups. These projects are similar to the organizing efforts that have led to large-scale behaviour changes among gay men at risk for AIDS (Adam, 1987; Coutinho, van Griensven & Moss, 1989), in which the members of the group consciously acted as influence agents to facilitate AIDS risk reduction both among group members and then among wider circles of their peers. These organized peer-group projects were particularly effective in increasing condom use among their members (Friedman *et al.*, 1991, 1992; Poole *et al.*, 1989).

Considering how much HIV antibody testing of drug injectors has already been conducted throughout the world, there have been surprisingly few studies of the effectiveness of counseling and testing at changing the sexual behaviour of IDUs or at maintaining their sexual risk reduction efforts. Existing studies do show a positive effect of counselling and testing on sexual behaviour (Roggenburg *et al.*, 1989; Schoenbaum *et al.*, 1989; Vanichseni *et al.*, 1992; Wyld *et al.*, 1991). The positive effects seem to be as great or greater for seropositive IDUs as for seronegatives. The data presented above from the Brooklyn network suggest that sexual risk reduction may be particularly great with partners who are not themselves drug injectors.

Models such as the health-belief model, that are usually applied from the framework of subjects' protecting themselves from illness, would predict greater behavioural change among those who know or suspect that they are seronegative (who could protect themselves against HIV infection). The finding that more behaviour change occurs among seropositives suggests that IDUs are more moti-vated to protect the health of others, specifically their sexual partners, than to protect their own health. Their efforts to protect others probably reflect a mixture of altruism and of enlightened self-interest. Similarly, drug injectors have engaged in altruistic behaviour regarding safer needle and syringe hygiene. For example, researchers in both Glasgow and Stockholm (McKeganey & Barnard, 1992; Olin, personal communication) report that HIV-positive drug injectors warn persons who want to borrow needles and syringes of their HIV-positive status. Research and risk-reduction programmes should build upon this altruistic concern for protecting others from HIV.

In summary, then, sexual behaviour change by IDUs and their sexual partners is possible. The present literature does not, however, provide a well-tested set of "how to" guidelines for establishing effective programmes for changing sexual behaviour. Nonetheless, what follows here is a tentative set of "preliminary principles" for programmes to reduce the risk of heterosexual transmission of HIV from injecting drug users. These principles are based on the literature reviewed in this paper, our own experience working in the area, and informal discussions with many others working in the area.

1. **A programme must legitimate candid public and private discussions of the risks of heterosexual and perinatal transmission of HIV.** Such legitimation facilitates social influence processes, which can in turn strengthen behaviour change among programme participants as well as spread the behav-iour change beyond the participants in a programme. Programme staff or peer volunteers who facilitate discussions of sexual behaviour will, of course, need to have "worked through" any emotional inhibitions regarding the frank discus-sion of sexual behaviour.

2. **There are a number of cultural values that can be invoked to overcome cultural restrictions on discussions of sexual behaviour.** These cultural values include concern for health, concern for sexual partners and concern for children. Programmes should not limit their appeals only to drug injectors' desires to protect themselves from HIV. In spite of common images of drug users as demons, altruism appears to be a major force behind their condom use and other behaviours that reduce the probability of HIV transmission.

3. **Programmes need to present accurate information about the risks of heterosexual and perinatal transmission of HIV.** Such information alone

is not likely to produce much behaviour change, but it is probably necessary for large-scale behaviour change. Further, providing accurate information may be critical for the overall credibility of the programme.

4. **Programmes should provide multiple services whenever possible.** Injecting drug users and their sexual partners typically raise multiple health and social service needs in discussions with programme staff. Programmes to reduce sexual HIV transmission risks should be integrated with programmes to reduce drug-injection HIV risks—except perhaps for some programmes that aim only at sexual partners who do not themselves inject drugs and who are unlikely to start drug injection. Programmes should also be able either to provide drug abuse treatment or complementary health and social services on site, or else be able to provide effective and successful referrals. Provision of multiple services can build credibility and good will for an AIDS prevention programme. For programmes aimed at changing sexual behaviour, such credibility and good will may have to be established before the topic of sexual behaviour change can be introduced.

5. **If the programme works, offer it again for the same people.** While little research has studied "relapse" back to unsafe sexual behaviour among IDUs and their sexual partners, there is good reason to expect such relapses to occur frequently. Relapse to unsafe sexual behaviour has been reported among homosexual men (Turner, Miller & Moses, 1989), as has relapse to unsafe drug-injection behaviour among IDUs (Des Jarlais, Abdul-Quader & Tross, 1991). In Amsterdam, widespread public concern about AIDS led for a time to a discernible decrease in sexually transmitted diseases among heterosexuals, but this concern was not maintained and the rates of sexually transmitted diseases subsequently returned to their previous levels (van den Hoek, personal communication).

   Furthermore, sexual behavioural patterns are characteristics of couples rather than simply of individuals. Thus, when drug injectors form new relationships, additional exposure to an effective programme may help ensure that condom use or other safer sex practices are implemented in the newly formed couple.

6. **If a programme works, repeat it frequently for the same target population.** Target populations are dynamic. People migrate to and from neighbourhoods; begin to inject drugs; and start having sex. Protecting newcomers to drug scenes, and protecting their sexual partners, is an ongoing process rather than a one-time event.

7. **Changing the sexual behaviour of injecting drug users is possible.** Almost all of the studies reviewed for this paper did report statistically significant changes in the sexual behaviour of IDUs and their partners. (There is the possibility, however, that studies showing a lack of change were less likely to be accepted for publication or presentation at conferences.) These changes in behaviour tended to be modest, and to require somewhat intensive work with the participants in the study. Nonetheless, based on what is now known, any programme that cannot produce evidence of changes in the sexual behaviour of IDUs and their sexual partners should be modified immediately.

REFERENCES

Abdul-Quader, A.S., Tross, S., Friedman, S.R. *et al.* (1990) Street-recruited intravenous drug users and sexual risk reduction in New York City. *AIDS*, 4: 1075–1079.

Adam, B. (1987) *The Rise of a Gay and Lesbian Movement.* Boston: Twayne.

AIDS Surveillance in Europe. (1991) WHO-EC Collaborating Center on AIDS. Quarterly Report No. 30. Geneva, World Health Organization, June 30, 1991.

Baxter, D.N. & Schlecht, B. (1990) Patterns of behaviour amongst injecting drug users—Implications for HIV. *Public Health*, 104: 321–325.

Becker M.H., Joseph J.G. (1988) AIDS and behavioural change to reduce risk: A review. *Am J Public Health*, 78: 394–410.

Bellis, D. J. (1990) Fear of AIDS and risk reduction among heroin-addicted female street prostitutes: Personal interviews with 72 Southern California subjects. *Journal of Alcohol and Drug Education*, 35: 26–37.

Boxaca, M., Libonatti, O., Muzzio, E., *et al.* (1990) HIV-1 prevalence and the role of other infectious diseases in a group of drug users in Argentina. Presented at the Sixth International Conference on AIDS, San Francisco, CA. Abstract #3141.

Calello, M., Libonatti, O., Boxaca, M., Weissenbacher, M. (1991) Increasing risk of heterosexual HIV-1 spreading due to intravenous drug use in Argentina. Presented at the Seventh International Conference on AIDS, Florence, Italy.

Centers for Disease Control. (1990) Risk behaviours for HIV transmission among intravenous drug users not in drug treatment—United States, 1987–1989. *Morbidity and Mortality Weekly Report*, April 27, 1990.

Centers for Disease Control. (1991) Drug use and sexual behaviours among sex partners of injecting drug users—United States, 1988–1990. *Morbidity and Mortality Weekly Report*. December, 13, 1991.

Chiasson, M.A., Hildebrandt, D., Ewing, W., *et al.* (1991) Similar risk of HIV infection through heterosexual transmission for men and women at a New York City sexually transmitted disease clinic. Presented at the Seventh International Conference on AIDS, Florence, Italy. Abstract #M.C.3093.

Choopanya, K. (1991) Substance use and HIV. Oral Presentation at the Panel on Communities Challenging AIDS, Seventh International Conference on AIDS, Florence, Italy.

Choopanya, K., Vanichseni, S., Plangsringarm, K., *et al.* (1991) Risk factors and HIV seropositivity among injecting drug users in Bangkok. *AIDS*, 5(12): 1509–1513.

Cohen, Judith. (1991) Why woman partners of drug users will continue to be at high risk for HIV infection. *Journal of Addictive Diseases*, 10(4):99–110.

Corby, N.H., Wolitsky, R.J., Thornton-Johnson, S., Tanner, W.M. (1991) AIDS knowledge, perception of risk, and behaviours among female sex partners of injecting drug users. *AIDS Educ and Prevention*, 3: 353–366.

Coutinho, R.A., van Griensven, G.J.P., Moss, A. (1989) Effects of preventive efforts among homosexual men. *AIDS* 3 (Suppl. 1): S53–S56.

Darke, S., Hall, W., Carless, J. (1990) Drug use, injecting practices and sexual behaviour of opioid users in Sydney, Australia. *Br J Addict*, 85: 1603–1605.

Deren, S., Davis, W.R., Tortu, S. (1990) The Harlem AIDS Project: Preliminary outcomes of a skills development intervention. Presented at the Second Annual National AIDS Demonstration Research Conference, Bethseda, MD.

Des Jarlais, D.C., Friedman, S.R. (1988). HIV infection among persons who inject illicit drugs: Problems and prospects. *J AIDS,* 1: 267–273.

Des Jarlais, D.C., Abdul-Quader, A., Tross, S. (1991). The next problem: Maintenance of AIDS risk reduction among intravenous drug users. *Int J Addict.* 26 (12): 1279–1292.

Des Jarlais, D.C., Choopanya, K., Wenston, J., *et al.* (1992) Risk reduction and stabilization of seroprevalence among drug injectors in New York City and Bangkok, Thailand. In: Rossi *et al.*, eds., *Science Challenging AIDS: Proceedings of the VII International Conference on AIDS. Florence, Italy. 1991*. Basel, Switzerland: S. Karger; pp. 207–213.

Des Jarlais, D.C., Freidman, S.R. (1992). The AIDS epidemic and legal access to sterile equipment for injecting illicit drugs. *Ann Am Acad Poli Soc Sci*, **521**: 42–65.

De Vincenzi, I., Ancelle-Park, R. (1991) Heterosexual transmission of HIV: Follow-up of a European cohort of couples. Presented at the Seventh International Conference on AIDS, Florence, Italy. Abstract #M.C.3028.

Donoghoe, M.C., Stimson, G.V., Dolan, K., Alldritt, L. (1989) Sexual behaviour of injecting drug users and associated risks of HIV infection for non-injecting partners. *AIDS Care* 1: 103–109.

Falciano, M., Ferri, F., Macedonio, A., *et al.* (1991) Heterosexual transmission of HIV: A 4-year follow-up. Presented at the Seventh International Conference on AIDS, Florence, Italy. Abstract #M.C.3070.

Fay, O., Taborda, M., Fernandez, A., *et al.* (1991) HIV seroprevalence among different communities in Argentina after four years of surveillance. Presented at the Seventh International Conference on AIDS, Florence, Italy.

Fazey, C.S.J. (1990)*Preventing the spread of HIV infection: A study of drug patients' syringe and condom use*. Mersey Regional Health Authority, Studies of Drug Issues: Report No. 4.

Feucht, T.E., Stephens, R.C., Roman, S.W. (1990) The sexual behaviour of intravenous drug users: Assessing the risk of sexual transmission of HIV. *J Drug Issues*. 20: 195–213.

France, A.J., Skidmore, C.A., Robertson, J.R., *et al.* (1988) Heterosexual spread of human immunodeficiency virus in Edinburgh. *Br Med Journal*. 296: 526–529.

Friedman S.R., Des Jarlais D.C., *et al.* (1987) AIDS and self-organization among intravenous drug users. *Int J Addict* **22**(3): 201–219.

Friedman, S.R., Des Jarlais, D.C. (1991) HIV among drug injectors: The epidemic and the response. *AIDS Care* **3**(3): 239–250.

Friedman, S.R., Lipton, D.S. (1991) Cocaine, AIDS and IV drug use. *Journal of Addictive Diseases*, **10**(4): 1–12.

Friedman, S.R., Jose, B., Neaigus, A., *et al.* (1991) Peer mobilization and widespread condom use by drug injectors. Presented at the Seventh International Conference on AIDS, Florence, Italy. Abstract #W.D.54.

Friedman, S.R., Neaigus, A., Des Jarlais, D.C. *et al.* (1992) Social intervention against AIDS among injecting drug users. *Br J Addict*, **87**: 53–64.

Friedman, Samuel R. (in press) Issues in the analysis of AIA and AFA data. *Proceedings of the Second National AIDS Demonstration Research Conference*. NIDA monograph.

Friedman, S.R., Young, P.A., Snyder, F.R., *et al.* (1993). Racial differences in sexual behaviours related to AIDS in a nineteen-city sample of street-recruited drug injectors. *AIDS Education and Prevention*. 5(3): 196–211.

Garcia, S., de la Loma, A., Romero, J. (1988) Non-blood heterosexual transmission of HIV infection. Presented at the Fourth International Conference on AIDS. Stockholm, Sweden. Abstract #4003.

Hart, G.J., Carvell, A.L.M., Woodward, N., *et al.* (1989) Evaluation of needle exchange in central London: Behaviour change and anti-HIV status over one year. *AIDS*, **3**: 261–265.

Huang, K.H.C., Watters, J., Lorvick, J. (1989) Relationship characteristics of heterosexual IV drug users. Presented at the American Public Health Association Annual Meeting, Chicago, IL.

Jain, S., Flynn, N., Bailey, V., *et al.* (1989) IVDU and AIDS: More resistance to changing their sexual than their needle-sharing practices. Presented at the Fifth International Conference on AIDS, Montréal, Canada. Abstract #W.D.P.79.

Johnson, A.M., Petherick, A., Davidson, S.J., *et al.* (1989) Transmission of HIV to heterosexual partners of infected men and women. *AIDS*, 3: 367–372.

Johnson, B.D., Goldstein, P.J., Preble, E., Schmeidler, J., Spunt, B., Miller, T. (1985). *Taking Care of Business: The Economics of Crime by Heroin Abusers.* Lexington, Massachusetts: D.C. Heath and Company.

Jose, B., Friedman, S.R., Neaigus, A., *et al.* (in press) Peer mobilization and widespread condom use by drug injectors. Revised version of a paper presented at the Seventh International Conference on AIDS, Florence, Italy.

Klee, H., Faugier, J., Hayes, C., Morris, J. (1991) Risk reduction among injecting drug users: Changes in the sharing of injection equipment and in condom use. *AIDS Care*, 3: 63–73.

Lewis, D.K., Watters, J.K., Case, P. (1990) The prevalence of high-risk sexual behaviour in male intravenous drug users with steady female partners. *Am J Public Health*, 80: 465–466.

Lima, E.S., Bastos, F. I. P. M., Friedman, S. R. (1991) HIV-1 epidemiology among IVDUs in Rio de Janeiro, Brazil. Presented at the Seventh International Conference on AIDS, Florence, Italy.

McCusker, J., Koblin, B., Lewis, B.F., Sullivan, J. (1990) Demographic characteristics, risk behaviours, and HIV seroprevalence among intravenous drug users by site of contact: Results from a community-wide HIV surveillance project. *Am J Public Health*, 80: 1062–1067.

McKeganey, N., Barnard, M. (1992). *AIDS, Drugs and Sexual Risk: Lives in the Balance.* Buckingham, UK: Open University Press.

Mesquita, F., Moss, A.R., Reingold, A.L., Ruiz, M., Bueno, R.C., Paes, G.T. (1991) Pilot study of HIV antibody seroprevalence among IVDUs in the city of Santos, Sao Paulo State, Brazil. Presented at the Seventh International Conference on AIDS, Florence, Italy.

Moore, L., Padian, N.S., Vranizan, K.M., *et al.* (1990) Sexual partners of intravenous drug users in San Francisco. Presented at the Sixth International Conference on AIDS, San Francisco. Abstract #Th.C.587.

Naik, T.N., Sarkar, S., Singh S.L., *et al.* (1991) Intravenous drug users—a new high-risk group for HIV infection in India. *AIDS* 5: 117–118.

National Research Council's Committee on AIDS Research and the Behavioural, Social, and Statistical Sciences, Commission on Behavioural and Social Sciences and Education (CBSSE) (1989). AIDS, sexual behaviour and intravenous drug use. In: C.F. Turner, H.G. Miller, & L.E. Moses (Eds.), *AIDS, Sexual Behaviour and Intravenous Drug Use* (pp 186–255). Washington, DC: National Academy Press.

Neaigus, A., Sufian, M., Friedman, S.R., *et al.* (1990) Effects of outreach intervention on risk reduction among intravenous drug users. *AIDS Education and Prevention*, 2: 253–271.

Neaigus, A., Friedman, S.R., Jose, B., *et al.* (1991) Social networks and HIV risk behaviour among IV drug users. Presented at the International Sunbelt Social Network Conference, Tampa, Florida, February 15.

Papetti, C., Mezzaroma, I., D'Offizi, G.P., *et al.* (1991) Risk factors for heterosexual transmission of HIV-1 in stable couples. Presented at the Seventh International Conference on AIDS, Florence, Italy. Abstract #W.C.3108.

Poole, L.E., Cohen, J.B., Lyons, C.A., *et al.* (1989) Behaviour changes to reduce HIV transmission risk in a prospective study of seropositive women. Presented at the Fifth International Conference on AIDS, Montreal, Canada. Abstract #W.D.P.53.

Roggenburg, L., Sibthorpe, B., Tesselaar, H., *et al.* (1989) The relation between HIV-antibody testing and HIV risk behaviours among intravenous drug users. Presented at the first Annual National AIDS Demonstration Research Conference, Bethseda, MD.

Schoenbaum, E.E., Hartel, D., Selwyn, P.A., *et al.* (1989) Low HIV seroconversion and change in high risk behaviour in intravenous drug users (IVDUs) from 1985–88 in the Bronx, NYC. Presented at the Fifth International Conference on AIDS, Montreal, Canada. Abstract #Th.D.P.59.

Smith, P.F., Mikl, J., Truman, B.I., *et al.* (1991) HIV infection among women entering the New York State correctional system. *Am J Public Health*, **81**(Suppl.):35–40.

Sogolow, E.D., Des Jarlais, D.C., Strug, D., *et al.* (1991) Heterosexual HIV risk reduction among women: The heterosexual AIDS transmission study (HATS). Presented at the Seventh International Conference on AIDS, Florence, Italy. Abstract #Th.D.58.

Sotheran, J.L., Friedman, S.R., Des Jarlais, D.C., *et al.* (1989) Condom use among heterosexual male IV drug users is affected by the nature of social relationships. Poster presented at the Fifth International Conference on AIDS, Montréal, Canada. Abstract #T.D.P.81.

Sotheran, Jo L. (1991) HIV risk and social relationships among IV drug users. Presented at the Annual Workshop on Psychosocial Factors in Population Change. Washington, D.C., March 19–20.

Sterk, C.E., Friedman, S.R., Sufian, M., Stepherson, B., Des Jarlais, D.C. (1989). Barriers to AIDS interventions among sexual partners of IV drug users. Poster presented at the Fifth International Conference on AIDS, Montréal, Canada.

Stimson, G.V. (1990) The prevention of HIV infection in injecting drug users: Recent advances and remaining obstacles. Presented at the Sixth International Conference on AIDS, San Francisco, CA.

Strug, D., Des Jarlais, D.C., Sogolow, E., *et al.* (1991) Types of sexual partner relationships and condom use among women in Brooklyn: A report from the heterosexual AIDS transmission study (HATS). Presented at the Seventh International Conference on AIDS, Florence, Italy. Abstract #W.C.3112.

Tor, J., Soriano, V., Muga, R. *et al.* (1991) HIV transmission in heterosexual partners of intravenous drug abusers: A follow-up study. Presented at the Seventh International Conference on AIDS, Florence, Italy. Abstract #M.C.3048.

Tross, S., Abdul-Quader, A., Silvert, H. & Des Jarlais, D.C. (1992) Condom use among male injecting-drug users—New York City, 1987–1990. *MMWR*, 41(34): 617–620.

Turner, C.F., Miller, H.G., & Moses, L.E. (Eds.), (1989). *AIDS: Sexual Behaviour and Intravenous Drug Use*. Washington, DC: National Academy Press.

Vanichseni, S., Sakuntanaga, P. (1990) Results of three seroprevalence studies for HIV in IVDU in Bangkok. Presented at the Sixth International Conference on AIDS, San Francisco, CA. Abstract #F.C.105.

Vanichseni, S., Choopanya, K., Des Jarlais, D.C., *et al.* (1992) HIV testing and sexual behaviour among drug injectors in Bangkok, Thailand. *J AIDS*, 5(11): 1119–1123.

Worth, Dooley. (1989) Sexual decision-making and AIDS: Why condom promotion among vulnerable women is likely to fail. *Studies in Family Planning*, 20: 297–307.

Wyld, R., Davidson, S., Brettle, R., *et al.* (1991) Changes in sexual behaviour amongst drug users: Edinburgh 1983–89. Presented at the Seventh International Conference on AIDS, Florence, Italy. Abstract #W.C.3106.

4

Preventing Transmission of HIV in Heterosexual Prostitution

DAVID WILSON

INTRODUCTION

Prostitution is commonly defined as "the exchange of sexual services for money or things of monetary value" (Darrow, Deppe, Schable *et al.*, 1989, p 18). Under this definition, anyone who buys, sells or mediates commerce in sexual services, is engaged in prostitution (Day, 1988). As with earlier STD epidemics, the global emergence of HIV has elevated interest in prostitution. It is inevitable, given that HIV is transmitted primarily through sexual intercourse, that attention will be focused on an activity in which many individuals trade in sexual services (de Zalduondo, 1991).

REGIONAL CHARACTERIZATION OF PROSTITUTION

Regional characterization of an activity as heterogeneous as prostituion is hazardous, but some cautious generalizations may be helpful.

Day (1988) notes that in much of the west, criminalization of commercial sex forced prostitutes underground, created scope for pimps, estranged prostitutes from society and led to the "professionalization" of prostitution. Western prostitutes emphasize their role as workers and pointedly separate work and home. At work, condoms provide a desirable psychological barrier between private self and work; at home, the same barrier may make condoms undesirable. In Africa, where punitive legislation is seldom upheld and is extrinsic to community concerns, prostitution is sometimes difficult to differentiate from other sexual relations. Prostitutes remain part of their communities, often engaged in petty trade and playing several societal roles. A professional working identity is eschewed and the passage in and out of prostitution may be fluid (Day, 1988; Stanning, 1989). Intermediaries are rare and African prostitutes in general possess greater independence than prostitutes elsewhere (Wilson, Sibanda, Mboyi, Msimanga, Dube *et al.*, 1990). The problems such "non-professionalization" poses to interventions include occupational fluidity and unwillingness to identify oneself as a prostitute.

In Asia, prostitution is often highly organized, with controlling, even coercive, management, but prostitutes seldom develop professional self-identities (Khan & Arafeen, 1988; Day, 1988; Gillies, Parker, de Moya *et al.* 1991).

EPIDEMIOLOGY OF HIV AMONG FEMALE PROSTITUTES

In the west, HIV seroprevalence among female prostitutes is primarily associated with injecting drug use (Darrow, 1990; Padian, 1988; Plant, 1990).

Johnson (1988) found no HIV infection among prostitutes in Copenhagen, London and Paris. However, 17 of almost 2,000 prostitutes (under one percent) tested in six German cities were HIV-positive: half of these injected drugs (Schultz *et al.*, 1986). Ten (71%) of 14 drug injecting prostitutes in Pordenone, Italy (Tirelle, Vaccher, Carboni *et al.*, 1985) and 14 (78%) of 18 drug injecting prostitutes in Zurich, Switzerland (Luthy, Ledergerber, Tauber *et al.*, 1987) were HIV-positive.

HIV seroprevalence levels among prostitutes are higher in North America, but vary markedly across regions. In a CDC multicentre study, 172 of 1,396 (12%) of female prostitutes were HIV-positive: infection levels varied from zero among women recruited from Nevada brothels, none of whom injected drugs, to nearly 50% among women largely enrolled through a methadone programme in New Jersey. In the sample as a whole, injecting drug use was the best predictor of HIV seropositivity (Darrow *et al.*, 1990). Darrow *et al.* (1990) concluded that although HIV seroprevalence among US prostitutes who do not inject drugs is relatively low, it is higher than that reported among other US women of reproductive age.

In developing countries, the picture is starkly different. In Africa, prostitutes have HIV infection rates that are three to 300 times higher than those of pregnant women in nascent epidemics and three to seven times higher than those of pregnant women in established epidemics (Mann, Tarantola & Netter, 1992). Among African prostitutes, 88% of 33 tested in Butare, Rwanda in 1984, 61% of 286 tested in Nairobi, Kenya in 1987, 56% of 265 tested in Blantyre, Malawi in 1986, 38% of 230 tested in Bamako, Mali in 1987, 35% of 1233 tested in Kinshasa, Zaire in 1989, 34% of 67 tested in Brazzaville, Congo in 1987, 29% of 225 tested in Dar es Salaam, Tanzania in 1986, 29% of 2091 tested in several Ethiopian towns in 1989, 26% of 264 tested in several Gambian site in 1988, 21% of 179 tested in Bangui, Central African Republic in 1989, 20% of 101 tested in Abidjan, Cote d'Ivoire in 1987, 16% of 50 tested in Juba, Sudan in 1989, 7% of 168 tested in Yaounde, Cameroon in 1989, 7% of 177 tested in Lagos, Nigeria in 1988 and 6% of 604 tested in several Niger sites in 1989 were HIV-positive (Nkowane, 1991;

Piot & Hira, 1990). Prostitutes in east, central and southern Africa, where HIV prevalence is higher, are worst affected (Mann *et al.*, 1992). HIV seroprevalence is also higher among prostitutes of lower socioeconomic status: in Nairobi, Kenya in 1985, 66% of low socioeconomic status prostitutes and 31% of high socioeconomic status prostitutes were HIV-positive (Kreiss, Koech, Plummer *et al.*, 1986).

The HIV epidemic among prositutes in parts of Asia, including areas of India and Thailand, is becoming equally serious. In Thailand, prostitutes have HIV infection rates 17 to 120 times higher than those of pregnant women (Mann *et al.*, 1992). In 1989, 44% of female prostitutes in Chiang Mai were tested HIV-positive. In longitudinal research over two months, a 10% monthly incidence was observed (Weninger, Limpakarnjanaart, Ungchusak *et al.*, 1991). Data for other Asian countries are more limited. However, HIV infection among prostitutes in Bombay, India has increased over ten-fold in three years, reaching 28% in 1989 (Pavri, 1991).

Several factors help to explain the different HIV infection rates between western prostitutes who do not inject drugs and those in affected developing countries. Western prostitutes have more education, which enlarges understanding, choice and health in the widest sense, work in an overall socioeconomic environment unconducive to HIV transmission, face fewer STD (particularly GUD) pathogens, have better STD services, often provide oral sex and very frequently use condoms. The vulnerability of prostitutes in many developing countries is amplified by poverty — personal and societal. They provide sexual services in social contexts ripe for HIV dissemination, have limited education and hence choice, are frequently exposed to STD, receive wholly inadequate STD care, provide vaginal intercourse to large numbers of clients and seldom use condoms.

In addition to situation factors, there may be important differences in the context of AIDS prevention.

PREVENTING HIV TRANSMISSION IN PROSTITUTION

Programmes to prevent HIV transmission in prostitution are found primarily in the west, Africa and latterly Asia, especially Thailand, but also India and the Philippines.

An important distinction — based on how prostitute interventions are initiated and organized — may be drawn between programmes in the west and the developing world.

Public health or research institutions have initiated prostitute programmes in several western countries, including Britain (Day & Ward, 1990; Kinnell, 1990; Matthews, 1990; Morgan Thomas, 1990; Morgan Thomas, Plant, Plant, & Sales, 1989; Plant, Plant, Beck & Setters, 1989), Plant, Plant & Morgan Thomas, 1990) Greece (Padaevangelou, Roumeliotou, Kallinkos, Papoutsakis, Trichopoulou & Stefanou, 1988), Holland (Venema & Visser, 1990), Germany (Gersch, Heckmann, Leopold & Seyrer, 1988) and the United States (Darrow, Deppe, Schable,

Hadler, Larsen, Khabbaz, Jaffe, Cohen, Wofsy, French, Gill, Potterat, Ravenholtd, Sikes & Witte, 1990; Freund, Leonard & Lee, 1989; Leonard, 1990).

However, many western prostitute programmes have either originated from prostitute organizations and activism, or been subject to prostitute activist involvement and scrutiny. Examples of prostitute-originated initiatives include the Association for Women's AIDS Research and Education (AWARE), a women's AIDS research and intervention programme, focusing especially on female prostitutes (Cohen, 1987), the California Prostitutes Education Project (CAL-PEP) (Alexander, 1988) and Call-Off-Your-Old-Tired-Ethics (COYOTE) in California, USA (COYOTE, 1989), the Prostitutes Safe Sex Project (PSSP) in Toronto, Canada (Prostitutes' Safe Sex Project, 1989), Red Thread in the Netherlands (Red Thread, 1989) and the Australian Prostitutes Collective and Scarlet Alliance in Australia (Bates, 1989; Over & Bates, 1989; Over & Hunter, 1989).

In contrast, almost all developing country prostitute programmes have been initiated by outside agencies, including public health departments, universities and NGOs. These programmes may operate at community-level, but they are not owned by prostitute communities and they remain dependent on outside funding and personnel. Examples may be found from several African countries, including Cameroon (Monny-Lobe, Nichols, Zeking, Salla & Kaptue, 1989), Ethiopia (Belete, Larivee, Gebrehidane & Fisehaye, 1990) Kenya (Ngugi & Plummer, 1989; Ngugi *et al.*, 1988); Nigeria (Soyinka, Hossain & Onayemi, 1989; Williams, Efem, Lamson & Lamptey, 1990), Senegal (Siby, Thior, Sankale, Ndoye & M'boup, 1989), Tanzania (Mhalu, Akim, Senge, Shao, Bredberg & Biberfield, 1989), Zaire (Laga, Nzila, Goeman, Tuliza, Manoka, Kivuvu *et al.*, 1992) and Zimbabwe (Wilson, Chiroro, Lavelle & Mutero, 1989; Wilson, Sibanda, Mboyi *et al.* 1990).

PROSTITUTE-OWNED INITIATIVES

Community initiatives differ from outside instigated projects in both ownership and who they primarily serve.

Prostitute-initiated programmes are community-owned. The importance of community ownership is best illustrated by the Stop AIDS campaign in San Francisco's gay community, which may confidently be called the most successful AIDS intervention yet reported. A variety of behavioural self-report, STD and HIV prevalence data document the extent of change in this group (McKusick, Wiley, Coates *et al.*, 1985; San Francisco Department of Public Health, 1986; Winkelstein, Samuel, Padian *et al.*, 1987). Reported rates of unprotected receptive anal were 27 times lower in 1985 than 1978 (Doll, Darrow, Jaffe *et al.*, 1987), rectal gonorrhoea incidence declined sharply (Pickering, Wiley, Padian *et al.*, 1986) and new HIV infections approached (Winkelstein *et al.*, 1987).

Notwithstanding the absence of proof in the narrowly positivistic tradition, case study analysis strongly indicates that community activism, ownership, involvement and accountability were integral to success (Bye, 1990). The community received little or no outside help. Widespread community mobilization at the outset ensured full community participation in the planning and review of the campaign. Extensive debate of strategies ensured continuous accountability. Involvement continued unabated throughout the campaign. Gay activists recruited large numbers of volunteers. Bartenders were organized and trained to engage patrons in discussion about AIDS. Gay physicians and psychologists lent authority to education. Hundreds of volunteers reached 25,000 gay men in personal street campaigns. Over 7,000 gay men participated in peer discussion in private houses (Bye, 1990).

Australia's community-owned prostitute campaigns are equally inspiring. Prostitution in Australia was recently legalized. Prostitutes have organized collectives, which resemble trade unions. Moreover, the Australian government funds prostitute collectives through state funds allocated for community initiatives, including injecting drug use programmes, gay organizations, haemophiliac associations and prostitute collectives (Commonwealth of Australia, 1989). Prostitute collectives are led and staffed by prostitutes, who in turn are chosen by, and answerable to, prostitute members. The Prostitutes' Collective of Victoria, Australia, which was founded in 1983, organizes the following programmes (Overs & Hunter, 1989):

Safe House Endorsement Scheme The vetting of legal brothels, provision, display and publication of "safe house" endorsements and education of brothel management to expand the scheme.

Sex Industry and AIDS Debate Workshops, attended by prostitutes, brothel managers, health and legal service providers and policy makers.

Poverty Action Programme Legal, financial assistance and training to empower prostitutes.

Prostitute Service Education, counselling, a drop-in centre and community visits for male and female prostitutes.

Needle Exchange A needle exchange, drop-in, education and counselling service for injecting drug users.

Worksafe/Playsafe A safe sex educational video for prostitutes, and medical professionals.

Hello Sailor An AIDS information and education service for visiting sailors.

Ugly Mug A description of dangerous clients.

As of 31 December, 1991, heterosexual transmission accounted for just 2.1% of all HIV infections in Australia (National Centre in HIV Epidemiology and Clinical Research, 1992). Remarkably, not a single case of HIV transmission in prostitution (indepedent of drug injection) has been documented in Australia (Harcourt & Philpot, 1990; National Centre in HIV Epidemiology and Clinical Research, 1992). None of a sample of 491 prostitutes tested at an STD centre in Sydney, Australia were HIV-positive (Philpot, Harcourt and Edwards, 1991).

In addition to formal, documented programmes, numerous less publicized efforts have prostitutes in western countries and substantial diffusion of safe sex knowledge and practices has occurred (Delacoste & Alexander, 1988). This is to be expected, as community-initiated and owned efforts do not require formal programmes and documentation and have great potential for spontaneous diffusion.

PUBLIC HEALTH INITIATIVES

Whereas prostitute-owned programmes axiomatically aim to protect prostitutes, public health initiatives usually aim to protect a wider audience–prostitutes, if possible, but certainly clients and their wives and partners.

Such initiatives usually have their origins in "core group" theory, originally formulated by Yorke, Heathcote and Nold (1978) to explain gonorrhoea epidemics. To sustain an STD epidemic, the basic reproductive rate, R_0 or number of secondary infections produced by one primary case must exceed one, $R_0 < 1$. R_0 is defined by the mean probability of transmission per contact, B, the duration of infectiousness, D and the mean number of sexual partners, c (Anderson, 1991).

$$R_0 = B\,D\text{c}$$

Plummer, Nagelkerke, Moses *et al.* (1991) note that, in the absence of potentiating factors, the transmissibility of HIV is low, probably between .001% and 1%. Thus, from 100–10,000 exposures to an infected person would be required to generate a new infection. Differences in HIV reproduction between the west and much of Africa are so great that, if mean number of partners were responsible, Africans would have to have 10-1,000-fold more sexual partners, a proposition for which there is no evidence whatever (Carballo, Tawil & Holmes, 1991).

However, variability in rate of partner change profoundly influences the reproductive rate. In circumstances where small sexually active subsets of men and women have large numbers of partners, variability is high and the reproductive rate is elevated (Anderson, 1992). Among the large numbers of partners, numerous sexually transmitted infections circulate. The small sexually active subset are differentially exposed to, and rapidly acquire, sexually transmitted infections. Thereafter, their many partners are exposed. Plummer *et al.* (1991) cites the example of a group of approximately 500 low-income prostitutes in Nairobi, who have approximately 1,000–1,200 clients annually. They rapidly acquire sexually transmitted infections from some clients, which they may then transmit to other clients. Other examples include military and long-distance truckers.

Mathematical models of HIV transmission support the following conclusions (Anderson, 1992; Over & Piot, 1992; Potts, Anderson & Boily, 1992; World Bank, 1991):

— The most sexually active subsets may play an important role in the initial growth and long-term continuation of an epidemic.
— Interventions introduced early have disproportionately greater effect than comparable ones introduced later.
— Where general HIV prevalence is "low" (under 1%), interventions among the most sexually active subsets may prevent an epidemic in the general population. (The successful prostitute-owned interventions in the west may illustrate precisely this principle).
— Targetting the most sexually active subsets is cost-effective. When the effects over 10 years of preventing a single case of HIV among the most sexually active subsets and among the general population are modelled, the former is estimated to avert approximately 10 times as many infections. Another model comparing

condom promotion to the most sexually active subset and to the general population suggests that the former averts 60–80 times as many HIV infections.
— In societies with widespread HIV infection, although the overall proportion of infections preventable by interventions targetting the most sexually active subsets diminishes, such as interventions remain highly cost-effective.

Public health specialists in developing countries, faced with spiralling epidemics and meagre resources, are understandably attracted by the cost-efficiency arguments of such analyses.

The models may have an unimpeachable mathematical basis and they do help to refine intuitive judgements and clarify options. However, effective solutions to AIDS cannot simply be defined by technical requirements, a temptation invited by narrowly mathematical approaches. Several concerns arise:

Evidence of the effectiveness of prostitute interventions in Africa is limited. In several studies, self-reported condom use increased sharply (Williams, 1992; Wilson, Nyathi, Lamson *et al.*, 1992), but the validity of these reports is unknown. A well evaluated prostitute intervention in Nairobi, Kenya has increased condom use and delayed HIV infection (Ngugi *et al.*, 1988), but 80% or more of prostitutes still contract HIV (Moses, Ngugi, Nagelkerke, Anzala & Ndinya-Achola, 1991). The best evidence is from Matonge suburb, Kinshasa, Zaire, where, in a cohort of 1226 prostitutes, over 22 months, regular condom use with clients increased from 4%–55%, GUD, gonorrhoea, chlamydia and trichomoniasis incidence diminished and annual HIV incidence declined from 18%–2.2% (Larga *et al.*, 1992). However, this occurred during an expensive research project, with a sophisticated laboratory and large staff. The project could not be sustained with the existing cohort, much less expanded to other prostitutes. In keeping with evidence that interventions in Africa offer prostitutes limited protection, models assume that all, or most, prostitutes in severely affected countries will acquire HIV infection, but that giving them education and giving or selling (adding insult to injury!) them condoms will protect many of their clients. The long-term commitment of prostitutes to projects that offer them marginal protection is uncertain. One may also ask how effectively, mathematical simulations aside, programmes that do not protect prostitutes, actually protect their partners.

Mathematical models are presented with scant attempt to prevent scapegoating, thus reinforcing the misogynistic tendencies of societies, which traditionally define STD as 'women's disease', spread, by definition, in one direction. In addition to conventional models, we should model and publicize the way in which professional sexual service providers, by educating clients and promoting condoms non-penetrative sexual alternatives, have helped to prevent heterosexual HIV epidemics in many western countries. Similarly, the primary role of men in perpetuating unsafe commerical sex must be persistently explained.

When prostitute interventions originate from technical agencies, not community activism, there is little pressure to revoke punitive legislation and policing practices. Unless prostitutes are free from arrest and harassment, it is hard to envisage how nationwide programmes reaching all or most prostitutes can even be contemplated.

Scrambler and Graham-Smith (1991) and DeCosas (personal communication) argues that health policies and programmes are supported not simply because they are technically correct, but because they are backed by effective constituencies. An excellent example is immunization: child survival has universal support, transcending political or religious divisions. Another is family planning, central to the feminist lobby, with broad sponsorship from those influenced by macroeconomic, environmental and strategic considerations. AIDS received rapid attention partly because of effective pressure from gay groups. The growing environmental lobby has transformed environmental policy and action.

Programmes to protect prostitutes currently have no effective lobby. Hence prostitute programmes in developing countries (except Thailand) lack champions among senior policy makers, have no concerted public support, receive little or no in-country funding and are modestly financed by external specialist research or technical agencies.

Lacking the sponsorship of effective pressure groups, prostitute programmes remain isolated and fragmentary. Potts *et al.* (1991) identified 14 prostitute interventions in seven African countries, reaching about 24,000 prostitutes. Yet there are over 100 African cities with populations above 100 000, each requiring prostitute interventions. Moreover, despite the need for immediate action, programmes took up to two years to initiate. Securing bureaucratic approval, usually from national AIDS committees, frequently accounted for nine-tenths of the time between project conception and implementation. In an east African country with very high HIV seropositivity among prostitutes, it took 18 months to obain approval for an intervention among prostitutes and clients. There was no influential domestic constituency to press for approval.

A more recent review by Ferencic, Alexander, Lamptey *et al.* (1991) identified 83 sex-work interventions in 38 developing countries (36 in Africa, 23 in the Americas and 18 in Asia). Some data were obtained for 45. Thirty (67%) used peer education and 12 (27%) provided STD services. Of 38 reporting on numbers reached, only 8 (21%) reached more than 2,000 prostitutes. Projects reported numerous constraints, including problems created by punitive law enforcement practices, lack of long-term financial support and inadequate numbers and quality of condoms. The authors concluded that projects were few in relation to need and small in scope, reaching only a small proportion of prostitutes, in certain categories of sex work.

If one accepts the view that effective programmes are buttressed by forceful constituencies and pressure groups, then simply increasing external support or further elucidating the cost-effectiveness of targetted interventions to ministries will not suffice. Effective sponsorship is needed and this can only be found in the feminist movement (DeCosas, personal communication; Scrambler and Smith, 1991). Unfortunately, there is no consensus within the women's movement. Radical feminists oppose prostitution as a form of violence against women (Dworkin, 1981). Liberal feminists emphasize women's freedom to work and live as they choose (Delacoste & Alexnader, 1988). Yet this is a western debate, remote from the survival needs of low income women in, say Nairobi or Harare, who deserve the support of women in their endeavour to earn a living in one of few ways they can, free from harassment, arrest or disease, organized in groups and unions and protected by the best possible STD and occupational safety services.

SOCIAL CONTEXT OF PROSTITUTES' VULNERABILITY

Larson (1989) provides a brilliant analysis of the social context of African prostitutes' vulnerability. She differentiates two patterns of partner relations. In one pattern, society is patriarchal, marriage is stable, women are highly dependent on their spouses, strong sexual double standards legitimize male, but not female, sexual experimentation and men frequently have extramarital relations, choosing from small numbers of women who have consequently have many partners. In the other pattern, marriage is unstable, women are often educated and engaged in commerce, may return home with their children and have greater independence and both men and women have extramarital relations. In the first pattern, prostitution is more extensive, women, including prostitutes, have lower status and fewer social and economic alternatives and HIV spreads rapidly. This pattern interacts with sociodemographic trends to increase the vulnerability of women, particularly prostitutes. In west Africa, indigenous African cities with authentic family and community life predated and survived colonization. In much of eastern and southern Africa, blacks, particularly women, were regarded as temporary interlopers in "white" cities, housed in single sex hostels in dormitory suburbs, with profoundly "anticommunity" environments. Women in such cities had low status and few commercial opportunities beside prostitution, for which there was a demographically fuelled demand. To this day, whereas the male:female ratio in the 20–39 age group averages 1:1 in most west African cities, it is 1.25:1 in eastern and southern African cities (Decosas, 1991).

The World Bank (Over & Piot, 1991) provide macroeconomic support for Larson's thesis. Using data from 12 African countries, they reported an association between an excess of males aged 20–39 and HIV prevalence among prostitutes. In an analysis of 11 countries, they obtained a strong correlation between the female:male secondary school enrollment ratio and HIV seropositivity in the general adult population and among prostitutes.

The regression coefficients obtained suggest that a five point reduction in adult seroprevalence could be achieved by increasing either the urban sex ratio by 35 women per 100 men or the secondary school sex ratio by 50 girls per 100 boys.

RECOMMENDATIONS

Socioeconomic Approaches

Socioeconomic approaches are essential to long-term strategies in developing countries. Decosas (1992) and Mann (1992) note that large development projects requiring the translocation of large migrant labour forces may increase HIV transmission. They propose subjecting development programmes to an AIDS impact audit. To those who argue this is unrealistic, they observe that the same was once said of environmental impact audits, which the environmental movement now has sufficient influence to impose. Such an audit needs to be designed not to terminate development projects, but to ensure adequate STD services, health education, condom promotion and where possible, provision for continued family life. For example, prostitutes in Lesotho currently have low HIV seroprevalence. Will this be true when the giant Lesotho Highlands Water Project to provide South Africa with water and hydroelectricity is completed in 1996?

In a remarkable convergence between development workers and macroeconomists, the World Bank recently argued that female education is the most cost-effective development investment any country can make, benefitting, inter alia, maternal and child health, sanitation, family planning, environmental conservation and the educational attainment and productivity of future generations. They recommend investment, including cost remission, in girls' schools, boarding places, teaching equipment, textbooks and uniforms, with safeguards to prevent diversion to males. Identification and advocacy of sound macroeconomic interventions is vital, not least because of the potential for leveraging non-health funds into activities that reduce HIV transmission. To underline this point, consider the fact that World Bank economic assistance to Ghana alone in 1992/1993 may exceed by 50-10-fold Ghana's National AIDS Programme budget and approach or surpass the global WHO/GPA budget.

The Women's Movement and Prostitution

This paper has argued that technical justifications will not lead to effective large-scale prostitute interventions, without the sponsorship of a committed, influential lobby, which can only be found in the women's movement. Notwithstanding the difficulties, dialogue between prostitute organizations and feminist groups to achieve such sponsorship is of paramount urgency. Funding women's groups to develop positions, strategies and programmes on prostitution should be considered.

Legalization

The experience of Australia and several continental European countries provides persuasive pragmatic grounds for the legalization of prostitution. Full legalization is probably a prerequisite for nationwide interventions reaching all or most prostitutes. Self-esteem may be a critical determinant of safe sexual behaviour and legalization is the first step to improved self-esteem and empowerment of prostitutes.

Prostitute Organizations

Australian examples underscore the need to follow legalization by support for prostitute activist organizations and unions. Membership of cohesive, effective organizations and unions will further enhance self-esteem and empower prostitutes and provide a springboard for community-owned AIDS prevention programmes. There are admittedly considerable problems. Unions may be chauvinistic: for example, South Africa's major union body recently dismissed a suggestion for prostitute unions without serious discussion (Wilson & Lavelle, in press). In many developing countries, the lack of professional self-identity — and concomitant disinclination to identify oneself as a prostitute — clearly hinders effective organization.

Prostitute Activism, Leadership and Ownership of Projects

Few would challenge the cardinal importance of community activism, leadership, ownership and accountability in successful community interventions. Yet the social context of most developing world prostitutes could scarcely be further removed from that of educated, affluent, articulate, highly cohesive gay men in San Francisco. Programmes must acknowledge this and pursue several approaches — some cautious and incremental, others experimental and risky — to foster activism, both working within existing externally conceived programmes and encouraging new activist initiatives.

Within existing programmes, desirable steps include developing increasingly democratic programme structures, progressively devolving growing responsibility to programme participants, providing medical, administrative and leadership training to senior participants and engaging current prostitutes as full-time staff, in increasingly senior prositions.

New activist initiatives could be fostered by developing activist training courses (including carefully chosen organizational placements) based, for example, on successful experiences in the feminist, gay, environmental and human rights movements and awarding scholarships to promising prostitute activists. Seed money and grants could be provided to prostitute organizations, as venture capital in an uncertain, but important, endeavour. Analysis of indigenous agencies may identify indigenous forms of activism and organization, based on different principles, that may be more likely to succeed. Linking fledgling prostitute groups to women's organizations may be feasible.

These approaches face enormous obstacles in developing countries, including the deplorable position of women, particularly prostitutes, in south Asia and the absence of activist tradition and culture in overwhelmingly rural Africa. In Africa, perhaps South Africa, whose urban society, powerful unions and culture of organized resistance are in some ways more reminiscent of Latin America than Africa, can spearhead prostitute activism.

CONCLUSION

Prostitute interventions, which lie at the confluence of two ordinarily divergent streams: the technology of mathematical modelling and the culture of activism, help to remind us of the perils of technical hubris. Technical guidance is vital, but AIDS prevention cannot be confined to technical prescription.

REFERENCES

Alexander, P. (1989). *Prostitutes and AIDS: Scapegoating and the law: an AIDS information packet.* San Francisco, California: National Task Force on Prostitution.

Alexander, P. (1988). *Prostitutes prevent AIDS: a manual for health educators.* San Francisco, California: California Prostitutes Education Program.

Alexander, P. (1988). Prostitution: a difficult issue for women. In F. Delacoste & P. Alexander (Eds). *Sex work: writings by women in the sex industry.* San Francisco: Cleo Press.

Anderson, R.M. (1991). The transmission dynamics of sexually transmitted diseases: the behavioural component. In J.N. Wasserheit, S.O. Aral, Holmes, K.K. & P.J. Hitchcock (Eds). *Research issues in human behaviour and sexually transmitted diseases in the AIDS era.* Washington, DC: American Society for Microbiology (pp 38–60).

Bates, J. (1989). Community development model for interventions with prostitutes. Fifth International AIDS Conferences, Montreal, June.

Belete, F., Larivee, C., Gebrehidane, A., Fisehaye. (1990). Report on pilot study to mobilize multi-partner sexual contact females to use condoms and provide peer education on AIDS. Paper presented at the Fifth International Conference on AIDS in Africa, Kinshasa, Zaire.

Bye L.L. (1990). Moving beyond counseling and knowledge enhancing interventions: A plea for community-level AIDS prevention strategies. In DG Ostrow (ed) *Behavioural aspects of AIDS.* New York: Plenum (pp 157–167).

Carballo, M. Tawil, O., Holmes, K.K. (1991). Sexual behaviours: temporal and cross-cultural trends. In J.N. Wasserheit, S.O. Aral, Holmes, K.K. & P.J. Hitchcock (Eds). *Research issues in human behaviour and sexually transmitted diseases in the AIDS era.* Washington, DC: American Society for Microbiology.

Cohen, J.B. (1987). Three year experience promoting AIDS education among 800 sexually active high risk group women in San Francisco. Presented at the National Institute for Mental Health/National Institute for Drug Abuse Research Conference on "Women and AIDS: Promoting Healthy Behaviors", Bethesda, Maryland, USA, September.

Commonwealth of Australia (1989). *National HIV/AIDS strategy. A policy information paper.* Canberra: Australian Government Publishing Service.

Conant, M., Hardy, D.., Sernatinger, J., Spicer, D. & Levy, J. (1986). Condoms prevent transmission of AIDS-related retrovirus. *Journal of the American Medical Association.* 25, 1706.

COYOTE (1989). Awful new prostitution laws — effective 1 January, 1989. *COYOTE Howls,* January, 1989, pp 1–2.

Darrow, W. Deppe, D., Schable, C., Hadler, S., Larsen, S., Khabbaz, R., Jaffe, H., Cohen, J., Wofsy, C., French, J., Gill, P., Potterat, J., Ravenholtd, O., Sikes, R., Witte, J. (1990). Prostitution, intravenous drug use and HIV-1 in the United States. In M. Plant (Ed) *AIDS, drugs and prostituion.* London: Tavistock.

Day, S. (1988). Prostitute women and AIDS: anthropology. *AIDS.* 2, 421–428.

Day, S., Ward, H. (1990). The Praed Street Project. A cohort of prostitute women in London. In M. Plant (Ed) *AIDS, drugs and prostitution.* London: Tavistock.

DeCosas, J. (1992) The impact of underdevelopment on AIDS. Eighth International Conference on AIDS, Amsterdam, Netherlands, July.

DeCosas, J. (1991) The demographic AIDS trap for women in Africa: Implications for health promotion. Seventh International Conference on AIDS, Florence, Italy, June.

Delacoste, F., Alexander, P. (Eds) (1988). *Sex work: writings by women in the sex industry.* San Francisco: Cleo Press.

de Zalduondo, B. (1991). Prostitution viewed cross-culturally: toward recontextualizing sex work in AIDS intervention research. *Journal of Sex Research.* 28, 223–248.

Doll, L., Darrow, W.W., Jaffe, H., Curran, L., O'Malley., Bodecker, T., Campbell, J., Francks, D. (1987). Self-reported changes in sexual behaviours among gay and bisexual men from the San Francisco City Clinic Cohort. Paper presented at the Third International AIDS Conference on AIDS, Washington, USA, June.

Dworkin, A. (1981). *Pornography: men possessing women*. London: The Women's Press.

Ferencic, N., Alexander, P. Lamptey, P., Slutkin, G. (1991). Review of coverage and effectiveness of current sex-work interventions in developing countries. Paper presented at the Seventh International AIDS Conference on AIDS, Florence, Italy, June.

Freund, M., Leonard, T.I., Lee, N. (1989). Sexual behaviour of resident street prostitutes with their clients in Camden, NJ. *Journal of Sex Research*, 26, 460–478.

Gersch, C., Heckmann, W., Leopold, B., Seyrer, Y. (1988). *Drug addicted prostitutes and their customers*. Berlin: Sozialpadagogisches Institut Berlin.

Gillies, P., Parker, R., de Moya, E.A., Sittitrai, W., Suwwannanond, U., Neequaye, A., Carael, M., Slutkin, G. (1991). Action research to facilitate intervention for prostitutes in developing countries.: first results. Paper presented at the Seventh International AIDS Conference, San Francisco, June.

Harcourt C., Philpot, R. (1990). Female prostitutes, AIDS, drugs and alcohol in New South Wales. In M. Plant (Ed) *AIDS, drugs and prostitution*. London: Tavistock.

Holmes, K.K., Aral, S.O. (1991). Behavioural interventions in developing countries. In J.N. Wasserheit, S.O. Aral, Holmes, K.K. & P.J. Hitchcock (Eds). *Research issues in human behaviour and sexually transmitted diseases in the AIDS era*. Washington, DC: American Society for Microbiology.

Kinnell, H. (1989). Prostitutes and their clients in Birmingham: action research to measure and reduce the risks of HIV. *Royal Society of Medicine AIDS Letter*, 19, 1–4.

Kreiss, J.K., Koech, D., Plummer, F.A., Holmes, K.K., Lightfoote, M., Piot, P. *et al.* (1986). AIDS virus infection in Nairobi prostitutes: spread of the virus to east Africa. *New England Journal of Medicine*, 314, 414–417.

Laga, M., Nzila, N., Goeman, J., Tuliza, M., Manoka, A., Kivuvu, M. *et al.* (1992). Condom promotion and STD diagnosis and treatment among female prostitutes in Kinshasa, Zaire. Paper presented at the World Health Organization Meeting on Strategies for Effective Intervention, May.

Lamptey, P., Potts, M. (1990). Targeting of prevention programmes in Africa. In P. Lamptey & P. Piot (Eds) *Handbook of AIDS Prevention in Africa*. Durham, NC: Family Health International.

Larson, A. (1989). Social context of HIV transmission in Africa: Historical and cultural bases of East and Central Africa sex relations. *Review of Infectious Diseases*, 11, 716–731.

Leonard, T.I. (1990). Male clients of female street prostitutes: Unseen partners in sexual disease transmission. *Medical Anthropology Quarterly*. 4, 41–55.

Luthy, R., Lederberger, B., Tauber, M., Siegenthaler, W. (1987). Prevalence of HIV antibodies among prostitutes in Zurich, Switerlands. *Klinische Wochenschrift*, 65, 287–288.

Mann, J. (1992) Plenary address. Eighth International Conferences on AIDS. Amsterdam, Netherlands, July.

Mann, J., Chin, J., Piot, P., Quinn, T. (1988). The International epidemiology of AIDS. *Scientific American*, 259, 60–69.

Mann, J., Tarantola, D.J.M., Netter, T.W. (Eds) (1992). *AIDS in the World*. Cambridge, Massachusett, Harvard University Press.

Matthews, L. (1990). Outreach work with female prostitutes in Liverpool. In M. Plant (Ed) *AIDS, drugs and prostitution*. London: Tavistock.

McKusick, L., Wiley, J.A., Coates, T.J., Stall, R., Saika, G., Morin, S., Charles, K., Horstman, W., Conant, M.A. (1985). Reported changes in the behaviour of men at risk for AIDS, San Francisco, 1982–1984. *Public Health Reports*, 100, 622–629.

Mhalu, F., Akim, C., Senge, P., Shao, J., Bredberg, R.U., Biberfield, G. (1989). Adoption of safer sexual behaviour by an HIV high risk group of bar and restaurant workers in Dar es Salaam, Tanzania. Paper presented at the Fifth International AIDS Conference, Montreal, June.

Monny-Lobe, M., Nichols, D. Zeking, L., Salla, R., Kaptue, L. (1989). The use of condoms by prostitutes in Yaounde, Cameroon. Paper presented at the Fifth International AIDS Conference, Montreal, June.

Morgan Thomas, R. (1990). AIDS risks, alcohol, drugs and the sex industry: a Scottish study. In M. Plant (Ed) *AIDS, drugs and prostitution*. London: Tavistock.

Morgan Thomas, R. Plant. M.A., Plant, M.L., Sales, D.I. (1989). AIDS risks, alochol, drugs and the sex industry: a Scottish study. *British Journal of Addiction*. 299, 148–149.

Moses, S., Plummer, F.A., Ngugi, E.N., Nagelkerke, N.J.D., Anzala, A., Ndinya-Achola, J. (1991). Controlling HIV in Africa: effectiveness and cost of an intervention in a high-frequency STD transmitter core group. *AIDS*, 5, 407–411.

National Centre in HIV Epidemiology and Clincial Research (1992). *Australian HIV Surveillance Report*, 6, 2.

Ngugi, E.N., Plummer, F.A. (1989). Health outreach and control of HIV infection in Kenya. *Journal of Acquired Immune Deficiency Syndromes*, 1, 566–570.

Ngugi, E.N., Plummer, F.A., Simonsen, J.N., Cameron, D.W., Bosire M., Waiyaki, P., Ronald, A., Ndinya-Achola, J. (1988). Prevention of Human Immunodeficiency Virus in Africa: Effectiveness of condom promotion and health education among prostitutes, *Lancet*, 2, 887–890.

Nkowane, B. (1991). Prevalence and incidence of HIV infection in Africa: a review of data published in 1990. *AIDS*, 5, S7–S15.

Nyathi, B.B., Wilson, D., Nhariwa, M., Lamson, N., Weir, S. (1991). Naturalistic evaluation of a community-based HIV prevention programme among vulnerable groups in Bulawayo, Zimbabwe. Paper presented at the Seventh International AIDS Conference, Florence, June.

Over, M., Piot, P. (1992). HIV infection and sexually transmitted diseases. The World Bank health sectors priorities review. In D.T. Jamison & W.H. Mosley (Eds) *Disease control priorities in developing countries*. New York: Oxford University Press for the World Bank.

Overs, C., Bates, J. (1989). The sex industry and the AIDS debate — Australian conference. Fifth International AIDS Conference, Montreal, June.

Overs, C., Hunter, A. (1989). AIDS prevention in the legalized sex industry. Fifth International AIDS Conference, Montreal, 4–7 June.

Padaevangelou, G., Roumeliotou, A., Kallinkos, G., Papoutsakis, G., Trichopoulou, E., Stefanou, T. (1988). Education in preventing AIDS in Greek registered prostitutes. *Journal of Acquired Immune Deficiency Syndromes*, 1, 386–389.

Padian, N. (1988). Prostitute women and AIDS: epidimiology. *AIDS*, 2, 413–419.

Pavri, K.M. (1991). Status of AIDS/HIV in India. *Virus Information Exchange Newsletter*, 8, 54–56.

Philpot, C.R., Harcourt, C.L., Edwards, J.M. (1991). A survey of female prostitutes at risk of HIV infection and other sexually transmissible diseases. *Genitourinary Medicine*, 67, 384–388.

Plummer, F.A., N.J.D., Moses, S., Ndinya-Achola, J. Bwayo, J., Ngugi, E. (1991). The importance of core groups in the epidemiology and control of HIV-1 infection. *AIDS*, 5, S169–S176.

Pickering, J., Wiley, J.A., Padian, N.S., Lieb, L., Ekenberg, D., Walker, J. (1986). Modelling the incidence of acquired immune deficiency syndrome (AIDS) in San Francisco, Los Angeles and New York. *Mathematical Modeling*, 7, 661–668.

Piot, P, Harris J. (1990). The epidemiology of HIV/AIDS in Africa. In P. Lamptey & P. Piot (Eds) *Handbook of AIDS Prevention in Africa*, Durham, NC: Family Health International.

Piot, P. Laga, M., Ryder, R., Perriens, J., Temmerman, M., Heyward, W., Curran, J. (1990). The global epidemiology of HIV infection: continuity, heterogeneity, *Journal of AIDS*, 3, 403–412.

Plant, M.L. (1990). Sex work, alcohol, drugs and AIDS. In M. Plant (Ed) *AIDS, drugs and prostitution*. London: Tavistock.

Plant, M.L., Plant, M.A., Beck, D.F., Setters, J. (1989). The sex industry alcohol and illicit drugs. Implications for the spread of HIV infection. *British Journal of Addiction*, 84, 53–59.

Plant, M.L., Plant, M.A., Morgan Thomas, R. (1990). Alcohol, AIDS risks and commercial sex. *Drug and Alcohol Dependence*, 29, 51–55.

Prostitutes' Safe Sex Project (1989). *Prostitution and Safer Sex Kit*. Toronto: Prostitutes' Safe Sex Project.

Red Thread (1989). *Tips and tricks for working girls*. Amsterdam: Red Thread.

Ronald, A.R., Ndinya-Achola, J.O., Plummer, F.A., Simonsen, M.D., Cameron, D.W., Ngugi E.N., Pamba, H. (1988). A review of HIV-1 in Africa. *New York Academy of Medicine Bulletin*, 64, 480–48.

Schultz, S., Milberg, J.A., Kristal, A.R., Stoneburner, R.L. (1986). Female-to-male transmission of HTLV-III. *Journal of the American Medical Association*, 255, 1703–1704.

Scrambler, G., Graham-Smith, R. (1991). *Female prostitution and the realities of social exclusion*. Unpublished paper.

Shedlin, M. (1990). An ethnographic approach to understanding HIV high-risk behaviours: Prostitution and drug abuse. *National Institute on Drug Abuse Research Monograph Series. AIDS and intravenous drug use: future directions for community-based prevention research*, 93, 134–149.

Siby, T., Thior, I., Sankale, J.L., Gueye, A., Ndoye, I., M'boup, S. (1989). Surveillance-education sanitaire des prostituees au Senegal. Paper presented at the Fifth International AIDS Conference, Montreal, June.

Soyinka, F., Hossain, M.Z., Onayemi, O. (1989). STD patients' and prostitutes' knowledge on AIDS: Modification of sexual practices, and education needs. Paper presented at the Fifth International AIDS Conference, Montreal, June.

Stanning, H. (1989). Sexual behaviour in sub-Saharan Africa: an annotated bibliography. London: ODA.

5

Discordant Couples

LORRAINE SHERR

An increasing number of couples currently countenance relationships in which one is HIV positive and the other is not. They are described as discordant couples. The term 'discordant' implies conflict, antagonism, disharmony and strife. It may be a misleading label under which to gather couples world wide who face the ravages of HIV and AIDS together. An emerging literature on these couples provides insight into the mysteries of AIDS and HIV infection. This chapter concentrates on heterosexual couples. Gay couples face similar situations, but the literature on heterosexual couples has focussed on problems at the 'virus spread' level. Studies of gay couples have moved towards an understanding of the psychosocial impact, setting the future agenda for studying discordant couples. The chapter will attempt to glean from the literature an overview of issues as they effect discordant heterosexual couples.

It is unclear whether discordant couples constitute a 'group'. They do not gather together, self identify or have common purpose. Their only defining characteristic is the fact that they are discordant for HIV and are drawn from the larger group of couples where both are infected.

Traditionally 'discordant couples' referred to those who have had sex in the presence of HIV, where one has remained uninfected. Yet the definition could extend to other possible dyads such as mother baby dyads where an HIV + ve mother has carried a pregnancy but her baby is subsequently uninfected; where injecting drug users (IDUs) have shared needles but one has remained uninfected or where couples live together in the presence of a single infection, not necessarily sharing a risk behaviour but still sharing the burden of illness, stigma or behaviour adjustments in the presence of HIV.

Studies of such discordant couples can provide some insight into male to female and female to male patterns of spread. They may illuminate aspects of viral transmission or resistance. They provide a key for understanding behaviour change patterns and the ability to sustain these over time. They also expose the many psychological and social ramifications this disease has on networks, in addition to the individual.

It is clear that as heterosexual HIV infection increases the chances of both concordant and discordant couples are also increased. The CDR (1992) reports that in the UK 417 cases of AIDS and 1,620 of HIV had been documented through sex between men and women. For the years 1986 to 1991 AIDS cases which were attributable to heterosexual transmission increased from 2% to 14% and of diagnosed HIV from 4% to 23%. The patterns of such increase are slowly moving from predominantly first generation (from partners who were not sexually infected) to second generation (from those who were sexually infected). Indeed of the 417 cases of AIDS through heterosexual contacts in the UK, 42 (10%) were first generation, 328 (79%) were second generation from abroad and 47 (11%) from contacts in the UK. Such patterns are similar in other Western countries which underlies the need to anticipate heterosexual spread and the increase in couples exposed to HIV infection. In other areas, such as Africa, spread has always been predominantly heterosexual and such couples have been present from the start of the epidemic.

The majority of studies of these couples have been dogged with methodological and sampling problems and a systematic overview is difficult. These difficulties include an over-representation of cross sectional and retrospective studies, limited follow up in many reports and a variety of factors accounting for HIV infection in the index subject which renders comparisons and generalisations problematic. These factors themselves may account for variation rather than concordance or discordance. Studies often describe small subject numbers, include different groups, extend over geographically diverse areas and monitor different behavioural factors (Feldblum, 1991). Discordant couples are often drawn from pre-existing groups such as injecting drug users and haemophiliacs. The latter group provides the most comprehensive data source given that infection source can often be traced and timed.

The bulk of the literature covers situations where the male is HIV positive and the female negative although there are growing numbers where the opposite is true. Discordant couple definitions are interpreted narrowly and although there is wide coverage of mother-baby infection this is usually more in the context of understanding vertical transmission than shedding light on them as a 'discordant' couple. The literature on father–baby dyads is exceedingly limited. Similarly despite an emerging literature on twins and levels of discordance between them, no studies have looked at the psychological and behavioural implications for such twins. This may well emerge in time as at present such studies are very new and many of the children are still comparitively young. Similarly sibling studies are few and far between.

At some point in time all concordant couples were discordant. It is challenging to assume that there may be something unique about those who remain discordant compared to those who become concordant and to document this. The literature tends to suggest that the outcome is a result of multiple rather than single factors most of which are poorly understood. Differences may occur at many levels involving possible resistance, host factors, virus strain and virulence, timing and circumstance of exposure and background social, medical and behavioural factors.

Some couple relationships are long term and some fleeting. The literature rarely differentiates between the two and mostly focuses on those in relationships of longer term. Transient couples could include casual and commercial sex situations and these should not be excluded. Sexual exposure is the route which is most exclusively studied in discordant couple literature. Sexual relationships are often complex and the role of power, particularly power imbalance must be examined.

EMPIRICAL STUDIES

The empirical studies can be examined in terms of the information they supply on transmission and also the information (often submerged) on psychological factors. This has direct implications for counselling intervention. A summary of findings on discordant couples worldwide can be found in table 5.1 below. This table shows clearly that at the initiation of a study a high proportion of partners are shown to be positive. Discordant couples who remain, then show a low rate of conversion. This rate, despite being low, is higher for female partners of infected males than male partners of infected females. Some studies do not give an indication of population prevalence rates prior to discordant couple selection. This may artificially infalte the high rate of partner positivity noted in the studies which do measure this.

TRANSMISSION RATES

Most studies claim that male to female infection is more efficient than female to male. Many studies suffer from the overriding problem that it is difficult to ascertain who was infected first. It is not necessary that the individual who was first identified is the individual who was first infected within a couple. Indeed, as HIV is less likely to be entertained as a diagnosis for women (Hankins, 1992), it is more likely that male index cases will be identified. Discordant couples in studies tend to be identified on examination of all the partners of an index case. A proportion are then noted who are both infected (concordant) and another where the partner is not infected (discordant). Factors that preclude initial infection may already be operational. Thus the selection biases are apparent in most studies from the start.

Haemophiliac men may be easier to identify, given the gender linked nature of their predisposing condition. It is difficult to generalise from this literature as there are double problems of the parallel haemophilia disease itself and other transfusion related phenomena.

Male to female infection rates are consistently reported as higher than female to male. Single exposures of the cervix to the semen of infected men during artificial insemination has transmitted the virus (Stewart *et al.*, 1985). On the other hand not all female partners become infected (Padian *et al.*, 1987) despite long term exposure.

TABLE 5.1
Summary of Findings on Discordant Couples

Study Author (Date)	Place	N	% Partner Convert Comment
1. *Female partners of HIV + ve Men*			
Belec *et al.* 89	Cent AF Republic	11 M	3/11 converted 30%
Sepulveda 90	Mexico City	58 F partners of + ve men	16/58 converted 27.5%
Kreiss 85		42 Haem	2 wives/21 converted 9.5%
Kim 1988	US	14 men Haem + spouse	1/14 wives converted 7%
Ragni 89	USA	45 Men	6 wives converted 13%
Latif 89	Zimbabwe	75 men	45/70 wives HIV + ve 60%
Avila 89	Mexico	23 + ve Husband blood donors	7/23 + ve women 30% 1 yr f/up 5 F + ve 21.7%
2. *Male partners of Female HIV + ve*			
Sion 90	Brazil	Female Blood tx n = 11	0/11 husbands converted 0%
3. *Couple studies*			
Moore 92	USA	86 couples	0 conversions
Gongora	Yucatan	n = 21	47% (8/17) F spouse +
Brachi 91		17 M + ve 4 F + ve	0% (0/4) male spouse +
Gala 89	Italy	11 + ve	4/11 converted 3 Females, 1 Male
Hira 89	Africa	71 couples 47 M + 24 F +	no converted 3 month f/up
Peterson 89	USA	54 couples 43 discord	79.6% converted overall
Vogler 89		31 couples	17 partners -ve at entry 0 conversions 45% seroconverted prior to study commencing
Papetti 89		43 couples 34 M + ve 9 F + ve	17 both + ve (39.5%) 1 yr f/up 2/26 + ve (7.7%)

TABLE 5.1
Summary of Findings on Discordant Couples *(Continue)*

Study Author (Date)	Place	N	% Partner Convert Comment
Vaira *et al.* 89	Africa	36 couples 13 + F 23 + M	All partners − ve. 0%
Mbyi *et al.* 89	Zaire	122 couples 67 M + 55 F +	
De Vincenzi 90	Europe	403 couples 69 170 fup	17.1% part + ve @ entry 6/170 converted 3.5%
Feldblum 90	Africa	85 couples 62M + ve 23F + ve	8 converted 12 pregnancies
Rehmet 90		184 couples 40 f/up	m-F 30% F-M 6%
Papetti 90		100 couples 76 M + ve 24 F + ve	44% converted
Tacconi 90		142 couples 36 F + ve 106 M + ve	0 males converted (0%) 6 females converted 7 pregnancies 4 terminations
Tice 90	Rwanda	46 couples 21 f + ve 25 M + ve	0 males converted 3 females converted 12%
Jingu 90	Zaire	175 D Couples 85 F + ve 90 M + ve	10 converted (5.7%) 6 M 4 F
DeVincenzi 91	Europe 9centre	541 couples 88 (16.3% disc)	10 converted 7/72 F 3/32 M
Moore 91	San Fran	86 Discordant couples	0 Conversions
Kamenga 91	Zaire	194 conc 160 DC 84 M + F − 76 M- F + plus 8 4M 4 F	 6 (4% conc @ fup) 2 F 4 M
Deschamps *et al.* 91	Haiti	148 89 Disc 50 Conc	3 (61%) 30 pregnancies
Moss 91	Kenya	70 couples	40 (57%) + ve 36 (43%) − ve
Carael 88	Rwanda	138 couples	124 (90%) both + ve

De Vincenzi (1990) studied 403 couples and presented follow up data for 170 of whom 6 converted (none of whom always used condoms). By 1991 this cohort comprised 504 couples with 10 partners seroconverting (7/72 female partners and 3/31 male partners – none of whom always used condoms).

Rehmet *et al.* (1990) studied 184 couples and prospectively monitored 40 discordant couples within this group. Male to female transmission was reported as 33% and female to male as 6%. In a 1991 follow up male to female transmission was 4 times higher than female to male (31% vs 8%).

Latif *et al.* (1989) studied 75 married men found to be HIV positive and their wives of whom 45 (60%) were positive. Johnson *et al.* (1989) studied 78 female partners of HIV + ve men and 18 male partners of infected women. 15/78 (19.2%) of the female partners were positive for HIV compared to 1/18 (5.5%) of the male partners of positive women. No differences between the seropositive and seronegative women were documented in terms of length of relationship, number of vaginal intercourse episodes, other sexual practices, stage of illness or numbers of outside sexual partners in the preceding 5 years. For 2 women seroconversion occurred after a single exposure.

Early haemophiliac couples in the USA were studied and showed low frequency of transmission (Kreiss *et al.*, 1985, Jason *et al.*, 1986). Kreiss showed that 2 of 21 haemophiliac wives were HIV positive (9.5%). Kim (1988) studied 14 HIV + ve haemophiliac men and their wives who were monogamous and practiced sex without condoms prior to 1986. At follow up only 1 of the 14 wives was HIV + ve. These gave rise to a rate of 0.1–1% per M–F sexual encounter (Plummer *et al.*, 1991). Gafa *et al.* looked at 13 sexual partners of ll HIV + ve subjects and found in the absence of condom use, 4 seroconverted (3 women and 1 man). Two of the partners of the 3 women were bisexual. Ragni (1989) studied 45 female partners of 45 HIV + ve haemophiliac men in the USA and found 6 (13%) seroconverted and documented an early seroconversion. The subsequent risk of HIV transmission in those who remained negative is essentially unknown. This data also tends to concentrate on figures from early exposure when men were newly infected. There is little insight into rates of transmission from sexual partners exposed later on in the disease course.

The low numbers of female index cases identified make such calculations difficult for male partners of infected females. In Africa where the epidemic has always been heterosexual, there is a sharp contrast in findings.

Moss (1991) studied female spouses of 70 HIV positive men and found 40 (57%) to be positive with cervical ectopy as the major predictor. Sion *et al.* (1990) studied 11 HIV positive women in stable sexual relationships and did not observe any male seroconversion. Gongora *et al.* (1991) studied 21 subjects (17 M and 4 F) and their spouses. Bisexuality was documented in 15 of the 17 males. Females were infected by transfusion (n = 2), IDU and prostitution. 8/17 female spouses were HIV positive compared to none in the four male spouses. The small numbers in this study make generalisations difficult.

TRANSMISSION FACTORS

Factors which promote vulnerability in the recipient must be studied as well as factors which promote transmission from the HIV + ve person. Plummer *et al.* (1991) identified 5 factors in an African context which were associated with
— increased transmission,
— past genito urinary (gu) disease history,
— current GU diagnosis,
— frequent prostitute contact,
— lack of circumcision,
— travel.

These studies conclude that an examination is needed of behavioural factors which increased exposure such as multiple exposures, limited protection, and specific behaviours. LaGuardia (1991) documents four key issues for transmission which are:
— partner selection,
— partner number,
— mode of sexual expression,
— condom use.

The literature also tends to suggest that for many women, the risk factors they carry is bound up with the behaviour of their male partners. This has vital implications for prevention and intervention. It is easier to modify within person behaviours, and more difficult, if not impossible in some circumstances, to modify sexual partners' behaviour. Careful partner selection is often advocated as a strategy against HIV infection, but if HIV status is kept a secret then partner selection will be ineffective in controlling personal subsequent risk exposure.

SEROCONVERSION PREDICTORS

Padian *et al.* (1990) point out that it is not simply number of exposures which account for infection but also the nature of the behaviour which may increase the likelihood of transmission. They highlight such issues as anal intercourse and the presence of bleeding.

The literature tends to suggest a variety of factors including:
— timing of exposure,
— routine condom usage,
— the presence of other sexually transmitted diseases (STDs).

Some conflicting evidence is presented for:
— sex during menses,
— circumcision,
— contraceptive pill use,
— crack use.

Lack of condom usage is consistently reported as a predictor for such seroconversion. Papetti *et al.* (1989) studied 43 couples (34 males and 9 females) and found 17 to be concordant with the remaining 26 discordant. After one year follow up 2 of the 26 (7.7%) were infected. 95% of couples where both were infected did not use condoms compared to 62% of those with only one infected.

De Vincenzi (1990) found that of 6 couples converting (from 170 followed up) all did not use condoms consistently. Rehmet *et al.* (1990) in a prospective study of 40 discordant couples found that more infectious patients deteriorated faster than less infectious patients and noted that the period of highest risk was soon after the initiation of the sexual relationship.

Childbirth without marriage was found to relate to higher rates of HIV than in the presence of marriage (Makuwa *et al.*, 1991) in a study of 2,000 pregnancies in Brazzaville.

In Zaire, Kamenga *et al.* (1991) noted that of the 6 couples (4% of the sample) who became concordant risks were: inconsistent condom use; urethritis; one occasion of breakage in regular condom usage; one claimed always using condoms yet wife was pregnant. None of the seroconverters reported extramarital sex.

Ryder *et al.* studied large cohorts (7,068 male workers) in Kinshasa together with 416 female employees and 4,548 wives. HIV rates were 3.6% for employees and 5.8% for wives. The presence of recent extramarital sex was related to a significantly higher incidence of HIV infection (2.8% vs 4.4% and rising to 8.7% for men with more than 5 partners). Essentially in this population there was a strong association between HIV infection and STDs generally, with Genital Ulcer Disease (GUD) specifically.

Latif (1989) showed that in a sample of 75 wives of HIV positive men, the 60% concordance rate was related to genital ulcers in the men or symptoms of illness.

De Vincenzi and Ancelle Park (1990) looked at predictors of seroconversion in partners of 403 identified heterosexual couples in Europe. They recorded that risk factors for male to female transmission included index case with full blown AIDS, recent STD, anal sex and older female (+ 45 years). Risk factors for female to male transmission include index case with full blown AIDS and sexual contact during menses.

Seidlin *et al.* (1991) examined couples with more than 10 episodes of vaginal sex with an infected index case. 61 partners were studied (mostly female with only 5 male) and 29 index cases – mostly male with only 4 female. 31 partners were HIV + ve and 28 were HIV-ve. The only significant predictors of partner positivity was crack use and anal intercourse. No gender differences were reported.

Carael *et al.* (1988) in a study of 150 couples (90% n = 124 concordant) seropositivty was associated with prostitute contact, history of STD and second marriages.

BEHAVIOUR DIFFERENCE : DOES THE MALE DECIDE?

Few studies set out specifically to examine gender differences. Gender relationships in HIV must acknowledge wider gender issues if true behavioural patterns are to be understood, let alone altered. For some women their major (and only) risk factors are associated with the behaviour of their male partner rather than their own behaviour. For some women the element of choice is limited and wider social circumstances may limit their willingness to implement and sustain changes. Indeed the notion of choice implies a freedom which may not be available to many women who are dependent on men for social and economic support given the gender structure of many societies. Countless studies report on the 'powerlessness' of women. Such assumptions are often demeaning and may endorse and perpetuate imbalances. Rather power differences should be studied and gender related reactions should be understood. For example women are less likely to abandon an HIV positive partner than the converse. They are less likely to withold knowledge of their own status but more likely to be kept in ignorance of a partner's status. They will often put the care of their partner or their children before their own care. Such behavioural patterns (often noted) may not simply reflect a lack of power, but may reflect alternative life styles and philosophy which could be admired rather than shunned and demeaned. Often studies look at change (or empowerment) of women as a solution – but perhaps a parallel educational effort geared towards their men could also be helpful. For example Kamenga found that pregnancy was more common if the male partner was positive than the female partner. This finding is rarely highlighted and is not translated into policy in worldwide ante-natal clinics where it is the women (rather than the men) who are engaged in the dialogue.

Most writers conclude that male to female transmission is more likely than female to male. This may be due to biological factors but may also involve behavioural factors. Carael *et al.* (1988) studied 150 couples with at least one HIV positive member and found that 90% (n = 124) were both positive and proposed that most of the risk factors for the couples were the risk factors for the husband raising the possibility that the male acquired HIV and passed it to his female partner.

Kamenga *et al.* (1991) documented that at risk males were more likely to protect themselves than at risk females. Infected males (n = 80) were more likely to place women at risk than the likelihood of an infected woman (n = 69) to place an uninfected man at risk. Positive wives were younger than negative wives. If the wife was the positive member then the marriage was usually of shorter duration. When the husband was negative they were more likely to abstain from sex than when the woman was negative (41.2% compared to 58.8%) despite the fact that for both groups the numbers of sexual episodes increased over time after notification of HIV status. Husbands who were abstinent from sex within their marriage as a result of their own HIV status reported extramarital sex which was invariably unprotected. Thus even when they did not expose their wife to risk, they did expose other women who included sex workers or casual partners. No women in this study reported extramarital sex in the presence of HIV infection. Condom use depends, to a great extent on male willingness. When men were at risk of infection (i.e. their wives are positive) 82% sustained condom use. When they were the positive partner, and risked infecting their wife, condom use was significantly lower (62%). Of the 149 couples, 18 suffered from psychological problems: 11 where the female was positive compared to only 7 where the male was positive. More negative males divorced their positive female wives than negative females divorced their positive husbands. Pregnancy was more common when the male was positive than when the female was positive.

Such findings were confirmed by Tice *et al.* (1990) who studied 46 couples in Rwanda. After extended follow up (mean of 316 days) unprotected sexual episodes were higher in couples with an HIV + ve male (11/99) compared to female (4/93). None of the men and 3 of the women seroconverted.

CONTINUING DISCORDANCE

Few studies examine entire populations and present the rate of discordancy or concordancy in any systematic way and rarely how this changes over time. Thus convenience samples are most often employed and it is difficult to work out accurate rates of seroconversion, let alone establish the direction of conversion in concordant couples unless clear primary risk or infection was established. Such is the case in some studies of haemophiliac couples but often there are no other groups in whom this is true.

The literature shows initial cohort descriptions with varying rates of concordant and discordant couples. Subsequently seroconversion in discordant couples is often reported as low, is often associated with specific behavioural factors and is often reported to predominate in female partners rather than male partners.

Deschamps *et al.* (1991) studied '148 sexually active couples' and found 89 to be discordant with 50 concordant over a 3 year period. Their data does not give insight into how many couples could possibly emerge from the pool who were not sexually active (abstinence is commonly recorded in couples after HIV diagnosis).

Papetti *et al.* (1991) studied 130 couples and found 41% to be concordant. After 12 months of follow up, 5 of the remaining 35 discordant couples seroconverted.

Carael *et al.* (1988) studied 150 couples with at least one HIV positive member and found that 90% (n = 124) were both positive.

REPRODUCTIVE BEHAVIOUR

Pregnancy in the presence of HIV is common (Sherr, 1991) and is documented in concordant and discordant couples alike (Kamenga 1991). Klimes *et al.* (1992) studied 17 couples where the male had haemophilia and HIV infection and compared them with 17 such couples without HIV infection. 2 (12%) with HIV had a newborn baby and 4 (24%) wanted more children. Jason *et al.* (1990) reported 24 completed pregnancies in 20 HIV + ve partners of HIV infected haemophiliac men.

Vogler *et al.* (1989) studied 31 couples and of whom 17 partners were HIV negative on entry to the study. 7 partners were pregnant at the time of their first test, 4 of whom were found to be HIV + ve. One of the HIV + ve partners and 3 HIV-ves completed their pregnancies. Two additional pregnancies occurred after HIV testing.

Deschamps *et al.* (1991) studied 148 sexually active couples of whom 89 were discordant and 50 were concordant. After counselling 17 couples ceased sexual activity, 77 couples continued sexual activity for the duration of the 3 year study, and 54 couples ceased sexual activity after a mean of 10 months. Within the latter two groups condom uptake was below half and pregnancy rates were high (close on 25% n = 30) in both concordant (n = 11) and discordant (n = 19) couples who continued sex for the entire study and those who abstained after a mean of 10 months. No data is given on seroconversion rates of infants or whether those who became pregnant were among the 3 (6%) who seroconverted over the three year period of the study.

Counselling often needs to help couples face these dilemmas when they desire a baby. Such a conception carries the risk of exposing the uninfected partner to HIV over and above the possible exposure risks for the baby. It is trite to assume that all couples will immediately decide not to procreate in the presence of HIV. Indeed, international evidence shows the opposite, despite the fact that many studies see 'failure to terminate pregnancy' or 'pregnancy conceived subsequent to HIV identification' as a negative outcome or evidence of failed behaviour change. Such biases show little understanding of the life goals and expectations of individuals, especially those faced with mortality or the loss of a beloved partner. Medical advice in the presence of such a situation poses a variety of ethical problems (Smith *et al.* 1991).

PSYCHOLOGICAL PROBLEMS

Psychological distress has been monitored generally in HIV infection (Carballo & Miller, 1989) and specifically in a few studies of discordant couples. Findings show high levels of reported sexual dysfunction, increased psychological symptomatology (such as anxiety, depression, mood fluctuations and suicidal ideation) with allied marital and relationship strain. Bereavement reactions have been monitored in those whose partners have died of AIDS though few studies particularly focus on discordant couples. Descriptive studies (e.g. Miller *et al.*, 1989) have outlined many issues facing such couples such as informing, secrets, stigma and unmittigating burdens. No empirical studies provide comprehensive prevalence and severity insight for this group. There is a growing literature on 'the worried well' (Miller *et al.*, 1989; Davey and Green, 1991). Within these groups there are those who are worried, well and have low HIV risks as well as those who are preferably described as 'AIDS anxious' who may well have exposure risks. Discordant couples would certainly fall into the latter category.

Klimes found sexual dysfunction among 29% HIV + ve discordant couples and 11% among HIV-ve couples prior to HIV testing. The proportions increased after HIV testing for both groups to 41% and 32% respectively. Sexual relationships had changed since HIV status for 41%, and 71% still reported sexual intercourse but not always with a condom (only 59% always). They found that women (regardless of partners' HIV status and bearing in mind that all were living with a partner with either one or two life threatening diseases) reported higher levels of symptomatology than their male spouses. Surprisingly this was not significantly raised if HIV was present.

These findings were confirmed by Dew (1991) who studied 36 women married to haemophiliac men, 17 of whom were HIV positive. Psychiatric symptoms of women did not differ according to HIV status of husbands.

Kamenga *et al*. (1991) described severe psychological trauma on HIV diagnosis for 18 of the 149 couples studied. 15/18 were able to use counselling to resolve the trauma and effect reconciliation within their relationships. Three couples divorced.

Mbuyi *et al*. (1989) studied 122 discordant Zairian couples (67 M and 55 F) and recorded that 17 (14%) experienced psychological distress. This was higher for females (n = 10) than males (n = 7) and resulted in 5 temporary separations and 2 divorces. Three suicide threats were recorded (2 F and 1 M).

Bromberg *et al*. (1991) studied 41 couples (6 HIV + ve females and 35 HIV + ve males). HIV + ve women reported more psychological symptoms than HIV positive men. However this study had small numbers and controls were not reported. The data may simply reflect well documented gender differences in the population generally.

PARTNER DISCLOSURE

Although some people with HIV do not inform their partners, many do divulge their HIV status. This is not always inevitable or immediate and some studies themselves initiate partner notification. Conversely when partners are not told, they rarely find their way into studies so the full extent of ignorance is simply unknown.

Divulgence of HIV status to sexual or sharing partners is difficult. There are documented cases of men and women in the sex industry who continue working in the presence of HIV given no alternative survival means. Manaloto *et al*. (1990) reported that 36 HIV + ve female prostitutes in the Philippines continued to work as prostitutes after HIV infection. Cochran and Mays (1990) noted that partners said they would lie if they were HIV positive. Wilkins *et al*. (1989) followed up 31 asymptomatic seropositive subjects identified in the course of a seroprevalence survey (13 male and 18 female) where only 3 discussed HIV with their partners and only 8 had used any of the condoms given to them at follow up.

Sepulveda *et al*. (1990) showed a protective effect associated with knowledge of partner's infection. Such knowledge was the trigger for safer sex and hence seroconversion was reduced.

This raises ethical and legal questions about the implications of withholding such knowledge and the extent to which an individual with HIV is duty bound to inform a sexual partner of his/her status, and the code of conduct for health care workers caught up within the process.

COUNSELLING AND BEHAVIOUR CHANGE

Behaviour change in the face of HIV infection in one partner has been dramatic and consistent in the majority of studies. Partners also seem to be able to sustain such behaviour over time. Behaviours monitored tend to focus specifically on condom uptake, frequency of sexual intercourse and more recently studies of the range of sexual behaviours reported by such couples.

There is clear evidence that condom use is protective in preventing seroconversion. Feldblum (1991) summarised findings from prospective studies and concluded that there was an overall lower cumulative incidence of HIV in condom users compared to non users. Variations in behaviour change were often associated with the place of study and characteristics of the groups under study.

Peterson *et al.* (1989) studied 54 couples and noted high levels of behaviour change after counselling. Behaviour comparisons between point of enrollment and 6 month follow up showed 43 couples discordant with only 3 not having intercourse, 30/43 having less intercourse and 10 having the same or more intercourse. Of the 40 having intercourse, condoms were used by 32. Nine couples practiced anal intercourse (4 with condoms) and this reduced to 2 at follow up, both protected with condoms.

Kamenga *et al.* (1991) showed condom uptake changed from 5% to 70.7% at one month and to 77.4% at 18 month follow up. Before notification frequency of sex was reported as 8 times per month. This reduced initially but increased with time from 4.1 episodes after the first month to 6.2 at 18 months. No couples were abstinent prior to notification yet 28% reported abstinence by the second month.

Moore *et al.* (1991) showed that intensive counselling was correlated with sustained behaviour change.

De Vincenzi *et al.* (1990) showed that only half of their discordant couples followed up for at least 1 year (n = 170) always used condoms. No seroconversion occurred in couples systematically using condoms.

Vogler *et al.* (1989) studied 31 couples and found 17 partners to be HIV negative on entry to the study. 29 reported changes in sexual behaviour after testing including abstinence and condom use (yet this was inconsistent over time). Although half of the couples reported anal intercourse prior to testing, only one couple continued this. Two of the couples reporting condom use also became pregnant. Tice *et al.* (1990) reported high uptake of condoms and spermicide in discordant Rwandan couples (n = 46).

Deschamps *et al.* (1991) studied 148 couples from Haiti of whom 50 were concordant and 89 were discordant for HIV. Prior to counselling condom uptake was 9%. After counselling 17 couples abstained from sexual intercourse, (of whom 19% were concordant and 7% were discordant). A further 52% of the sample (51 Discordant and 26 concordant) continued their sexual activity and 54 couples (32 discordant and 22 concordant) discontinued sexual activity after a mean of 10 months. In the continuous sexually active group, there were no significant differences between concordant and discordant couples in the rate of regular condom use (49% of discordant couples and 39% of discordant couples always used condoms). Seroconversion was observed in 3 of the 51 discordant couples (6%), all of whom were drawn from the group which did not use condoms consistently. Of the consistent condom users (n = 25) no subjects seroconverted. Condom use in the group who gave up sexual activity was reported at 31%.

Skurnick *et al.* (1991) reported that New Jersey couples reduced frequency of vaginal sex and dramatically increased condom use in a longitudinal study of 35 couples whose relationship began prior to knowledge of HIV status. At this time vaginal sex occurred on average twice per week. After HIV knowledge, over half reduced the frequency of sexual activity and 20% abstained completely. Condom use was low prior to knowledge of HIV (6%) and increased to 89% in the following year.

Moss *et al.* (1991) studied 65 couples from an STD clinic (male n = 38, female n = 27). Again after counselling and testing condom uptake increased from 5% to 54% and frequency of intercourse decreased from 9.9 to 4.5 occasions per time interval. Yet seroconversion occurred in 18% of the sample per year (slightly higher for women than men – 19% compared to 16%).

Thus it seems clear that sexual behaviour change occurs and is maintained for this group as a whole. It is unclear why such changes are sustained (compared to reported difficulties in other groups (Ostrow, 1991)). Studies all discuss counselling as an ingredient, but few describe the content of such counselling and monitor specific elements which may account directly for behaviour change and maintenance. Few studies examine factors associated with couples whose behaviour does not change or where such change is not maintained over time.

OTHER DYADS

The literature coverage overlooks many other 'couples' who share risk behaviours. Most are overlooked because of the fleeting nature of their interaction such as sex workers and their partners or rape victims whose attackers cannot be found; because their linkage is not recognised such as infected doctors or dentists and their uninfected patients; because their mode of transmission is not sexual such as mother to child or idus who share needles or syringes. For others the fear of infection may link them rather than actual exposure such as those who are raped, those who are sexually abused, those who received blood or body products or even those who share in the lives of the infected such as carers or siblings.

This underscores the need to examine HIV in its wider context and to place individual infection within its familial and societal setting.

Procreation

HIV positive mothers face the dual possibility of infecting their unborn or newly born infants and their sexual partners. Similarly HIV positive fathers may infect their partners and their infants in turn. Breast feeding mothers also face this possibility (Dunn *et al.*, 1992). HIV positive infants may infect their mothers whilst being breast fed (Pokrovsky, 1990). The act of conceiving may expose a man or woman to HIV infection either directly through unprotected sex, or through such procedures as artificial insemination by an infected donor. The rate of vertical transmission varies according to place of study, nature of samples, and length of follow up (Peckham, 1990). As most pregnancy studies are concentrated on underlying themes of understanding vertical transmission few studies examine the emotional reactions and behaviour for parents whose babies are not infected, or differences between those children who are infected with those who are not.

Twins

A high twinning rate has been noted in HIV positive births. Furthermore, international cohort studies have revealed that discordant twins are common, with a greater propensity for infection in the first delivered twin (Twin A) compared to the second. This data is in the early stages of completion and provides no insight into the trauma that the individual twins may face where one is positive and the other is not. The often noted special relationship between twins may be altered in the presence of HIV or AIDS and development in the presence of a sick and needy twin may be influenced.

Siblings

Uninfected siblings have been overlooked despite the fact that they carry many of the same burdens. Harris (1990) studied 14 HIV positive children and their siblings who were residing with their biological mothers. The study identified behavioural problems in just under half of the young siblings (43%). Such siblings also constitute the potential groups of orphans if and when their parents succumb to opportunistic infections. Studies in Africa have also highlighted that siblings are commonly dispersed despite the fact that strong sibling relationships are protective against psychological symptomatology in those who lose parents. The worldwide literature tends to focus on the ramifications of HIV from the male point of view which has meant a lag in understanding for women (see Hankins, chapter 2) and especially children whose point of view and disease experience has still not received the international attention it deserves.

COUNSELLING DISCORDANT COUPLES

Counselling challenges for such couples encompass the wide range of counselling issues that any individual with HIV faces (Green & McCreaner, 1989) compounded by the complexity of the relationships and potential transmission of HIV within that relationship. The threads of counselling need to follow themes of support, decision making, emotional expression and address trauma associated with telling, unremitting stressors and illness/death in a loved one.

Specific issues in counselling have centred around risk reduction, safe sex and reproduction in the literature. This needs to be expanded. In addition there is a growing awareness that couples need to be treated as separate individuals with differing, and at times conflicting, needs. Roy (1990) studied 20 haemophiliac couples and found differences in support needs from women to men with a high endorsement of groups and couple assistance and a need for dialogue (particularly on the part of the women) about safe sex.

Studies clearly document an initial period of trauma and stress in relationships at the point of HIV disclosure or diagnosis. Many couples are able to utilise their own strengths or counselling support to overcome these. Yet others may need support if their relationship does not survive this trauma.

Counselling needs change over time and may become greater at points of illness, stress, decision making or bereavement. Family work has often been used to incorporate whole families into care (see chapter 9, Bor). Individual, couple and group work may also be adapted to this client group.

BEREAVEMENT WORK AND MULTIPLE BEREAVEMENT

HIV and AIDS invariably involve a catalogue of losses and bereavement is often a heavy burden. There may well be multiple bereavements and this may set unprecedented levels of emotional trauma within family and friendship networks (Sherr *et al.*, 1992).

BURDEN OF BEING A CARER

Both concordant and discordant couples entail a need for constant caring. The stigma and social burden of HIV and AIDS may often mean that such tasks are unaided and unsupported. Family members may compete for caring resources and carers may be exhausted and drained with little provision for respite or support. Group interventions have been shown to alleviate some of the stresses (Reidy, 1992) but many carers keep HIV a closely guarded secret and cannot share the burden (Mok, 1990). In some centres this may result in an overreliance on health care rather than community resources – some of which are stretched to breaking point. Often the immediate needs of the person with AIDS overshadows the needs of the carer and their plight can go unrecognised (Church *et al.*, 1989).

SUBSEQUENT RELATIONSHIPS

There are no comprehensive studies which detail the course of subsequent relationships after an AIDS death. Those that do exist focus on the potential HIV transmission problems rather than the difficulties survivors may have in initiating and maintaining relationships after a previous AIDS bereavement.

CONCLUSION

HIV infection after sexual exposure is not automatic. Despite the fact that many individuals are infected by one off exposures, there are also those who remain uninfected after prolonged exposure. The reasons for this are unclear. Much of the literature focuses on the rate of such transmission, predisposing factors and correlates. Yet there is also a need to understand the psychological burden experienced by such couples through the course of infection and to develop theoretical and empirical understanding of interventions which are effective at minimising such trauma and maximising coping and adjustment.

Many couples sustain long term relationships in the presence of HIV and AIDS and the literature on such couples, be they concordant or discordant, sheds lights on biological, social and psychological elements of HIV spread and the burdens of illness. The literature clearly points to protective and facilitative factors which account for infection with HIV in couples who are initially discordant but who continue to be exposed to HIV.

Condom usage appears to be the most important factor and proper counselling also has a strong effect. Counselling needs to take on board the diverse nature of this population group, the high motivation they have for addressing behaviour change and sustaining this over time, and the background upheaval that they face during the course of infection. Particular attention should be focussed on the unequal balance of outcomes for male and female partners.

REFERENCES

Belec, C., Georges, A.J., Steenman, G., Martin, P. (1989) Antibodies to HIV in the Semen of Heterosexual Men *Jnl of Infect Diseases* **159** (2), 325–27

Bromberg, J., Grijalva, K., Skurnick, J., Cordell, J., Wan, J., Cornell, R., Louria, D. (1991) Psychologic differences betwen HIV + ve women and HIV + ve men in discordant couples. 7th Int AIDS Conf Abst WD 4128, p 420

CDR (1992) Heterosexually acquired HIV 1 infection cases reported in England wales and NI 85–91 CDR Review Communicable Disease report vol 2 review 5 24 April 92.

Carael, M., Van de Perre, P., Lepage, P., Allen, S., Nsengumuremyi, F., Van Goethem, C., Ntahorutaba, M., *et al.* (1988) HIV transmission among heterosexual couples in Central Africa *AIDS* **2**(3), 201–5

Church, J., *International AIDS Conference* Abstract

Cochran, S.D., Mays, V.M., (1990) Sex, Lies and HIV. *New England Journal of Medicine* **322**, 774–775

Davey, T. and Green, J. (1991) The worried well – ten years of a new face for an old problem *AIDS Care* **3**(3), 289–294

Deschamps, M., Pape, J., Haffner, A., Hyppolite, R., Johnson, W. (1991) Heterosexual activity in at risk couples for HIV infection. 7th Int AIDS Conf WC 3089, p 318

De Vincenzi, I., Ancelle Park, R. (1990) Heterosexual transmission of HIV follow up of a European cohort of couples. Int AIDS Conf 6, abst ThC 100 p 158.

Dew, M., Ragni, M., Nimorwicz, P. (1991) Correlates of psychiatric distress among wives of haemophiliac men with and without HIV infection AM. *Jnl of Psychiatry* **148**, 1016–1022

Dew, M., Ragni, M., Nimorwicz, P. (1990) Infection with HIV and vulnerability to psychiatric distress. Archives of General Psychiatry 47, 737–44

Dunn, D., Newell, M., Ades, A., Peckham, C. (1992) Risk of HIVtype 1 transmission through breastfeeding *The Lancet* 340, 585–8

Feldblum, P. (1991) Results from prospective studies of HIV discordant couples *AIDS* 5(10), 1265–6

Gafa, S., Giudici, M., Vezzani, F., Tuzza, A. (1989) A retrospective study of the heterosexual transmission of HIV infection in couples with unprotected sexual intercourse. *Giornale di Malattie Infe. e Parass.* 41(9), 928–29

Gongora Biachi, R., Gonzales Martinez, P., Puerto, F., Franco, J. (1991) Heterosexual transmssion of HIV in a group of couples residing in the Yucatan Peninsula. *Rev Invest Clin* 43(2) 128–32

Green, J., McCreaner, A. (1989) Counselling in HIV Infection and AIDS, Blackwell Scientific Publications, Oxford

Hankins, C. (1991) Public policy and Maternal Foetal HIV transmission. *Psychology and Health* 6(4), 287–296

Harris, A. (1990) Treating the non infected sibling an AIDS Dilemma. VI International Conference on AIDS, San Francisco, THD 123

Jason, J., Evatt, B. (1990) Pregnancies in HIV infected sex partnrs of haemophiliac men AM, *Jnl of Diseases of Children* 144(4), 485–90

Jason, J., McDougal, J., Dixon, G. (1986) HTLV III/LAV antibody and immune status of household contacts and sexual partners of persons with haemophilia. *J Amer Med Assoc* 255, 212–5

Johnson, A., Petherick, A., Davidson, S., Brettle, R., Hooker, M., Howard, L., McLean, K., Osborne, L., Robertson, R., Sonnex, C. (1989) Transmission of HIV to heterosexual partners of infected men and women *AIDS* 3(6), 367–72

Kamenga, M., Ryder, R., Jingu, M., Mbuyi, N., Mbu, L., Behets, F., Brown, C., Heyward, W., (1991) Evidence of marked sexual behaviour change associated with low HIV 1 seroconversion in 149 married couples with discordant HIV 1 serostatus – experience at an HIV counselling centre in Zaire *AIDS* 5, 61–7

Kim, H., Raska, K., Clemow, L., Eisele, J., Matts, L., Saidi, P., Raska, K. (1988) HIV Infection in sexually active wives of infected hemophilic men *Am J Med* 85(4), 472–6

Klimes, I., Catalan, J., Garrod, A., Day, A., Bond, A., Rizza, C. (1992) Partner of Men with HIV infection and Haemophilia *AIDS Care* 4(1), 149–157

Kreiss, J., Kitchen, L., Prince, H. (1985) Antibody to HTLVIII in wives of haemophiliacs. Evidence of heterosexual transmission *ANN Intern Med* 102, 623–6

La Guardia, K. (1991) AIDS and Reproductive Health Womens Perspectives ed. Amor J.S. and Segal S.J., Plenum Press New York

Latif, A., Katzenstein, D., Bassett, M., Houston, S., Emmanuel, J., Marowa, E. (1989) Genital ulcers and transmission of HIV among couples in Zimbabwe. *AIDS* 3(8), 519–23

Makuwa, M., Miehakanda, J., Nsimba, B., Bakouetela, J. (1991) Study of heterosexual couples in Central Africa of children born outside the marriage and risk of HIV. *Med. d Afrique Noire* 38(3), 180–82

Manaloto, C., Hayes, C., Padre, L. (1990) Sexual Behaviour of Filipino female prostitutes after diagnosis of HIV infection *Southeast Asian Jnl of Tropical Medicine and Public Health* 21(2), 301–5

Mbuyi, K., Jingu, M., Mbu, M., Nzila, M., Ryder, R. (1989) Intensive HIV counselling following serostatus notification is associated with low divorce rate in 122 discordant Zairian couples 5 Int AIDS Conf Abst WDP 2 p 743

Miller, D., Carballo, M. (1989) HIV Counselling Problems and Opportunities Defining the New Agenda for the 1990s in *AIDS Care* 1(2),

Miller, D., Acton, T., Hedge, B. (1988) The worried well: their identification and management. *Journal of the Royal College of Physicians* 22(3), 158–65

Miller, R., Bor, R. (1989) AIDS A guide to clinical counselling. Science Press

Mok, J. (1990) VI International Conference on AIDS, San Francisco, THD 813

Moore, L., Padian, N., Shiboski, S., OBrien, T. (1991) Behaviour change in a cohort of heterosexual couples with one HIV infected partner Int AIDS Conf 7, WC 103 p 49

Moss, G., Clemetson, D., Costa, L., Plummer, F., *et al*. (1991) Association of cervical ectopy with heterosexual transmission of HIV. *J Infect Dis* **164**(3), 588–91

Ostrow, D. (1991) Behavioural Aspects of AIDS Plenum Press Medical, New York and London

Padian, N. (1987) Heterosexual transmission of Acquired Immunodeficiency Syndrome. Int Persp and National Projections. *Rev Infect Dis* **9**, 947–60

Padian, N., Shilboski, S., Jewell, N. (1990) The Effect of number of exposures on the risk of heterosexual HIV transmission. *Jnl of Infect Disease 90* **161**, 883–7

Papetti, C., Pesce, A., Mezzaroma, I., Pinter, E., D'Offizi, G., Luzi, G., Aiuti, F. (1989) HIV 1 transmisison in heterosexual couples 5 Int AIDS Conf abst TAP 103 p 116

Papetti, C., Mezzaroma, I., DOffizi, G., Campitelli, G., *et al*. (1991) Risk Factors for heterosexual transmission of HIVl. 7 Int AIDS Conf Abst WC 3108 p 323

Peckham, C., Newell M.L. (1990) HIV-1 Infection in mothers & babies AIDSCARE, vol 2, no 3 p 205–12.

Peterson, H., Padian, N., Glass, S., Moreno, A., AJaniku, I., Wofsy, C. (1989) Behaviour modification in couples enrolled in a study of heterosexual transmission Int AIDS Conference 5, abst TAP 100 p 115.

Plummer, F., Moses, S., Ndinya, Achola, J.O. (1991) Factors affecting female to male transmission of HIV 1 Implications of transmission dynamics for prevention AIDS and Womens Reproductive Health ed, L. C. Chen *et al*. Plenum Press New York

Pokrovsky, V. (1990) VI International Conference on AIDS, San Francisco, FC 648

Ragni, M., Kingsley, L., Nimorwicz, P., Gupta, P., Rinaldo, C. (1989) HIV heterosexual transmission in haemophilia couples lack of relation to T4 number *J Acquire Immune Defic Synd* **2**(6), 557–63

Rehmet, S., Staszewski, S., Von Wangenheim, I., Bergmann, L., Helm, E., Doer, H., Stille, W. (1990) HIV transmission rates and co factors in heterosexual couples. 6 Int AIDS Conf Abst ThC 582 p 270

Reidy, M., Taggart, M.E., Asselin, L. (1992) Psychosocial needs expressed by the natural caregivers of HIV infected children. *AIDS Care* **3**(3), 331–345

Roy (1990) Haemophila and HIV: an assessment of psychosocial needs of couples. 6 Int AIDS Conf Abst ThD 821 p 331

Ryder, R., Hassig, S., Ndilu, M., Behets, F., Nanlele, K., Malele, B., Bishagara, U., Kashamuka, M. (1989) Extramarital prostitute sex and GUD are important HIV risk factors in 7,068 male Kinshasa factor workers and their 4,548 wives, Int AIDS Conf Abst MAO 35, p 51.

Seidlin, M., Dugan, T., Vogler, M., Bebenroth, D., Krasinski, K., Holzman, R. (1989) Risk factors for HIV transmission in steady heterosexual couples. 5 Int AIDS Conf abst TAO 17.

Sepulveda, J., Hernandez, M., Herrera E Avila, C. (1990) Heterosexual HIV transmission: a multicentre partner study in Mexico City Int AIDS Conf 6, abst ThC 568 p 267

Sherr, L. (1991) HIV and AIDS In Mothers and Babies, Blackwell Scientific Publications, Oxford.

Sherr, L. (1992) Unique Patterns in Bereavement among people with HIV and AIDS G U Medicine December 1992

Sion, F., Santos, E., Salerno Goncalves, R., Almeida, M., Morais de Sa, C., Vanderborght, B., Carvalho, M., Brandao, A., Rocha, J. (1990) Lack of female to male transmission in husbands of HIV infected women Int AIDS Conf 5, Abst ThC 567, p 266

Skurnick, J., Bromberg, J., Grijalva, K., Cordell, J., Louria, D., Monto, A., Weiss, S. (1991) Behaviour changes in heterosexual couples discordant for HIV VII Int AIDS Conf Abst WC 3094 p 319

Smith, J.R Reginald, P.W Forster, S.M (1990) Safe sex and conception: a dilemma. *The Lancet* 335, 359

Stewart, G., Tyler, J., Cunningham, A., Barr, J., Driscoll, G., Gold, J., Lamong, B. (1985) Transmission of HTLVIIII by artificial insemination by donor. *Lancet* 2, 581–4

Tice, J., Allen, S., Serufilira, A., van de Perre, P., Ziegler, J., Hulley, S. (1990) Impact of HIV testing on condoms: spermicide use among HIV discordant couples in Africa, 6Int AIDS Conf abst SC 694 p 262

Vogler, M., Dugan, T., Seidlin, M. (1989) Changes in sexual and reproductive behaviour in heterosexual couples after HIV testing 5 Int AIDS Conf Abst TAP 101, p 115

Wilkins, H., Alonso, P., Baldeh, S., Cham, M., Corrah, T., Hughes, A., Jatteh, K., Oelman, B., Pickering, H. (1989) Knowledge of AIDS, use of condoms and results of counselling subjects with asymptomatic HIV2 infection in the Gambia, *AIDS Care* 1(3), 247

6

Heterosexual Issues in Haemophilia

RIVA MILLER AND ELEANOR GOLDMAN

INTRODUCTION

Issues related to heterosexual HIV transmission required attention in the haemophilic population very soon after the disease was recognised, because it appeared that the majority of sexually active haemophilic men were involved in heterosexual relationships.

Haemophilia is a life long, inherited bleeding disorder for which there is treatment but no cure. It is a sex-linked recessive condition carried by females and passed on to their male offspring. Treatment for bleeds is by intravenous infusions of the missing factor VIII or IX derived from pooled donations of blood. It was through this replacement therapy that haemophiliacs in the UK became infected with HIV prior to 1985. Since then all blood donations have been tested for HIV and the resulting blood products treated to inactivate viruses.

In the UK at least 1,206 haemophiliacs were infected with HIV (Lee et al., 1992). The ages of those infected ranged from young children to old men. Those who were children in 1985 have reached adolescence, and those who were adolescents then are now young men. Some haemophilia carriers with low levels of clotting factor required replacement treatment for surgery or after injury and ran the same risk of infection as haemophilic men. Both men and women needed counselling about the possible risks to partners from 1983 onwards and about the HIV antibody test when it became available in 1985. The factors that influence HIV transmission are varied and complex ranging from sexual practises to the stage of HIV infection of the haemophilic (Eyster et al., 1989), (European Study Group on Heterosexual Transmission of HIV).

Before HIV there was a pre existing structure in place in haemophilia centres for genetic counselling, work with families and providing medical care. Patients were seen at regular intervals as part of comprehensive care. Those severely affected were seen six monthly, and mildly affected patients were reviewed annually. At these reviews not only their medical care was discussed but also their social and psychological circumstances. There had long been recognition of the risk of transmitting viral diseases, especially hepatitis through blood and sexual contact.

Heterosexual issues in haemophilia emerged with recognition of the virus, before there was a reliable antibody test. When it first became apparent that HIV could be spread through blood products the reviews, already in place for regular counselling and medical care, incorporated advice about safer sex, handling of blood products and disposing of used equipment, particularly needles. This information was given by treatment centres and disseminated more widely through the Haemophilia Society in the UK (Haemofact). Thus throughout the epidemic information about transmission, particularly from man to woman, and the risks of vertical transmission to children has been offered to this population. In addition because of the structure of haemophilia care, patients have regular blood tests. Thus dates of seroconversion are known in the majority of cases and valuable information has emerged from the cohort studies on progression to disease, death and infectivity (Phillips *et al.*, 1991).

In considering heterosexual issues it is important to remember that there are different approaches and different attitudes amongst patients and staff that are dependent on cultural and social attitudes, beliefs and economic forces. Attitudes to revealing secrets, marriage customs, relationships between parents and children, family structure may vary, for example in India, Greece, New York.

COUNSELLING APPROACH

Haemophilia affects not only the individual but the whole family. When addressing heterosexual issues we consider that it is more effective to counsel couples. Adolescents under the age of 16 are interviewed with their parents.

The method of counselling developed by the authors is based on techniques of the Milan Associates who use the systemic approach (Bor *et al.*, 1992). Every individual is part of a wider system. Every action taken by an individual has repercussions in and reactions from the wider systems which he or she inhabits. The systemic approach takes these relationships into account. The technique uses questions to elicit and transmit information and to stimulate communication between individuals. Questions are used which link people and ideas by asking them what they think others views may be. Thus when interviewing one individual absent members in the system can be included by the use of questions about their perceived views. This approach is particularly useful for addressing heterosexual issues which affect couples, their children, and relationships with the partners' family. Generally families with haemophilia have had close family relationships because of the inheritance pattern, and added dependence of affected children on their parents.

Haemophilia is an uncommon condition so there are not many people outside the family who understand the problems. In spite of this haemophilia and HIV have caused distancing in some families.

ISSUES TO BE ADDRESSED

There are particular heterosexual issues that need to be addressed in haemophilia which include:

Disclosure of diagnosis. The patients themselves have always had the problem of how and when to disclose haemophilia to a potential partner, and HIV has added a new dimension to this dilemma. At the time of diagnosis the defence reaction of some haemophilic patients was denial and reluctance to disclose the diagnosis. Disclosure may be inhibited by the fear of not making a relationship or losing a developing relationship, fears of breaches in confidentiality or an inability to start the discussion.

Safer sexual practice is of universal concern. How this will be negotiated differs according to the age and stage of life of the individual. Many have had to consider the use of condoms and contraceptive methods for the first time.

Other transmission risks existed for partners and household contacts. The safe handling of blood products, needles and other used equipment is essential. Those parents who treated children before sterilization and screening of concentrate might have been at risk of becoming infected through needle stick injuries and then transmitting the disease to their sexual partners.

Relationships are profoundly affected both by haemophilia and HIV infection. The haemophilic may fear infecting a sexual partner, and the partner may have unspoken fears that impede easy communication and inhibit sexual relations. These fears can prevent some haemophilics from making relationships, while others are more closely bound to partners who, through caring or feelings of guilt are unable to leave them. In some cases fear of HIV destroys the relationship.

Whether or not to have children. Some of the issues about childbearing are common to all couples having children. The genetic transmission of haemophilia was always an additional issue for couples to consider. Now they also have to take into account specific issues related to HIV such as transmission to the partner and the child, and the changed life expectancy of one or both parents.

Follow-up for those who have children. Since there are many unanswered questions, the HIV status and health of mother and child or children, (where couples have had children), should be monitored regularly even when both have been diagnosed as HIV negative, to add to the body of information about HIV transmission. For the HIV negative female partners, regular HIV testing may provide reassurance about the safety of sexual practises, but each visit may reawaken anxieties which need to be addressed. Regular monitoring of the physical and cognitive development of the children of positive haemophilic men is an essential part of the follow-up. If either the mother, or the mother and child should be infected specialist HIV care must be offered in the same way as for all others infected with HIV.

Reversal of hopes and expectations may result from HIV. Some may no longer envisage having close sexual relationships. Hopes for continuation of the family through children may be lost. Plans for the future may seem futile if the life expectancy is drastically reduced.

Self image is often affected by peer group pressures which focus on sexual relationships. Amongst adolescents the questions asked may be 'why are you a virgin?' or 'how often have you scored?' Pressure may come from family and others in their social circle for haemophilics to find partners or for couples to have children. Inability to fulfil these expectations may diminish self esteem which can also be damaged by the perception of being 'dirty', not 'manly', or unable to be 'normal'.

ADDRESSING THE MAIN ISSUES

Issues of heterosexual spread have to be addressed in different ways for those in different situations. There is a need to rehearse the possible ways of disclosing HIV and negotiating safer sex. This negotiation is equally necessary for the HIV negative haemophiliacs and indeed for all who are establishing new relationships.

Young Adolescents who are Beginning to Think about Sexual Relationships (Miller and Bor, 1988).

In adolescence, under the age of 16, parents' wishes must be respected and counselling carried out with the parents' permission, and in their presence. Counselling that is initially in general terms facilitates the introduction of sensitive topics. Discussion of hypothetical situations, until an atmosphere of trust has been built up, enables more free communication between the adolescent, his parents and the counsellor. An example is given of a 15 year old haemophilic boy with HIV infection who is being seen with his parents for a review by the doctor and a counsellor. They have recently told him that he is HIV positive.

> Counsellor: John, your mother says you are showing an interest in girls. Do you and your friends discuss girls?
> John: Sometimes.
> Counsellor: What are the kinds of things that you talk about?
> John: (*Smiles and looks at mother but does not answer*).
> Counsellor: Mrs Smith, what sort of things do you think they talk about?
> Mrs Smith: Dad has talked to John about what happens between girls and boys. We talk openly in our family and he knows it is important to protect girls from becoming pregnant.
> Counsellor: Do you know what Mum means by 'protecting'?
> John: Yes – condoms and all that.
> Counsellor: Mr Smith – do you think there are other reasons for using condoms?

(*The counsellor involves the whole family and does not take all the responsibility for giving information*).

> Mr Smith: There are infections that can be passed on through sex.
> Counsellor: Have you discussed some of these at home or has John learned about them at school?
> Mr and Mrs Smith: (*Look uneasy*).
> John: (*bursts out with*) It's AIDS, but I can't have a girl friend because I could give her AIDS.
> Counsellor: Mr and Mrs Smith did you know that John felt like this?
> Mrs Smith: We guessed. It is so hard for him and we don't know what to do. That is what makes it so difficult to talk to John. We all get upset.
> Counsellor: Yes it is hard and it is very important not to infect anyone else. But there are other people like you who have managed to make relationships. We can talk about some of the ways to have relationships with girls without putting them at risk. In your family you have already begun to talk about these things and we can talk about them in more detail if Mum and Dad agree.

This session was aimed at opening up discussion between the boy and his family about the realities of HIV transmission. When boys are 16 or over it is possible to see them alone and speak more frankly about how they might deal with a sexual encounter. Most adolescents do not wish to discuss their sexual lives in front of their parents. This is the most difficult group to deal with in view of the legal implications if the girl friends are under age, and also because the boys with haemophilia are only just emerging into sexual activity. It is hard to place them under restricted conditions and to create other problems for them amongst their peers. However, health care workers always have to keep in mind not only the patient but the health of the public.

Sexually Active Men

Sexually active men who are not yet in a stable relationship are faced with similar difficulties when seeking to make a new relationship. They have the dilemma of deciding how and when to disclose their HIV infection. The task of the counsellor is to ensure that they recognise their responsibility to others and that they understand what constitutes safer sex. Explicit discussion is essential.

For those who have succeeded in making a relationship new issues arise. Partners who may be willing to comply with the wish for penetrative sex to consummate the relationship may have different views after the 'honeymoon' is over. Realistic fears of infection may surface for one or both partners and require renegotiation. The counselling task is to identify concerns and explore ways of dealing with them. The following example is taken from an interview with a couple who have been living together for some time.

> Counsellor: What do you think Jane might be concerned about today?
> Andrew: Nothing—she just came along for moral support.
> Counsellor: Is that how you see it Jane?

> Jane: Yes, but I would like to know more about his health and I am a bit
> worried.
> Counsellor: Andrew what do you think Jane is worried about?
> Andrew: Well HIV I suppose.
> Counsellor: Is that right Jane?
> Jane: Yes. We are very careful but I sometimes worry about it.
> Counsellor: Andrew is there anything that you think you two could do to
> make Jane worry less?
> Andrew: No.
> Counsellor: If you are worried about sex with condoms have you thought
> that there could be ways of achieving satifaction without penetrative sex.
> You could use imagination to find ways to please each other.

Couples may feel that they need to have penetrative intercourse to maintain a
successful relationship. The idea that this is not essential when introduced by the
counsellor, may serve as 'permission' to consider alternatives.

Those who were already in established relationships and had been having
unprotected sex up to the time of their diagnosis of HIV required counselling about
HIV testing. Fortunately, this situation has not arisen since the introduction of heat
treated factor concentrates in the Western world. Counselling about safer sex and
fears of infection was similar to that offered to couples making new relationships
now. Some couples do not always maintain safer sexual practises and the need to test
their partners remains.

DISCUSSION ABOUT HAVING CHILDREN

Some couples already had children before the test was available and needed to know
whether the infection had been transmitted to the partner and the child. They
needed pre- and post- test counselling first. Decisions about having more children
were influenced by the result of the test. For them, and for those who had not yet had
children, fear of transmission was not the only factor that dominated the discussion.
The possible effect on their relationship of not having children had to be addressed
first. Such discussions included where the most pressure came from to have children
– the haemophilic man, the sexual partner, their parents, cultural, religious or peer
group pressures. For example, Mr and Mrs A, who had been married for 5 years
learned of the diagnosis two years after their marraige. They initially had decided to
wait to have children until their economic situation was stable, but after the
diagnosis of HIV fear of transmission became a deterrent. Gradually the pressure to
have children led them to seek counselling to discuss the issues.

> Mr A: My wife is nagging me to have a baby. I want you to help me to
> explain to her what the risks are.
> Counsellor: What happened that made you decide to come today?
> Mr A: There are pressure from all directions.
> Counsellor: Mrs A do you agree with your husband that the pressures are
> from all directions?

Mrs A: Yes. My parents and his parents keep asking why we don't have children. My sister thinks we are only interested in money and asks why we don't have children. All my friends are having babies and don't talk about anything else. We live in a community where young couples are expected to have children. They think that there is something wrong with us.

Counsellor: Mr A, you have heard what your wife has told us. Which of these things do you think is most difficult for her?

Mr A: Her parents because they don't know about the HIV, and her sister.

Counsellor: Mrs A, do you agree with your husband?

Mrs A.: Yes, I have to keep making up stories about not having children. He doesn't want me to tell them.

Counsellor: What do you think is the biggest pressure for your husband?

Mrs A: He is most worried about infecting me, and what would happen if my parents knew about HIV.

Counsellor: Is your wife right about this?

Mr A.: She is right, but it is not only her. I'm worried about passing it on to the child. The reason I don't want to tell her parents is that they wouldn't understand about HIV and it would make things even more difficult.

(The couple have introduced a number of issues. The counsellor must avoid being overwhelmed by the multiplicity of the problems, and to use time effectively must choose which issues to deal with first).

Counsellor: Do you think that if you found a way of telling Mrs A's parents it would be easier for you to think about how having or not having children affects you as a couple.

(The couple were to go home and think about ways of telling Mrs A's parents while the rest of the session was devoted to discussing transmission of infection). The following scenarios were offered for their consideration (Goldman *et al.*, 1992):

1. Mrs A would conceive without becoming infected and would have an uninfected child. She would have the risk of being a single parent and the child might lose a father earlier than normally expected.
2. Mrs A could become infected with HIV, but have an uninfected child (the risk of vertical transmission being between 13 and 39% (European Collaborative Study, 1991). The child could then be left an orphan.
3. Mrs A and the child could be HIV positive and there could be more than one of them ill at the same time with problems about who would be caring for who.
4. Mr and Mrs A might wish to investigate the possibility of artificial insemination from a screened donor so that Mrs A could have a baby and they could enjoy the child together while Mr A was well. The issues of being a single parent would be the same as in scenario 1. However, female offspring would not carry the haemophilic mutation.

(They decided to go home and discuss the risks again. At a later session they reported that they had told her parents of the diagnosis and the dilemma that they faced. The

couple had agreed between themselves that neither of them were ready to take such a risk and would help each other deal with outside pressures.)

Other couples faced with the same scenarios have decided to have children. Among those couples who had taken the risk and not transmitted the infection to mother and child there have been some that wished to have a second child. In this situation it is important for them to take into account the responsibility to the child they already have, and how the child's future may be affected by any risks they wish to take. When considering the risk of transmission the stage of HIV disease of either infected parent has a significant influence on the outcome. For example, HIV antigenaemia and advanced immunodeficiency increases the risk of HIV transmission.

DILEMMAS FOR HEALTH CARE PROFESSIONALS

Dealing with heterosexual issues and transmission of HIV cannot be accomplished effectively in the traditional linear way of working — defining cause and effect and seeking a cure. HIV disease is a condition which at present has no cure and therefore represents 'failure' for the person who is expected to heal.

Caring for the patients has to be balanced with the health care worker's responsibilities for the community as whole. The discussion of transmission of infection to sexual partners always involves more than just the index patient. The welfare of the patient, both psychological and physical, is traditionally paramount. There may be conflicts about upsetting patients dealing with two life threatening conditions, which may inhibit free discussion and the raising of issues that obviously have no solution. The only certain way to avoid sexual transmission of HIV is to abstain from penetrative intercourse. It is particularly difficult to say this to young people. However health care workers must make them aware of the risks of transmission and the means of prevention. Frank discussion by the counsellor of the risks of infection may be inhibited by being unaccustomed to discussing intimate sexual details with patients; by their own moral assumptions about what constitutes a problem; by the difficulties of keeping and revealing secrets; by the fear that raising issues may create new problems or that giving information will disrupt relationships or in some way damage the patient.

Haemophilic patients have a life long need for medical care and for a continuing relationship of trust with their haemophilia centres. This adds to the stress for the staff when balancing their responsibilities to the patient and others. For example:

> Patient: I am the only one in my crowd who is still a virgin. They think I am peculiar and I'm not. I've met a girl and we both want to lose our virginity together.
> Counsellor: Does she know about haemophilia or HIV?
> Patient: She knows about haemophilia but not about HIV. I will never tell her or anyone else and I want to have sex. It is normal.
> Counsellor: Yes having sex is normal. But you have a complicating factor because you have HIV which can be passed on to others. I feel a

responsibility not only for you but for your girl who does not know what risks she is taking. She has not been offered a choice.

Patients: So how can I make it safe?

Counsellor: You can't make it safe, you can only make it less risky. She already has an extra risk because she told you she is a virgin. Where there is bleeding it is easier to pass on HIV infection.

At this point it becomes clear to the counsellor that D intends to, or is likely to have sex. The task of the counsellor is to ensure as far as possible that:

He is aware of the risk of transmission of HIV to his partner.

He is aware of the risks of pregnancy and transmission of infection to a child.

He knows how to reduce the risks as far as possible.

Telling him to use a condom is not sufficient without ensuring that he knows how to do so correctly and understands about the need for contraception. Reduced incidence of penetration reduces the risk of transmission so that other ways of achieving sexual satisfaction should be discussed.

Counsellor: Do you know how to use a condom?

Patient: Not exactly.

An explicit discussion followed demonstrated with condoms. All that the counsellor can hope to achieve is to pass on all available information and check that the patient has heard and understood what was said. After that each individual will make his own decisions which must remain his responsibility. In view of the public health issues and for the protection of the health care worker it is recommended that such discussions are fully recorded and that the accuracy of the record is agreed by the patient.

CONCLUSION

From the moment that haemophilia is diagnosed in the UK, patients and their families are offered comprehensive care at designated haemophilia centres where health care workers have a unique opportunity of studying and addressing HIV problems. This experience and the counselling techniques that have been developed can be applied to other heterosexual groups.

REFERENCES

Bor, R. Miller, R. Goldman, E. (1992) Theory and practise of HIV counselling: A Systemic Approach. Cassell, London.

European Study Group on Heterosexual Transmission of HIV (1992) Comparison of female to male and male to female transmission of HIV in 563 stable couples. *British Medical Journal*, **304**, 809–813.

European Collaborative Study (1991) Mother to child transmission of HIV infection. *Lancet*, **2**, 1039–42.

Eyster, M. Ballard, J. Gail, M. *et al.* (1989) Predictive markers for the acquired immune deficiency syndrome (AIDS) in haemophiliacs: persistence of p24 antigen and low T4 cell count. *Annals of International Medicine*, 110, 963–9.

Goldman, E. Miller, R. Lee, C. A. (1992) Counselling HIV positive haemophilic men who wish to have children. *British Medical Journal*, 304, 329–830.

Haemofact 1–10. Haemophilia Society, London.

Lee, C. A. Phillips, A. Elford, J. Griffiths, P. Bofill, M. Swaden, L. Janossy, G. Kernoff, P.B.A. (1992) Applications of CD4 counts in a cohort of HIV-1 seropositive patients with haemophilia. Chapter in Janossy, G. *et al.* editors. Immunodeficiency in HIV infection and AIDS. Basel, Karger, 32–45.

Miller, R. Bor, R. (1988) AIDS: A Guide to Clinical Counselling. Science Press, London.

7

The Challenge of AIDs in Children

K. M. BARLOW AND J. Y. MOK

INTRODUCTION

Two percent of all cases of acquired immune deficiency syndrome (AIDS) reported to the World Health Organization (WHO) are accounted for by children under 13 years of age. In the UK over 400 children are currently infected by the Human Immunodeficiency Virus (HIV), approximately one third of these have acquired the virus from their mother. The other two thirds are those who have been infected mainly via blood products, the largest group being haemophiliac boys. With the routine screening and deferral of donors, as well as heat treatment of blood products, no further infection should occur via this route, in the developed world. As the number of women infected by HIV increase so will the number of children infected by mother-to-infant transmission. Recent surveys of maternal HIV infection in the United Kingdom revealed variations in seroprevalence throughout the country – 0.59 per 1,000 in Scotland as a whole with 2.4/1000 in Edinburgh (Tappin *et al.*, 1991). In three Thames regions in London, the seroprevalence was found to have risen from 1 in 2,000 in 1988, to 1 in 500 in 1991 (Ades *et al.*, 1991).

TRANSMISSION OF HIV

Children acquire HIV usually by either mother-to-infant transmission (vertically) or via infected blood or blood products, such as coagulation factors (horizontally). Vertical transmission accounts for almost 80% of paediatric HIV infection worldwide (CDC, 1992). Household transmission is extremely rare indicating that HIV is not transmitted through close non-sexual contact (Rogers, 1990).

The rate for mother-to-infant transmission in the European Collaborative Study was 12.9% (95% confidence interval 9.5–16.3%) (European Collaborative Study, 1991). The mechanisms involved as well as the exact timing are still being debated. Infection may occur in utero, during birth or via infected breast milk. In developed countries breast feeding is not recommended for children of infected mothers, however, the World Health Organization (WHO) recommends that breast feeding should continue in developing countries because of the known benefits of breast milk compared to the theoretical but apparently small risk of HIV infection through breast milk (Cutting, 1992; Dunn & Newell, 1992).

Although it is currently impossible to predict if a given mother will transmit the virus to her child, some factors which increase the likelihood are emerging such as: a low maternal CD4 T-cell count (<700 cell/mm^2) or the presence of p24 antigenaemia. Infants born before 34 weeks of gestational age are more likely to be infected as they may be born before the passive transfer of some maternal protective factor (European Collaborative Study, 1992). Maternal antibodies to a gp120 epitope may have a protective role although conclusive proof of the exact protective antibody is still lacking (Rossi *et al.*, 1989; Devash *et al.*, 1990; Parekh, 1991; Robertson *et al.*, 1992).

The method of delivery may also influence the risk of infection, although it is too soon to recommend caesarean section routinely. In the International Twin Register, the first born twin was more likely to be infected, suggesting that a large proportion of infection occurred during delivery (Goedert *et al.*, 1991).

The incubation period for adults is between 7.8 to 11.0 years (Berkelman *et al.*, 1989). While the incubation period of HIV infection in children is shorter than that for adults, there is a bimodal age distribution of children manifesting symptoms and signs of HIV infection. Of infants born to infected women in the European Collaborative Study, about 13% were truly infected. By 12 months, 26% had developed AIDS and 17% died of HIV related disease. After the second year of life, symptoms and signs diminished and some children can therefore remain undiagnosed for several years (European Collaborative Study, 1991).

The survival time after an AIDS defining condition is shorter for children especially during the first year of life. The commonest condition is Pneumocystis carinii *pneumonia* and those presenting with this have the worst prognosis, with the mean survival time being less than one month (Scott *et al.*, 1989). For children with less specific signs and symptoms, the prognosis is better. The Italian Register has demonstrated that lymphocytic interstitial pneumonitis, generalised lymphadenopathy, hepatosplenomegaly, parotitis and skin disease are compatible with a favourable outcome (Tovo *et al.*, 1992).

DIAGNOSIS OF HIV INFECTION IN CHILDREN

Diagnosing HIV infection in infants and young children differs from adults and remains a challenge. It is in the first year of life that diagnosis is the most difficult, but also the time when it is of greatest importance because during this period mortality due to HIV infection is the highest. Infants born to HIV infected women acquire maternal antibodies transplacentally and so a positive HIV antibody test in a child less than 18 months old does not necessarily imply infection. Therefore, other methods of diagnosis have to be employed, such as HIV culture, detection of the proviral DNA sequence using a gene amplification technique (polymerase chain reaction, PCR) and HIV p24 antigen detection, after acid dissociation of immune complexes.

HIV culture and PCR can identify half of infected infants at birth. This increases to greater than 90% of infants after two months of age. Detection of p24 antigenaemia although almost 100% specific is less sensitive than culture or PCR especially in the first few months of life (Borowsky *et al.*, 1992). This is because many infected children do not have p24 antigen until later on in the illness. There are other markers which although less specific, should alert the paediatrician to the possibility of HIV infection. These include raised gammaglobulin levels which by six months of age has been shown to indicate infection (Mok *et al.*, 1989; European Collaborative Study, 1991) and markers of immune activation e.g. beta-2-microglobulin. The measurement of HIV specific IgA or IgM are also emerging as early sensitive and specific markers of infection.

CLASSIFICATION OF HIV INFECTION

Table 7.1 shows a classification system of HIV infection in children proposed by the Centers for Disease Control.

TABLE 7.1
Classification System for HIV Infection in Children <13 Years of Age

P - 0	Indeterminate infection in children <15 months old, with perinatal exposure to HIV
P - 1	Asymptomatic infection
	A. Normal immune function
	B. Abnormal immune function
	C. Immune function not tested
P - 2	Symptomatic infection
	A. Non specific findings
	B. Progressive neurologic disease
	C. Lymphoid interstitial pneumonitis
	D. Secondary infectious diseases
	1. Those listed in surveillance definition
	2. Recurrent serious bacterial infections
	3. Other infections
	E. Secondary cancers
	1. Those listed in surveillance definition
	2. Others
	F. Other diseases possibly caused by HIV, e.g., hepatitis, cardiopathy, nephropathy, haematological and dermatological diseases.

Symptomatic Infection

Non-Specific Features

The clinical manifestations of HIV disease are varied, many of the symptoms and signs are non-specific and frequently occur in uninfected children. Symptoms include recurrent fever, repeated upper respiratory infections, chronic or recurrent diarrhoea and failure to thrive. Parents may notice enlarged lymph nodes or parotid glands, and further examination reveals hepatosplenomegaly. Considering that many of the children come from areas of social deprivation it is difficult to determine if HIV infection is the cause of the symptomatology.

Children may present with a variety of more serious illnesses, particularly severe bacterial infections such as pneumonia, osteomyelitis and septicaemia, which if recurrent, should alert the clinician to the presence of immune deficiency.

Progressive Neurological Disease

HIV encephalopathy may present as developmental delay or regression in milestones. The course can be rapidly progressive, or there may be a slower deterioration. Gross motor and language development seem to be particularly affected (Belman et al., 1988). The frequency of central nervous system (CNS) involvement varies according to different studies from 90% (Belman et al., 1988) to 30% (European Collaborative Study, 1991). Opportunistic infections of the CNS are rare in children, but must be considered in the differential diagnosis (Epstein & Sharer, 1988). The presence of HIV antigen in the cerebrospinal fluid in excess of 25 pg/ml confirms the diagnosis although no correlation exists between CSF antigen levels and neurological signs. Cerebral atrophy can be shown by imaging studies (CT or NMR). Most reports on CNS involvement have concentrated on young children who commonly present with delayed development, or more distressingly, lose milestones which have been acquired. In these circumstances, it is essential to involve the services of a physiotherapist, occupational therapist, speech therapist in a multidisciplinary team. Little attention has focussed on the school–aged child, who is likely to present with difficulties with writing or learning. Special educational input will be required from learning support staff and an educational psychologist. At all times, the family as well as the affected child will require emotional support to cope with the insight into losses experienced.

Lymphoid Interstitial Pneumonitis (LIP)

LIP is commonly present in cases of paediatric AIDS, approximately 50% (Rogers et al., 1987), but only rarely present in adults. Clinical symptoms and signs vary from the child who is asymptomatic, to the one who is severely debilitated and dependent on oxygen. A chest X-ray shows bilateral nodular infiltrates with or without mediastinal thickening due to perihilar lymphadenopathy. Infective causes must be excluded. Although LIP is presently an AIDS-defining diagnosis, the prognosis is good with low mortality. However, the morbidity is significant as children present with repeated respiratory infections and become more short of breath, relying on supplemental oxygen for normal activities such as dressing.

Pneumocystis carinii pneumonia (PCP)

PCP is the commonest opportunistic infection in AIDS patients affecting 80% of adults and 39% of children (Rogers, 1990). It is often the first presentation of HIV infection in children (Ades *et al.*, 1991). The symptoms and signs are non-specific and include cough, tachypnoea, feeding difficulties and fever. Infants may become apnoeic. Signs include cyanosis, subcostal recession, decreased breath sounds, rhonchi and rapidly increasing respiratory distress. A chest X-ray may initially be normal but quickly changes to rapid opacification of the entire lung field due to alveolar and interstitial infiltrates with air bronchograms.

The key to diagnosis is a high index of suspicion and demonstrating the organism in respiratory secretions or tissue. Open lung biopsy is rarely performed in children because of the operative risks involved. Bronchoscopy and bronchoalveolar lavage are preferred, although the use of monoclonal antibodies has allowed *Pneumocystis* antigen to be demonstrated in nasopharyngeal secretions obtained in a non-invasive way (Hague *et al.*, 1991). The outcome following an episode of PCP is poor, with most survivors developing further HIV or AIDS-related illnesses. It is therefore important to discuss with parents whether or not the child should be put on a ventilator, with a limited, poor quality of life.

HIV INFECTION AND THE FAMILY

It is important to remember that when HIV has been transmitted from the mother to her infant the family will have at least two members who are infected and who may be ill simultaneously. Whether the parents are seeking refugee status or are drug users, the social characteristics of HIV affected families are similar. The families are often disadvantaged prior to the onset of AIDS, with economic and social deprivation. They may be financially dependent on income support and live in inadequate accommodation. Many are single parent families or the parental relationship is unstable. The extended family network is often poor, because of drug use or emigration. Also, the reluctance to disclose the diagnosis of HIV effectively blocks off support from family and friends. The secrecy and stigma of HIV lead to social isolation and place the families under extreme psychosocial stress.

The mother is expected to be the major carer, struggling to come to terms with her own ill health and the prospect of a premature death at the same time. If she transmits the virus to her child she will also have to cope with feelings of guilt. When the mother is a drug user, she must control her drug habit with occasional withdrawal symptoms as she copes with caring for the children. If she fails to do this adequately the children may be taken into the care of another family member or the social services. If the woman has been infected by her partner she will probably have ambivalent feelings towards him. Those of love and compassion, but also ones of anger and hurt that he has infected her and her family.

Counselling the Family

The diagnosis of HIV in a child implicitly reveals that the mother may be infected, as well as infection in other members of the family. The time of testing for HIV infection is one of extreme anxiety for the family and often exacerbates pre-existing psychosocial problems. This opportunity is often used to try to assess the social situation including family supports and ongoing coping mechanisms. A careful explanation about HIV testing must be given to the family including the advantages and disadvantages of knowing the infection status. When the child is found to be infected with HIV, the parents will experience shock, guilt, anger and fear. Plenty of time should be allocated when breaking the news to allow a careful explanation of the difference between HIV infection and the development of AIDS. Hope should be instilled by explaining about careful follow-up, treatments which may slow the progression to AIDS and of the increasing survival times. Parents need time to come to terms with this news and frequent meetings to answer their questions will be necessary. Sensitivity to the kinds of problems the families encounter is important.

Many families may find they can not cope with the added burden of having an HIV infected child. This may occur near the time of diagnosis, or when the health of either the child or another family member deteriorates. The children must then be cared for by extended family members such as a grandparent or are received into foster care.

Foster and Adoptive Care

There is significant anxiety among the foster and adoptive families with regard to their personal safety. Detailed information regarding the transmission of HIV is required for potential foster families. Currently in the Lothian region, children coming into foster care are not routinely screened for HIV, but the carers are required to understand that any child placed with them may be infected. Because of the co-existent infection with Hepatitis B which is more easily transmitted, vaccination against Hepatitis B is offered to all foster carers. Regular training and education about HIV and AIDS is given, including universal good hygiene practices which should be taken with any child. If the Social Work Department has been informed about a child's HIV status, then the foster parents will be informed. It is important that foster families are supported with regular counselling (Mok & O'Hara, 1990).

Testing a child for HIV infection should never be done solely at the request of foster or adoptive parents. Prospective adoptive parents should be given as much information as is available on the medical and social background of the child's natural family. Where the natural mother has a lifestyle suggesting the possibility of HIV infection, or comes from an HIV prevalent area, this information should also be given to prospective adopters who may then seek more detailed investigation when the adoption order has been granted.

Schools and Nurseries

With time, more and more children infected by HIV will reach school age and will be integrated into local schools and nurseries. The parent has no obligation to inform the school of their child's diagnosis. All schools should now be adopting universal hygiene procedures with every child, such as wearing gloves during wound toilet, during contact with blood and making sure the wound is covered afterwards. Ideally all parents should be informed about any illness in the school such as measles or chickenpox. To an HIV infected child these diseases may be fatal.

The decision as to whether school staff need to be informed rests entirely with the parents, who should also be warned against breach of confidentiality should the information leak beyond the people who need to know. Parents of other children attending the school may well react negatively to the presence of an HIV infected child in their child's school.

At school HIV infected children may have learning difficulties. Language and developmental delay may be noticed for the first time. School progress may be affected because of neurological sequelae of HIV infection, frequent illness and hospital admissions with resultant absence from school, as well as non-attendance for social reasons. Children affected by HIV will be teased at school, and may also be severely stressed by parental ill health and death.

If the teacher is made aware of the child's or parent's diagnosis then he/she may be more understanding, alert to these problems and supportive. Special educational facilities may be required, and the need assessed on an individual basis. Staff working with all children will have to be prepared to cope with children living with HIV and AIDS who struggle through multiple losses, and who may turn to their teacher for comfort and advice.

Children and Illness

It has been shown that children with chronic health impairments are 1.5 to 3 times more likely than their peers to experience emotional, behavioural and educational difficulties (Cadman *et al.*, 1987; Gortmaker *et al.*, 1990). This may be due to the child's reaction to his illness or the reaction of his family and peers. Perhaps because of his illness, less is expected of him and so he may 'internalise' this vision of himself which may lead to problems and underachievement. With HIV infection this is compounded by the neurological sequelae of encephalopathy and also the increased frequency of social problems. Children who live with HIV and AIDS will also have experienced illness and death in many family members; may take on the care of younger siblings while parents are ill and are consequently inappropriately mature for their age.

Telling the Child

As a child becomes older, more aware and asks more questions, carers face the difficult decision of whether to tell their child about the diagnosis, when the opportune time should be, as well as what to say. Many parents have the very real fear that the risk of stigmatization outweighs any advantages, if the secret should leak out at school. Some feel that the child would not be able to cope with the diagnosis. Other parents may not be able to plan for the future, as they have not come to terms with their own diagnosis, or their child's. Uninfected children may suspect the presence of HIV in the family, but are also painfully aware of the need to keep the family secret.

Usually children have a greater awareness of their illness than the carers or professionals believe. Often a 'wall' is built up because of the lack of communication and the lack of explanation for the frequent tests and episodes of hospitalization. Disclosure often bridges this gap, it reduces the sense of isolation and fear that families experience (Lewert, 1990). Sharing and communication strengthens the family unit and eases the pain. The decision must lie entirely with the family and must be respected. If the family does decide to explain the illness to the child it is important that this is done on a developmentally appropriate level, meeting each child's individual requirements. Professional counselling during this period is a great advantage, and must involve all family members who are close to the child.

Helping the Family Cope with Death

As families are helped to face their own feelings about death, so can the child (Kubler-Ross, 1981). When a child dies there is a greater need for support and counselling than ever before. Specific bereavement counselling may be utilized especially when a carer is not coping. Every person manifests his grief in a different way. Parents may need help to appreciate this, especially if their reactions differ greatly.

As the number of families having to cope with the loss of a child grows, so does the number of children who experience the loss of a parent or sibling. A child's idea of death varies according to his age. Preschool children cannot yet comprehend death, but do experience loss. As the child gets older he gradually comprehends more, but may still have misconceived ideas of death.

Often children experience extreme guilt, imagining that they are the cause of the loss of their parent. Siblings, who have often been jealous of the attention the ill brother or sister has had, will also feel guilty when that sibling dies. The siblings commonly are neglected, the parents may feel they are 'too young to understand' and so these feelings remain hidden and lead to emotional, social and behavioural problems.

FOLLOW-UP

Advances in therapeutic interventions for a child with HIV infection have high-lighted the necessity for early diagnosis. This can only be achieved where the HIV infected pregnant woman can be identified. In Edinburgh any child born to a known HIV positive mother will be enrolled with parental consent, into the Edinburgh Perinatal Study and monitored closely from birth if possible. Referrals can be made by medical practitioners, health visitors, clinics and self-referrals (Mok *et al.*, 1989).

The existence of a family clinic in Edinburgh, since January 1986, has allowed close liaison between adult physicians and the paediatrician, enabling a high enrolment of infants.

The pregnant woman is referred to a member of the paediatric team in the antenatal period if possible, for information on the risk of mother to child transmission of HIV, the benefits of close monitoring of the infant to enable an early diagnosis to be made, and plans are also made for where the child might be seen. Most women welcome the medical attention for their child, during the early months when anxiety levels are highest regarding the outcome for their infant.

In many centres, pregnant women are first discovered to be HIV positive when they attend for antenatal care. There may also be unnecessary precautions and procedures which stigmatise the woman, who will then, understandably, refuse to have further contact with medical staff including the paediatrician.

Infants are seen at birth and then every six weeks until six months of age, then they are seen every three months until the age of two years. Thereafter children are seen every six months if they are 'presumed uninfected'. Infected children are seen every three months or as clinically indicated. At every visit a careful history is obtained regarding the health of the child, recent immunisations and the current social situation at home. A detailed examination and venesection is then performed. The children are seen either in hospital, at home, in medical centres or at nursery school. Most parents wish to be seen at home.

The medical team consists of a Consultant Paediatrician with a special interest in HIV infection, a Paediatric Registrar and a Specialist Health Visitor. There should be close liaison with community professionals such as the social worker, general practitioner and community health visitors. Each of the professionals involved should be aware of the social circumstances and psychosocial stresses of the families. The keys to effective working in a multi-disciplinary team are good communication, the identification of a key person, and working in partnership with the family.

Medical Management

The clear aim of medical management of these children is to make the diagnosis of HIV infection as early as possible. This enables close monitoring so that problems can be anticipated, identified and treated promptly. It is important that the growth of the children should be optimized and the advice of a Paediatric Dietitian sought if there is evidence of failure to thrive or weight loss.

At present, no cure exists for children infected with HIV. However, every attempt should be made to prevent and treat infections which are likely to cause further deterioration of the immune system. Good practice should include prophylaxis against common childhood illnesses, recurrent bacterial infections, and PCP, as outlined below:

1. *Immunizations*

   Definite guidelines regarding immunization of HIV infected children have been issued by Joint Committee on Vaccination and Immunization (1992). Children with or without symptoms should receive live vaccines (measles, mumps, rubella, polio) and inactivated vaccines (whooping cough, diphtheria, tetanus, polio, typhoid, cholera, HIB, hepatitis B). They should be given according to the current immunization schedule. Where possible the child's response to the vaccine should be checked by monitoring antibody levels as it may be less than optimal, especially when immune function deteriorates. Polio vaccine may be given in the live or inactivated form according to the discretion of the paediatrician. BCG vaccination should not be given in this country as there are risks of disseminated infection following vaccination compared with the low risk of tuberculosis.

2. *Recurrent Bacterial Infections*
   For children who suffer recurrent bacterial infections, regular infusions of immunoglobulin can be given. This has been shown to be effective with a reduction in the number of hospitalizations especially in those children with CD4 + cells >200/mm^3 (Mofenson, 1991). Other paediatricians prefer the use of long-term broad spectrum antibiotics.

3. *Pneumocystic Carinii Pneumonia*
   Many HIV infected children present with fatal PCP as the first indication of illness, and this has led several paediatricians to commence primary prophylaxis against PCP from birth. Prophylaxis against PCP should commence when the absolute CD4 + count is less than that appropriate for the age of the child. Guidelines from MMWR (1991) suggest the following cut-off, below which prophylaxis is recommended:

1–11 months	1,500 cell/mm^3
12–23 months	750 cell/mm^3
2–5 years	500 cell/mm^3.

   If at any time the CD4 + T cell percentage is less than 20%, prophylaxis should also commence. Suggested prophylaxis is Trimethoprim 150 mg/m^2 and Sulphamethoxazole 750 mg/m^2 per day given in two divided doses three times a week.
   Any child who has had an episode of PCP should be started on secondary prophylaxis.

Specific Antiretroviral Therapy

Currently Zidovudine is the only antiretroviral agent licensed for children. There are no guidelines as yet regarding when to start treatment. Most clinicians start Zidovudine when the child develops an AIDS defining illness. A multicentre European trial has just commenced assessing the effects of early versus deferred use of AZT in asymptomatic HIV infected children. Although the drug is generally well tolerated, side effects include haematological toxicity, nausea, vomiting and myositis (McKinney *et al.*, 1991). Other antiretroviral drugs are currently under trial, for use in children.

THE WAY FORWARD

Preventing the spread of HIV throughout the population must be the main aim. In the absence of a cure, education is the only form of prevention. For children and young people, information should be provided on healthy lifestyles, harm avoidance, sex and sexuality, drugs and alcohol. Young people should also be taught assertiveness in relationships. All schools should incorporate HIV awareness into their sex education programmes.

More information is needed about the transmission of HIV from the mother to her infant. Without this knowledge, treatment protocols interrupting this transmission cannot be developed. A role may exist for antiretroviral agents during pregnancy or in the newborn period. For those infected with HIV, therapies which may delay the progression of the disease are needed. Accurate predictors of disease are required so that earlier treatment and prophylaxis can be offered.

Staff working with children and families must be supported and trained to cope with needs of the HIV affected family, as well as come to terms with their own emotions and feelings towards people with AIDS. The co-ordination of policies on children and HIV require a collective effort from public health, health care, education and social service support systems, and pose a major challenge to statutory as well as voluntary agencies.

REFERENCES

Statistics from the Centers for Disease Control. (1992) *AIDS* 6(3), 343–345.

Department of Health Welsh Office. Immunisation against infectious disease. HMSO. 1992.

Guidelines for prophylaxis against Pneumocystis carinii pneumonia for children infected with human immunodeficiency virus. (1991) *MMWR* **40 RR 2**, 1–13.

Statistics from the World Health Organization and the Centers for Disease Control. (1989) *AIDS* 3, 863–867.

Ades, A.E., Parker, S., Berry, T., *et al.* (1991) Prevalence of maternal HIV-1 infection in Thames regions: results from anonymous unlinked neonatal testing. *Lancet* **337**, 1562–1565.

Belman, A.L., Diamond, G., Dickson, D., *et al.* (1988) Pediatric acquired immunodeficiency syndrome. Neurologic syndromes [published erratum appears in *Am J Dis Child* 1988 May; 142(5):507]. *Am J Dis Child* **142**, 29–35.

Berkelman, R.L., Heyward, W.L., Stehr-Green, J.K., Avvian, J.W. (1989) Epidemiology of HIV infection and acquired immune deficiency syndrome. *Am J Med* **86**, 761–770.

Borkowsky, W., Krasinski, K., Pollack, H., Hoover, W., Kaul, A., Ilmet-Moore, T. (1987) Early diagnosis of Human Immunodeficiency Virus infection in children <6 months of age: Comparison of Polymerase Chain Reaction, culture and plasma antigen capture techniques. *JID* **166 (Supp)**, 616–619.

Cadman, D., Boyle, M., Szatmari, P., Offord, D.R. (1987) Chronic illness, disability, and mental and social well-being: findings of the Ontario Child Health Study. *Ped* **79(5)**, 805–813.

Cutting, W.A.M. (1992) Breast feeding and HIV infection. *BMJ* **305**, 788–789.

Devash, Y., Calvelli, T.A., Wood, D.G., *et al.* (1990) Vertical transmission of human immunodeficiency virus is correlated with the absence of high-affinity/avidity maternal antibodies to the gp120 principal neutralizing domain. *Proc Natl Acad Sci U S A* **87**, 3445–3449.

Dunn, D., Newell, M.L. (1992) Vertical transmission of HIV. *Lancet* **339**, 364–365.

Epstein, L.G., Sharer, L.R., Goudsmit, J. (1988) Neurological and neuropathological features of human immunodeficiency virus infection in children. *Ann Neurol* **23 Suppl**, S19–S23.

European Collaborative Study. (1992) Risk factors for mother-to-child transmission of HIV-1. *Lancet* **339**, 1007–1012.

European Collaborative Study. (1991) Children born to women with HIV-1 infection: natural history and risk of transmission. *Lancet* **337**, 253–260.

Goedert, J.J., Duliege, A.M., Amos, C.I., *et al.* (1991) High risk of HIV-1 infection for first-born twins. The International Registry of HIV-exposed Twins. *Lancet* **338**, 1471–1475.

Gortmaker, S.L., Walker, D.K., Weitzman, M., Sobol, A.M. (1990) Chronic conditions, socioeconomic risks, and behavioural problems in children and adolescents. *Ped* **95(3)**, 267–176.

Hague, R.A., Burns, S.E., Mok, J.Y.Q., Yap, P.L. (1991) Diagnosis of Pneumocystis carinii pneumonia from non-invasive sampling of respiratory secretions. *Arch Dis Child* **65**, 1365–1367.

Kubler-Ross, E. (1981) Death is of vital importance! *Nord-Med* **96(2)**, 39–40.

Lewert, G. (1990) Psychosocial needs of HIV-infected children and their families. *Pediatric AIDS HIV Infection: Fetus to Adolescent* **1(6)**, 141–144.

McKinney, R.E.,Jr., Maha, M.A., Connor, E.M., *et al.* (1991) A multicentre trial of oral zidovudine in children with advanced human immunodeficiency virus disease. The Protocol 043 Study Group. *N Engl J Med* **324**, 1018–1025.

Mofenson, L.M., Burns, D.M. (1991) Passive immunization to prevent mother-infant transmission of human immunodeficiency virus: Current issues and future directions. *Pediatr Infect Dis J* **10**, 456–462.

Mok, J., O'Hara, G. (1990) Placement of children from HIV-affected families: the Edinburgh experience. *Pediatr AIDS and HIV Infect* **1(3)**, 20–22.

Mok, J.Y., Hague, R.A., Yap, P.L., *et al.* (1989) Vertical transmission of HIV: a prospective study. *Arch Dis Child* **64**, 1140–1145.

Mok, J.Y., Hague, R.A., Taylor, R.F. *et al.* (1989) The management of children born to human immunodeficiency virus seropositive women. *J Infect* **18**, 119–124.

Parekh, B.S., Shaffer, N., Pau, C.P., *et al.* (1991) Lack of correlation between maternal antibodies to V3 loop peptides of gp120 and perinatal HIV-1 transmission. The NYC Perinatal HIV Transmission Collaborative Study. *AIDS* **5**, 1179–1184.

Robertson, P., Burns, S.M., Yap, P.L., Mok, J.Y.Q., Parry, J.V. (1992) The use of saliva and urine for the detection of HIV infection in children: Preliminary report. *Pediatr AIDS and HIV Infect* **3**, 12–14.

Rogers, M.F., White, C.R., Sanders, R., *et al.* (1990) Lack of transmission of HIV from infected children to their household contacts. *Ped* **85**, 210–214.

Rogers, M.F., Thomas, P.A., Starcher, E.T., *et al.* (1987) Acquired Immunodeficiency Syndrome in children: report of the Centers for Disease Control National Surveillance, 1982 to 1985. *Pediatrics* **79**, 1008–1014.

Rossi, P., Moschese, V., Broliden, P.A., *et al.* (1989) Presence of maternal antibodies to human immunodeficiency virus 1 envelope glycoprotein gp120 epitopes correlates with the uninfected status of children born to seropositive mothers. *Proc Natl Acad Sci U S A* **86**, 8055–8058.

Scott, G.B., Hutto, C., Makuch, R.W., *et al.* (1989) Survival in children with perinatally acquired human immunodeficiency virus type 1 infection. *N Engl J Med* **321**, 1791–1796.

Tappin, D.M., Girdwood, R.W.A., Follett, E.A.C., *et al.* (1991) Prevalence of maternal HIV infection in Scotland based on unlinked anonymous testing of newborn babies. *Lancet* **337**, 1565-1569.

Tovo, P.A., de Martino, M., Gabino, C. *et al.* (1992) Prognostic factors and survival in children with perinatal HIV-1 infection. The Italian register for HIV infections in children. *Lancet* **339**, 1249–1253.

8

Adolescents

LEE STRUNIN AND RALPH HINGSON

INTRODUCTION

Since the first cases of AIDS were identified in the United States, prevention activities for adolescents in the USA and other countries have focused on educating adolescent populations about modes of Human Immunodeficiency Virus (HIV) transmission. A variety of studies of adolescent populations have explored whether there have been changes in adolescents' AIDS related knowledge, beliefs, and behaviours. These studies have been conducted within school settings (Anderson *et al.*, 1990; DiClemente, Zorn & Temoshok, 1986; Holtzman, Anderson, Kann *et al.*, 1991; Michaud & Hausser 1992; Moore, Daily, Colins, *et al.*, 1991; Hingson, Strunin, Grady, *et al.*, 1991; Price, Desmond, & Kulkula 1985; Walter, Vaughan, & Cohall, 1991) other settings such as clinics (Goodman, & Cohall, 1989; Forman, & Chilvers, 1989; Kegeles, Adler, & Irwin, 1988; Stiffman & Earls 1990), centres for runaways (Rotherum-Borus & Koopman, 1991) and juvenile detention centres (DiClemente, Lanier, Horan, *et al.*, 1991; Lanier & McCarthy, 1989). Other studies of adolescents have used quota sampling (Bowie & Ford, 1989) and random digit dial telephone sampling (Hingson, Strunin & Berlin, 1990; Hingson, Strunin, Berlin & Heeren, 1990; Strunin & Hingson, 1987).

In the first part of this chapter we will explore the behaviours of adolescents that pose risk for HIV infection. The second part of the chapter will focus on findings from four telephone surveys of adolescents and findings from other adolescent studies in order to determine whether there have been changes over time in HIV risk taking behaviours and the implications of the findings for interventions. We will review behaviour change theories that have been utilized in studies and will discuss issues that may not have been considered but which could prevent HIV infection among adolescents.

ADOLESCENTS' RISK BEHAVIOURS

Prior to the AIDS epidemic, surveys of adolescents indicated that half of the 25 million adolescents in the US had sexual intercourse by age 16, and over 70% by age 19 (Zelnik & Kanter, 1979, 1980). The age of first intercourse in the US differs by racial and ethnic background, socioeconomic status, and school attendance, with earlier onset of sexual intercourse among poor youth, minority youth and school dropouts (Pratt, Mosher, Bachrah & Horn, 1984; Zelnik & Kanter, 1980). The rate of unprotected sexual behaviour is high among adolescents. More than one million teenage girls in the US become pregnant each year, just over 400,000 have abortion, and almost 470,000 give birth (Hayes, 1987). Each year teenagers comprise one quarter of all sexually transmitted diseases (STDs) in the USA (Aral & Holmes, 1984) including chlamydia, gonorrhoea, genital herpes, condylomata, and other manifestations of Human Papilloma Virus. Studies also suggest that the earlier the first sexual experiences the greater the risk of contracting a sexually transmitted disease (STD) (Bell & Holmes, 1984; Irwin, Shafer & Millstein, 1985). Since the behaviour that leads to STDs is the same as for HIV infection, heterosexual AIDS cases are expected to occur disproportionately among groups at risk for other STDs (Miller, Turner & Moses, 1990; Chirgwin, DeHovitz, Dillon & McCormack, 1991). The danger of adolescents becoming infected with HIV is closely tied to the increasing rate of other STDs in this age group.

Alcohol and other drug use are also risk taking behaviours for HIV infection because mood-altering drugs can impair judgement and lead to risky behaviour for HIV infection. Adolescents' drinking may echo peer sentiment, their drinking may reflect non-normative peer behaviour, or their own norms or preferences may predict drinking practices (Biddle, Bank & Marlin, 1980).

A longitudinal national study of US high school seniors indicated that in 1987 64% of seniors reported alcohol use in the preceding month, with 4% reporting daily use and 35% reporting drinking five or more drinks on a single occasion (Johnston, O'Malley & Bachman, 1988). More recently, the study suggests that although other drug use has declined during the 1980s, rates of alcohol use have not decreased (Bachman, O'Malley & Johnston, 1991). In a 1990 random digit dial telephone survey of 1,152 16–19 year olds in Massachusetts, 82% of adolescents reported drinking alcoholic beverages, with 7% drinking 5 or more drinks daily (Hingson, Strunin & Berlin, 1991). One in five reported usually consuming five or more drinks on typical drinking occasions. A 1990 cross-sectional study of alcohol and other drug use among 2,127 9th-11th grade students in Massachusetts suggests high use of alcohol, with 85% of students reporting using alcohol at least once in their lifetimes and 51% reporting using alcohol at least once in the past 30 days (MDPH, 1990).

According to an ongoing National Household Survey on Drug Abuse of individuals aged 12 and older who live in households, the use of marijuana, hashish and hallucinogens decreased among 12 to 17 year olds between 1979 and 1985 although cocaine use fluctuated and has stabilized at 4% of teenagers. Other national drug use surveys suggest that marijuana and cocaine use increase by year in school with, for example, 5% of 8th graders and 15% of 12th graders reporting using cocaine at least once (Miller, Turner & Moses, 1990). A nationwide study of HIV instruction, HIV knowledge and drug injection among high school students in the US found that 2.7% of students reported ever injecting drugs with significantly more males than females reporting having injected drugs. Reported rates of ever injecting drugs declined from grades 9 to 12 but no significant differences were found by age group (Holtzman, Anderson, Kann, *et al.*, 1991). Other studies also suggest that there are gender differences in use of psychoactive drugs with earlier age of first alcohol and marijuana use for males than females and differences in patterns of substance use between males and females with higher levels of alcohol and marijuana use found among males (Ensminger, Brown & Kellam, 1982; Yamaguchi & Kandel, 1984).

Some studies about adolescents' knowledge, attitudes and behaviours concerning AIDS and HIV infection have found an association between perceived personal risk and behaviour (Chitwood & Comerford 1990; Connell, Turner & Mason, 1985; DiClemente, 1989; Jemmott, Jemmott & Fong, 1992; Sonenstein, Pleck & Ku, 1989), while others have not found such an association (Kegeles, Adler & Irwin, 1988; Rickert, Jay, Gottlieb & Bridges, 1989; Rotherum-Borus, Koopman & Bradley, 1989; Weisman, Nathanson, Ensminger, Teitelbaum *et al.*, 1989).

CHANGES IN ADOLESCENTS' KNOWLEDGE, ATTITUDES, AND BEHAVIOURS

During the period 1986–1991, four independent cross sectional statewide Massachusetts random digit dial telephone surveys of adolescents aged 16–19 examined exposure to AIDS education, knowledge of HIV transmission, health beliefs about AIDS, drug use, sexual behaviour and condom use. Each survey used identical sampling. Households were randomly selected using methods developed by Waksberg. Questions in the 1988, 1990 and 1991 surveys were identical to those in the 1986 survey although more questions were added concerning other sexually transmitted diseases, pregnancies and HIV testing. Within each household, one teenager was randomly selected (Kish, 1965). Response rates varied from 82%–87%. Potential respondents were told that the survey would ask about their own opinions and their own behaviours to help plan educational campaigns. They were also told that their answers were confidential and that their names and addresses were unknown and that their telephone number was drawn at random. At the end of the interview the interviewers gave the teenagers a toll free AIDS hotline to call if he/she had any questions about AIDS.

Some but not all beliefs about HIV have changed over time (table 8.1) In 1986 the first survey (N = 825, response rate 86%) revealed that 46% were worried

TABLE 8.1
Massachusetts Adolescent AIDS Surveys
Selected Beliefs About AIDS
1986–1991

	1986 N = 825	1988 N = 1762	1990 N = 1152	1991 N = 903
Worry you will get AIDS				
A great deal	8%	14%	14%	15%
Somewhat	14	31	28	31
Likelihood you will get AIDS				
Very likely	1	2	1	1
Somewhat likely	7	16	10	15
There is a cure for AIDS		1%	3%	2%
If infected a person is very likely to die		83	80	81
Very likely a female will be infected during sex with an infected male		70	74	82
Very likely a male will be infected during sex with an infected male		80	81	86
Very likely a male will be infected during sex with an infected female		64	67	73
Condoms very – extremely effective in preventing infection		65	71	67
Condoms reduce pleasure (very true)	18	22	20	
Condoms are difficult and embarassing to get (very – somewhat true)		38	36	34
Would be embarrassed if asked to use a condom (somewhat – very)		9	8	5
Very likely to use condom if partner wanted		78	79	85
Upset if partner wanted to use condom (somewhat – very)		8	8	5
Asked partner to use condom in past 6 months		32	44	47

Comments:
1) In the last 5 years the proportion of teens who believe they could acquire AIDS has doubled as has the proportion who say they worry about getting AIDS
2) Almost all teens know there is no cure for AIDS
3) Increasing proportions of teens believe sexual transmission is very likely if a partner is infected
4) Fewer teens over time believe
   • condoms are difficult and embarrassing to obtain
   • would be embarrassed or upset if partners wanted condoms used
5) More teens are asking partners to use condoms

about becoming infected with HIV and 9% thought it likely they will get AIDS in their lifetime (Strunin & Hingson, 1987). Our subsequent 1988 telephone survey of 1,762 adolescents (response rate 87%) the proportion of respondents doubled who indicated that they were worried about AIDS (74%) and who thought it likely they will get AIDS in their lifetime (18%) (Hingson, Strunin & Berlin, 1991). However, there has been little change since 1988. Similarly since 1988 there has been little change in the proportions who believe there is a cure for the disease or who believe infected people are very likely to die.

Exposure to information about AIDS increased significantly from 1986 to 1988 but changed little from 1988 to 1991 (table 8.2). In 1986 only 44% had discussed AIDS with their parents, 69% with friends and 52% in school. In 1991 over two thirds of 16–19 year old adolescents had discussed AIDS with their parents, 85% with friends, and 89% were taught about AIDS in school. Further the proportion of adolescents who had discussed AIDS with a physician increased sharply from 13% in 1988 to 22% in 1991 (p < .01) with twice the proportion of females than males reporting that their physician initiated counselling about AIDS (26% vs 13%, p < .01).

Among female respondents there were no differences between those counselled and not counselled regarding age, education, race or ethnicity. Among males, age was a significant factor with 19 year old male respondents more likely to have received counselling (p < .01). Physicians who had counselled both male and female adolescents about AIDS were more likely to have also discussed alcohol use, drug use, pregnancy and family planning, and prevention of sexually transmitted diseases. Fifteen percent of respondents reported receiving tests for HIV status and those counselled by physicians were more likely than those not counselled to receive an HIV test (p < .01). Although knowledge about the modes of HIV transmission did not vary between those receiving and not receiving physician counselling, both males and females who were counselled were more likely than other respondents to worry about getting AIDS, and to believe condoms are effective in preventing transmission of AIDS and STDs.

Since the first 1986 survey knowledge about HIV transmission has increased. In 1986, 89% did not know about heterosexual transmission risk of infection or when

TABLE 8.2
Massachusetts Adolescent AIDS Surveys
Results: Exposure to AIDS Education

	1986 N = 825	1988 N = 1762	1990 N = 1152	1991 N = 903
Discussed AIDS				
Parents	44%	65%	63%	69%
Friends	69	86	85	85
In school	52	82	83	89
Mass Media Exposure		65	56	
Counseled by MD		13	15	22

Comments:
1) Exposure to education about AIDS increased
2) Though 85% saw a MD, only 22% were counselled
3) Media exposure declined in 1990

sharing needles. By 1991 over 99% of all teenagers surveyed knew about transmission during sex between two men, a man and a woman and when injecting drugs (table 8.3). The proportion who believed in erroneous modes of transmission, such as toilet seats or sharing eating and drinking utensils declined with each successive survey (p < .01). However, the proportion of respondents who thought the virus could be transmitted while giving blood actually increased from 51% in 1988 to 55% in 1991.

There has been significant increase in the perceived likelihood of sexual transmission. From 1988 to 1991 there was an increase in the proportion who responded that it is very likely that a female will become infected during sex with an infected male (71% to 82%, p < .01). The proportions who believed it very likely that a male will become infected during sex with an infected male also increased (80% to 86%, p < .01) as did those who believed that a male would become infected during sex with an infected female (64% to 73%, p < .01).

Concerning condom use the proportions believing that condoms reduce sexual pleasure and/or are very or extremely effective in preventing HIV transmission have remained constant. However, there has been a decline from 1988 to 1991 in the proportion of respondents who thought condoms are difficult and embarrassing to obtain (38% to 34%, p < .05); who would be embarrassed if asked to use a condom (9% to 5%, p < .05), or upset if a partner wanted to use a condom (8% to 5%, p < .01).

In 1986, 55% of 16–19 year old respondents reported that they had had sexual intercourse but only 2% had adopted condom use specifically because of AIDS. By 1991, 28% of sexually active adolescents said they adopted condom use specifically because of AIDS. Nonetheless, despite increases in knowledge about HIV transmission and in the perceived likelihood of sexual HIV transmission the proportion of teenagers who had sex actually rose from 55% in 1986 to 61% in 1991. Even

TABLE 8.3
Massachusetts Adolescent AIDS Surveys
Changes in Adolescent Knowledge About AIDS

	1986 N = 825	1988 N = 1726	1990 N = 1152	1991 N = 903
Can you get AIDS from:				
Sex between 2 males	98%	99%	99%	99%
Sex male and female	91	99	99	100
Injecting drugs	91	99	100	99
Toilet seats	15	5	2	3
Sharing eating/ drinking utensils	38	11	10	8
Giving blood	61	51	54	55

Comments:
1) Knowledge increased 1986–1991
2) Most know the major modes of transmission
3) Some still believe AIDS is transmitted in ways it is not

though the proportions of sexual active adolescents who always use condoms rose from 1988-1991, even in 1991 only 37% of adolescents consistently used condoms.

An analysis of respondents beliefs about AIDS as structured in the Health Belief Model (Janz & Becker, 1984) revealed that respondents who believed condoms are effective in preventing HIV transmission and worried they can get AIDS were 3.1 and 1.8 times more likely to use condoms all the time. Those who believed condoms do not reduce sexual pleasure and would not be embarrassed if asked to use them were 3.1 and 2.4 times more likely to use them. Respondents who carried condoms and who had discussed AIDS with a physician were 2.7 and 1.7 times respectively more likely to use them. Adolescents who were heavy drinkers and marijuana users were less likely to use condoms (Hingson, Strunin & Berlin, 1991). From 1986 to 1988 media exposure, knowledge about HIV transmission and increases in condom use among sexually active adolescents were reported not only in Massachusetts but also nationwide (Forrest & Singh, 1990; Mosher, 1990). Nonetheless, despite almost all adolescents knowing the principal modes of HIV transmission, most of the sexually active are not using condoms, and, as in our surveys, the proportions of adolescents engaging in sexual intercourse actually increased. Studies have now found that beliefs about AIDS can influence sexual risk taking and condom use among adolescents and adults (Allard, 1989; Hingson *et al.*, 1990).

SUBSTANCE USE, HIGH-RISK SEXUAL BEHAVIOUR AND AIDS

The changes in beliefs found over time in the Massachusetts' studies were accompanied by reductions in the proportion of teenagers who drank alcohol (from 89% in 1988 to 77% in 1991, $p < .01$) and a slight reduction in marijuana use over the same period. The proportion who used drugs other than alcohol or marijuana has continued to drop and is about half about what it was in 1986 (6% compared to 13%, $p < .01$) (table 8.4). Unfortunately one quarter of adolescents said that they usually consumed five or more drinks per occasion which represents a 5% increase since 1988 ($p < .01$).

In the 1990 telephone survey of Massachusetts' adolescents, 66% of teenagers reported sexual intercourse in the past year and 83% reported drinking alcohol. Among the sexually active, 64% reported having sexual intercourse after drinking, and among those who drank 72% had sex after drinking. Significantly more sexually active adolescents said they were less likely to use condoms after drinking than said they were more likely to use them. Seventeen percent reported using condoms less often after drinking, 74% reported condom use as often whether drinking or sober, and 1% reported more frequent use after drinking. Adolescents who experienced intercourse at an earlier age were more likely to be in the group using condoms less often after drinking. On numerous other characteristics or beliefs about AIDS, STDs or pregnancy there were no significant differences between those who used or did not use condoms less often after drinking. That is, regardless of perceived susceptibility and concerns about AIDS, other STDs and pregnancy, after

TABLE 8.4
Massachusetts Adolescent AIDS Surveys
Behaviour Changes 1986–1990

	1986 N = 825	1988 N = 1762	1990 N = 1152	1991 N = 903
Drug use other than:				
Alcohol and marijuana	13%	9%	7%	6%
IV drugs	1	<1	<1	1
Sexual behaviour				
Sexual intercourse	55	61	66	63
Adopted condom use				
because of AIDS	2	19	14	28

Comments:
1) Adolescent drug use declined
2) Condom use increased because of AIDS, but the number of sexually active teens increased as well

drinking 17% of sexually active adolescents were less likely to use condoms when they had been drinking than when they were sober (Strunin & Hingson, 1992).

Other studies of adolescents also indicate how drugs pose a potential risk for HIV infection. For example, ethnographic studies of adolescent crack users in San Francisco found that 96% were sexually active and that 51% reported combining sex with drug use. One quarter of boys and girls said they had exchanged sexual favours for drugs or money (Fullilove & Fullilove, 1989; Fullilove, Fullilove, Bowser & Gross, 1990). Although 41% of the teenagers reported having had an STD, only 18% of girls and 26% of boys reported using a condom at last intercourse.

ADOLESCENTS AND THEORIES OF BEHAVIOUR CHANGE

Researchers of adolescent behaviour change within the context of AIDS have utilized a number of psychosocial behaviour change theories to explain why adolescents continue to engage in unprotected sexual intercourse. The Health Belief Model suggests that people who have engaged in a rational cost benefit analysis may change their behaviour after considering their susceptibility, the consequences, and the effectiveness of minimal measures taken. However, even studies supportive of the Health Belief Model concerning AIDS have been able to explain only a small part of the variance in condom use. It has been suggested that other beliefs such as those about sexually transmitted disease or pregnancy need to be considered as well as other factors such as partners' or peers' beliefs (Hingson, Strunin, Berlin & Heeren, 1990; Strunin & Hingson, 1992). The Theory of Reasoned Action suggests that both the importance of the desire to please friends or partners and what the individual believes are those preferences can influence adoption of a new behaviour (Fishbein & Ajzen, 1975). According to Social Learning Theory, behaviour can be influenced by social reinforcement for anticipated behaviour based on what has been learned from observing others (Bandura, 1977, 1984). And a theory concerning self-efficacy suggests that before attempting any new behaviour the individual must feel capable of success. All these theories of behaviour change imply that people weigh the costs and benefits of a behaviour before acting to adopt the behaviour. However, adolescents' sexual encounters are frequently not planned and alcohol and other drug use can affect all these judgements and influence sexual behaviour (Flanigan & Hitch, 1986; Hingson, Strunin & Berlin, 1990; Hingson, Strunin, Berlin & Heeren, 1990; Robertson & Plant, 1988; Strunin & Hingson, 1992). Furthermore, these theories do not address the importance of the environment on behaviour. Adolescents' responses to the environment can be a reflection of individual experience and cultural background (Strunin, 1991) and interventions emphasizing disease-related knowledge and beliefs of adolescents that do not consider the context of the individual's life may only have small effects on motivations to initiate preventive actions (Walter, Vaughan, Gladis, *et al.*, 1992). Studies of premature sexual intercourse have suggested the behaviour is one element of a syndrome of problem behaviours including drug and substance use, minor delinquency, and school difficulty (Donovan & Jessor, 1985; Jessor & Jessor, 1977; Ingersoll *et al.*, 1989). However, other studies have suggested that the concept of a problem behaviour syndrome is relatively unimportant for most adolescents in the US because the problem behaviours are isolated behaviours for the majority of US teenagers (Mott & Haurin, 1988) or because sociodemographic factors are important correlates of such behaviours (Velez & Ungemack, 1989). Within the context of HIV infection, whether or not there are links between behaviours needs further study particularly from a cross-cultural perspective.

CONCLUSIONS

In studies of adolescents it has been suggested that other beliefs such as beliefs about sexually transmitted disease or pregnancy need also to be considered as well as other factors such as partners' or peers' beliefs (Hingson, Strunin, Berlin, Heeren, 1990; Strunin & Hingson, 1992). The impact of context of the individual's life on motivation for preventive behaviour and the cultural factors that may affect sexual behaviour and alcohol use or other drug use also need to be considered (Leigh & Morrison, 1991; Stall *et al.*, 1986; Strunin & Hingson, 1992; Walter *et al.*, 1992). For example, it has been suggested that education and counselling to dissuade adolescents from having unprotected sex should target not only condom use but increased sexual activity among adolescents (Strunin and Hingson, 1992). However, such programmes must recognize that the adolescent population is a heterogeneous one comprising adolescents from different racial and ethnic backgrounds who do not necessarily share the same system of norms and values about sexual activity.

STD and family planning clinics should query patients about their alcohol and drug use and stress the risk of unprotected sex, HIV infection, other STDs and unplanned pregnancy after drinking or other drugs and alcohol abuse prevention and treatment programmes should discuss the risk of unprotected sex and HIV infection after drinking or drug use. School educational programmes about HIV infection and AIDS, other STDs, and pregnancy should all stress the disinhibiting features of alcohol and other drugs. Adolescents should be made aware that if they drink or use other drugs they may be likely to do things they may not do when sober. Yet programmes need also to recognize that this consequence may be desirable for some adolescents. For example, not using a condom could result in a desirable outcome. Desire for pregnancy may mitigate against birth control including using condoms and may also mitigate against pregnancy counselling. Such programmes also need to address the cultural context of HIV related behaviours.

Finally, because behaviour can be influenced by beliefs, attitudes and anticipations, the specific physiologic effects of alcohol and drugs are not the only factors of importance. Just as perceived reduction in sexual pleasure has been associated with adolescents being less likely to use condoms, education programmes might want to emphasize that alcohol and drug use can reduce sexual pleasure. At the same time the societal acceptance of alcohol as a sexual disinhibitor may hamper the progress and application of research because if drinking is assumed to cause sexual risk taking then other possible contributing factors may be overlooked (Leigh, 1991).

In order to address the behavioural chain of HIV transmission we need better to understand HIV-related risk. Culturally specific concerns, beliefs and taboos, language constraints of new immigrants affect and influence behaviour. These behavioural influences need to be taken into account not only for interventions designed for the adolescent population but also for interventions for the adult population. Alcohol and other drug use may contribute to some people being more likely to have sexual intercourse and to some being more likely to engage in unsafe sexual practices. Effective interventions to reduce sexual risk taking among adolescents must be tailored for specific audiences and address differences in drinking and other drug use behaviour, in cultural understandings and in context of behaviour.

REFERENCES

Allard, R. (1989) Beliefs about AIDS as determinants of preventive practices and support for coercive measures. *American Journal of Public Health* 79, 448–452.

Anderson, J.E., Kann, L., Hotzman, D., Arday, S., Turman, B., Kolbe, L. (1990) HIV AIDS knowledge and sexual behaviour among high school students. *Family Planning Perspectives* 22(6), 252–255.

Aral, S.O., Holmes, K.K. (1984) Epidemiology of sexually transmitted diseases. In K.K. Holmes, P.A. Mardh, P.F. Sparling, P.J. Wiesner (eds.) *Sexually Transmitted Diseases* New York: McGraw-Hill.

Bachman, J.G., Wallace, J.M., O'Malley, P.M., Johnston, L.D., Kurth, C.L., Neighbors, H.W. (1991) Racial/ethnic differences in smoking, drinking, and illicit drug use among American high school seniors, 1976–89. *American Journal of Public Health* 81,372–377.

Bandura, A. (1984) Self-efficacy: Toward a unifying theory of behavioural change. *Psychological Review* 84, 191–215.

Bell, T.A., Holmes, K.K. (1984) Age specific risks of syphilis, gonorrhoea, and hospitalized pelvic inflammatory disease in sexually experienced U.S. women. *Sexually Transmitted Diseases* 11, 291–295.

Biddle, B.J., Bank, B.J., Marlin, M.M. (1980) Social determinants of adolescent drinking: What they think, what they do and what I think and do. *Journal of Studies on Alcohol* 41, 3.

Bowie, C., Ford, N. (1989) Sexual behaviour of young people and the risk of HIV infection. *Journal of Epidemiology and Community Health* 43(1), 61–65.

Chirgwin, K., Eltovitz, J.A., Dillon, S., McCormack, W.M. (1991) HIV infection, genital disease and crack cocaine use among patients attending a clinic for sexually transmitted diseases. *American Journal of Public Health* 81(12), 1576–1579.

Chitwood, D.D., Comerford, M. (1990) Drugs, sex and AIDS risk. *American Behavioural Scientist* 33, 465–447.

Connell, J.B., Turner, R.R., Mason, E.F. (1985) Summary of the findings of the school health education evaluation: Health promotion effectiveness, implementation and costs. *Journal of School Health* 55, 316–323.

DiClemente, R.J. (1989) Adolescents and AIDS: An update. *Multicultural Inquiry and Research on AIDS* 3, 3–7.

DiClemente, R.J., Lanick, M.M., Horan, P.F., Lodico, M. (1991) Comparison of AIDS knowledge, attitudes and behaviours among incarcerated adolescents and a public school sample in San Francisco. *American Journal of Public Health* 81(5), 628–630.

DiClemente, R.J., Zorn, J., Temoshok, L. (1986) Adolescents and AIDS: A survey of knowledge, attitudes and beliefs about AIDS in San Francisco. *American Journal of Public Health* 76, 1443–1445.

Donovan, J.E., Jessor, R. (1985) Structure of Problem Behaviour in Adolescence and Young Adulthood. *Journal of Consulting and Clinical Psychology* 53(6), 890–904.

Ensminger M.E., Brown C.H., Kellam, S.G. (1982) Sex differences in antecendents of substance use among adolescents. *Journal of Social Issues* 38, 25.

Fishbein, M., Ajzen, I. (1975) Belief, attitude, intention and behaviour: An introduction to theory and research. Reading, MA: Addison-Wesley.

Flanigan, R., Hitch, M. (1986) Alcohol use and sexual intercourse and contraception: An exploratory study. *Journal of Adolescent Health Drug Education* 31–6–40.

Forman, D., Chivers, C. (1989) Sexual behaviour of young and middle-aged men in England and Wales. *British Medical Journal* 298(6681), 1137–1142.

Forrest, J.D., Singh, S. (1990) The sexual and reproductive behaviour of American women, 1982–1988. *Family Planning Perspective* 22, 206–14.

Fullilove, M.T., Fullilove, R.E. (1989) Intersecting epidemics: black teen crack use and sexually transmitted disease. *Journal of the American Medical Association* 44, 146–153.

Fullilove, R.E., Fullilove, M.T., Bowser, B.P., Gross, S.A. (1990) Risk of sexually transmitted disease among black adolescent crack users in Oakland and San Francisco, California. *Journal of Amerian Medical Association* 263, 851–855.

Goodman, E., Cohall, A. (1989) Acquired Immunodeficiency Syndrome and adolescents: Knowledge, attitudes, beliefs, and behaviours in a New York City adolescent minority population. *Pediatrics* 84, 36–42.

Hayes, C.D. (ed.) (1987) *Risking the future: Adolescent sexuality, pregnancy, and childbearing.* Vol. 1. Washington,D.C.: National Academy Press.

Hingson, R., Strunin, L., Berlin, B. (1990) Beliefs about AIDS, use of alcohol, drugs and unprotected sex among Massachusetts adolescents. *American Journal of Public Health* 80, 259–300.

Hingson, R., Strunin, L., Grady, M., Strunk, N., Carr, R., Berlin, B., Craven, D.E. (1991) Knowledge, beliefs and behavioural risks for HIV-1 infection of Boston Public School students born outside the United States Mainland. *American Journal of Public Health* 81(12), 1638–1641.

Holtzman, D., Anderson, J.E., Kann, L., Arday, S.L., Truman, B.I., Kolbe, L.J. (1991) HIV instruction, HIV knowledge, and drug injections among high school students in the United States. *American Journal of Public Health* 81, 1596–1601.

Ingersoll, G., Wilbrand, M., Brack, C., Orr, D. (1989) Self-esteem and coitus among young adolescents – a replication. *Journal of Adolescent Health Care* 10(3), 253.

Irwin, C.E., Schafer, M.A.S., Millstein, S.G. (1985) Pubertal development in adolescent females: A marker for early sexual debut. *Pediatric Research* 19, 112A.

Jemmott, J.B., Jemmott, L.S., Fong, G.T. (1992) Reductions in HIV risk-associated sexual behaviours among black male adolescents: Effects of an AIDS prevention intervention. *American Journal of Public Health* 82(3), 372–377.

Jessor, R., Jessor, S.L. (1977) Problem Behaviour and Psychosocial Development: *A Longitudinal Study of Youth*. New York: Academic Press.

Johnston, L.D., O'Malley, P.M., Bachman, J.G. (1988) *Illicit Drug Use, Smoking and Drinking by America's High School Students, College Students and Young Adults 1975–1988*. DHHS Pub No. (ADM) 89–1602. Rockville, MD: ADAMHA.

Junz, N.K., Becker, M.H. (1984) The Health Belief Model: A Decade Later. *Health Education Quarterly* 11, 1.

Kegeles, S., Adler, N., Irwin, C. (1988) Sexually active adolescents and condoms: Changes over one year in knowledge, attitudes and behaviour. *American Journal of Public Health* 78, 460–462.

Kish, L. (1965) *Survey Sampling*. New York: John Wilez and Sons.

Lanier, M.M., McCarthy, B.R. (1989) AIDS awareness and the impact of AIDS education in juvenile corrections. *Criminal Justice and Behaviour* 16(4), 395-411.

Massachusetts Department of Public Health (1990) *Alcohol and other drug use among Massachusetts adolescents: A preliminary report*. Boston MA: Division of Substance Abuse Services.

Michaud, P.A., Hausser, D. (1992) Swiss teenagers, AIDS and sexually transmitted diseases: presentation and evaluation of a preventive exhibition. *Health Education Research* 7, 79–86.

Miller, H.G., Turner, C.F., Moses, L.E. (1990) AIDS: The Second Decade. Washington, D.C.: National Academy Press.

Moore, J.R., Daily, L., Collins, J., Kann, L., Dalmat, M., Truman, B.I., Kolbe, L.J. (1991) Progress in Efforts to Prevent the Spread of HIV Infection Among Youth. *Public Health Research* 106(6), 678–686.

Morris, R., Baker, C., Stuscrott, S. Incarcerated Youth at Risk for HIV infection. In Diclemente, R. (ed.) *Adolescents and AIDS* Newbury Park, CA: Sage.

Mosher, W.D. (1990) Contraceptive Practice in the United States, 1982–1988. *Family Planning Perspectives* 22(5), 198–205.

Mott, F.L., Haurin, R.J. (1988) Linkages between sexual activity and alcohol and drug use among American adolescents. *Family Planning Perspectives* 20, 128-136.

Pratt, W., Mosher, W., Bachrach, C., Horn, M. (1984) Understanding U.S. fertility: Findings from the National Survey of Family Growth. *Population Bulletin* 39, 5.

Price, J.H., Desmond, S., Kukulka, G. (1985) High school students' perceptions and misperceptions of AIDS. *Journal of School Health* 55, 107–109.

Rickert, V.K., Jay, M.S., Gottlieb, A., Bridges, C. (1989) Adolescents and AIDS: Female attitudes and behaviours toward condom purchase and use. *Journal of Adolescent Health Care* 10, 313-316.

Robertson, J.A., Plant, M.A. (1988) Alcohol, sex and risks of HIV infection. *Drug and Alcohol Dependence* 22, 75–78.

Rotherum-Borus, M.J., Koopman, C. (1991) Sexual risk behaviours, AIDS, knowledge and beliefs about AIDS among runaways. *American Journal of Public Health* 81(2),206–208.

Rotherum-Borus, M.J., Koopman, C., Bradley, J.S. (1989) Barriers to successful AIDS programmes with runaway youth. In J.O Woodruff, D. Doherty and J.G. Athey, (eds.) *CASSP Technical Assistance Center: Gerogetown University Child Development Center.*

Sonenstein, F.L., Pleck, J.H., Ku, L.C. (1989) Sexual activity, condom use and AIDS awareness among adolescent males. *Family Planning Perspectives* 21, 152–158.

Stiffman, A.R., Earls, F. (1990) Behavioural risks for human immunodeficiency virus infection in adolescent medical patients. *Pediatrics* 85(3), 303–310.

Strunin, L. (1991) Adolescents' perceptions of risk for HIV infection: Implications for future research. *Social Science and Medicine* 32, 221–228.

Strunin, L., Hingson, R. (1987) AIDS and adolescents: Knowledge, beliefs, attitudes and behaviours. *Pediatrics* 79, 825–828.

Strunin, L., Hingson, R. (1992) Alcohol, drugs and adolescent sexual behaviour. *International Journal of the Addictions* 27(2), 129–146.

Yamaguchi, K., Kandel, D.B. (1984) Patterns of drug use from adolescence to young adulthood: III predictors of progression. *American Journal of Public Health* 74, 673.

Velez, C.N., Ungemack, T.A. (1989) Drug use among Puerto Rican youth: An exploration of generational status differences. *Social Science Medicine* 293(6), 779–789.

Walter, H.J., Vaughan, R.D., Cohall, A.T. (1991) Risk factors for substance use among high school students – implications for prevention. *Journal of the American Academy of Child and Adolescent Psychiatry* 30(4), 556–562.

Walter, H.J., Vaughan, M.S., Gladis, M.M., Ragin, D.F., Kasen, S., Cohall, A.T. (1992) Factors associated with AIDS risk behaviours among high school students in an AIDS Epicenter. *American Journal of Public Health* 82(4), 528-532.

Weisman, C.S., Nathanson, C.A., Ensminger, M. (1989) AIDS knowledge, perceived risk and prevention among adolescent clients of a family planning clinic. *Family Planning Perspectives* 21, 213–217.

Zelnik, M., Kanter, J.F. (1979) Reasons for nonuse of contraception by socially active women aged 15–19. *Family Planning Perspectives* 111, 286–289.

Zelnik, M., Kanter, J.F. (1980) Sexual activity, contraceptive use and pregnancy among metropolitan teenagers 1971–1979. *Family Planning Perspectives* 12, 230–237.

9

The Family and HIV Disease

ROBERT BOR

INTRODUCTION

The family, a person's primary social system, may be profoundly affected by illness, and specifically by HIV disease. For every person infected with HIV, there is a family or support system that is also affected. Since the beginning of the epidemic, HIV disease has been viewed as a social problem that has repercussions for relationships by virtue of the social stigma and isolation experienced by those affected, as well as the fact that HIV is transmitted through sexual contact. HIV disease may be viewed as both a chronic illness, and a specific illness in view of its unique social connotations (Rolland, 1987). This illness is a signal as it brings into focus relationship issues (Miller & Bor, 1988). The study of the family provides a context or frame through which to view the impact of illness on individuals and some of their most significant relationship systems.

Most published research in the 1980s has described the impact of HIV disease on the individual. The absence of family-oriented research may have perpetuated a belief that, in the West, gay men have been most affected by HIV and they are not connected to families. Recent interest in the topic of the impact of HIV disease on the family may stem from growing awareness of the global problem of heterosexually acquired HIV, the inference being that 'family' and 'heterosexual' are coterminous. While the study of the impact of illness on the family is still in its infancy, it is also clear that HIV has had a significant impact on the extended family in Africa (Barnett and Blaikie, 1992) and on same-sex relationships, mainly between men. Indeed, the study of the impact of HIV disease on the family raises the question: What constitutes the family? This chapter addresses the question of the definition of 'family' and reviews research describing the impact of HIV disease on the family. Some guidelines are also included for counselling people affected by HIV disease about family and relationship problems.

This chapter defines the family and reviews key studies describing the impact of HIV/AIDS on the family. This is discussed in the context of communication within the family, how the family copes with illness, and changes in roles and structure in the family. Distinctions can be drawn between theoretical writings and research studies, and between qualitative and quantitative research methods. The 'Scientific' literature comprises case studies, clinical reports, process research and empirical studies. Even though the results of these are included in this chapter, it should be possible to distinguish between these approaches by the way in which the research is described and reported.

DEFINING 'THE FAMILY'

The advent of HIV disease has prompted researchers to re-examine accepted definitions of the family and to take into account the diverse social networks affected by the disease. The meaning conveyed by the term 'family' probably relates to the setting or culture in which the family is studied (Gibb, Duggan & Lwin, 1991). The extended family in Africa, for example, is viewed not merely a large social network, but has important functions with regard to production, economic and social support, as well as socialization of new members (Kayongo-Male & Onyango, 1984). Illness and death in the family have a profound effect on all spheres of family life in Africa including social, economic, reproductive and political functioning (Ankrah, 1993). A popular perception of African families is that the extended kin network provides material and emotional support where a family member is unwell. HIV disease directly threatens this pattern as whole families and, in some cases, a large number of people living in the same village or community become infected. Recent studies of the impact of HIV disease on African families have revealed that the extended family is 'a safety net with holes' (Barnett & Blaikie, 1992; Sealey *et al.*, 1993). An epidemic, such as HIV disease, has a ripple effect throughout the family and kin system threatening their capacity to adapt, sustain one another physically and emotionally, and to replace some of the functions and roles lost by those members who become ill and die.

A sizeable number of gay men in the West have been affected by HIV disease, and this has brought into focus same-sex relationships. While same-sex partnerships may be *de facto* marriages, in almost all countries, same-sex relationships are not legally defined as a family and there is no legal protection or obligations for either partner. In some spheres, same-sex relationships may be similar to heterosexual relationships. In particular, economic, social and sexual activities are broadly similar (Hart *et al.*, 1990; McCann & Wadsworth, 1992). While same-sex relationships do not fulfil reproductive functions, some gay people including a proportion in same-sex relationships, may be married, have their own family, or use artificial insemination by donor or enter into heterosexual relationships with a view to having children and becoming parents (Geis, Fuller & Rush, 1986; Ussher, 1991).

Attempting to define the 'family' in HIV research places one in double jeopardy. On the one hand, some traditional definitions tend to be narrow as they focus either on blood relationships or the idea of a common household; other definitions emphasize the social network, which come to include any provider of social support. There are, in addition, both legal and sociological definitions of the family. It is clear that there is neither consensus as to what constitutes the family nor a concept of a 'traditional' family. For the purposes of this discussion, both biological (blood) relationships and social (chosen) relationships will be viewed within the context of family functioning, whether or not they are legally defined as a family. The following broad definition of the family that incorporates these ideas serves as a yardstick by which other views of the family can be gauged:

> 'Family members are individuals who by birth, adoption, marriage, or declared commitment share deep, personal connections and are mutually entitled to receive and obligated to provide support of various kinds to the extent possible, especially in times of need' (Levine, 1990).

THE IMPACT OF HIV ON RELATIONSHIPS IN THE FAMILY

Social Stigma, Isolation and Secrecy

It is common knowledge that people react differently to the threat or confirmation of illness. What is striking about families affected by HIV disease is that, among many of the issues that most families face in dealing with an ill member, the additional issue of social stigma associated with the diagnosis will also arise (Cates *et al.*, 1990). The marginalization of people with HIV disease is as a direct consequence of their sexual orientation, sexual behaviour or drug use, fear of an infectious disease, as well

TABLE 9.1
The impact of HIV disease on family relationships

- fear of loss and death
- social stigma
- fear of isolation, rejection, abandonment
- fear of becoming infected
- anxiety about talking about sex, sexuality, illness
- fear of betrayal or disclosure
- guilt arising from infidelity and past relationships
- blame
- shame
- secrets between family members, and between the family and others
- over-protectiveness or emotional disengagement
- exacerbation of 'normal' family problems
- fear of a loss of sexual freedom
- facing multiple losses
- loss of a sense of future

as social unease with death and dying. Some people view infection with HIV as the fault of the individual and AIDS as punishment for immoral or offensive behaviour (Blendon & Donelan, 1988). Disclosure of the diagnosis in the family may confront it's members with revelations about lifestyle or behaviour, such as homosexuality, infidelity or intravenous drug use. Even though there is some evidence of more enlightened views towards this stigmatized population, King (1990) notes that on a global scale there is increasing discrimination against people with HIV infection. Family members are also affected by social stigma and may experience rejection from friends, loss of jobs and harassment (Powell-Cope & Brown, 1992), as well as more subtle gestures such as neighbours not visiting and children not being invited to parties.

Social isolation resulting from a fear of stigma is one of the most challenging problems faced by these families. On the one hand, family members may draw a boundary between the family and others outside this system by not disclosing the diagnosis to more distant relatives, friends, close colleagues and others who comprise the social support system. There may also be secrets within the family unit where children are not told the diagnosis or elderly parents are 'protected' from the news where there is a belief or myth that this would compromise their health.

Secrets may have both positive and negative consequences. The aim of protecting others from adverse consequences may be viewed as a positive or functional aspect of secrets. On the other hand, secrets in families may reveal dysfunctional relationships and be physically or psychologically damaging (Bor, Miller & Salt, 1989). Where an HIV infected man refuses to inform his wife of his diagnosis, for example, and to take precautions during sexual activities to protect her, the destructive sequelae of secrets clearly outweigh any positive consequences. It remains to be seen whether secrecy-related problems stemming from HIV diminish as social stigma towards those affected decreases.

Stress and Coping

Stress is commonly seen in family members who may react to news of the diagnosis with disbelief, shock and confusion. The feelings experienced by family members where someone is dying may include guilt, helplessness, depression, anger, confusion and despair. There may be more rules prohibiting emotional expression, greater anxiety about illness and less trust in families affected by HIV disease (Atkins & Amenta, 1991). This may be a further manifestation of pre-existing relationship problems in the family in addition to the stress arising from illness in the family and a fear of social stigma. For this reason, it is reasonable to conclude that families affected by HIV/AIDS may face more complex problems in their adjustment to, and coping with, illness than other families having to deal with death and dying.

Many families affected by HIV disease experience similar concerns or fears. Urban families in Uganda (McGrath *et al.*, 1993), and patients attending a London hospital (Bor *et al.*, 1989) were asked to describe and rank their main fears about illness in the family. The fear of the death of a loved one, concern over the burden of care (both physical and psychological) of a sick family member and a sense of despondency and failure about the future were commonly raised. Fear of becoming infected (through social or intimate contact), and helplessness may also be experienced at different stages in the course of illness (Frierson, Lippmann & Johnson, 1987).

Some family members may become immobilized by not being able to identify the challenges and problems facing them and to assign priority in dealing with them. Stress of this kind can become 'infectious' and others may start to doubt their ability to cope and manage their stress (Murphy & Perry, 1988). A cycle of symptomatic behaviour may follow in which depression in one family member either triggers the same or its complement in another (Bor, Prior & Miller, 1990). This in turn may be exacerbated by secrets about how family members appear to be coping. Some families function best by 'putting on a brave face' and concealing their hurt, anger, disappointment or anxiety. Others may become overwhelmed by their reaction and seek counselling and psychotherapy in order to manage their anxiety and to find more adaptive ways of coping with stress.

Family members may display the same psychological symptoms as the infected person ranging from fear, anger, agitation and withdrawal to anxiety and depression (Beckett & Rutan, 1990). Some family members may also feel as if they are 'toxic' and resist getting emotionally close to others (Gambe & Getzel, 1989), which may serve as a protective mechanism against a fear of rejection. In contrast, the need for social support and close emotional attachments may be at its greatest at times of personal stress, misfortune and for those affected by illness (Rolland, 1990). Obstacles to adjustment, acceptance and reconciliation between family members may arise at different stages in the course of illness as issues about lifestyle and blame re-emerge. The stress that emanates from these conflicting forces can lead to suicidal thoughts, paranoid beliefs and even psychosis (Lovejoy, 1989). Arguments, threats, accusations, alcohol and drug abuse, and treatment non-compliance may be symptoms of psychological problems in families arising from ambivalent feelings between its members.

Periods of stress and anxiety in a family do not automatically lead to symptoms of psychopathology. However, some families may experience ongoing stress and may lose the capacity to differentiate between adaptive and dysfunctional coping. Behaviour in the family may become dysfunctional where reality is denied (for example, in a family where both parents are infected with HIV, the parents make no provision for the future care of their children), or where illness becomes the only reality that they attend to (for example, day to day activities are neglected). As with all families which experience or are threatened by rapid and profound change, there is an increased risk of psychological problems. This risk is probably greater where external support networks, such as the extended family and friends, have been not been told the diagnosis and are therefore excluded from providing a supportive and normalizing experience for the family. Studies which compare stress and coping in families affected by HIV who have engaged external support systems with those who have not, will throw light on this important issue.

Social Support

Studies of social support and emotional well-being have demonstrated that people with HIV report less feelings of depression and helplessness if they have close friends or relatives to talk to about emotional and illness-related problems (Ostrow *et al.*, 1989; Zich & Temoshok, 1987). People with HIV who fear disclosing their diagnosis to others and who are socially isolated may be at increased risk for psychological problems. Many gay men are dependent on a gay support network rather than on parents or siblings (Namir *et al.*, 1987). In some urban centres where there are larger concentrations of gay men infected with HIV, an increasing number of men will suffer multiple losses in their social support networks. The number of losses experienced is positively correlated with sedative use, traumatic stress responses and uptake of psychological services (Martin, 1989).

Contact with friends and other caregivers may decrease with the onset of illness (Donlou *et al.*, 1985). Even though social support may act as a buffer against stress for people with HIV, caregivers may themselves require support in order to carry out their tasks (Reidy, Taggart & Asselin, 1991). A sizeable proportion of gay men (54%) in one study reported that their relationships and social functioning had deteriorated since being diagnosed with HIV infection (Kaisch & Anton-Culver, 1989). In some cases, the physical manifestations of illness, including fatigue, weight loss and skin complaints, may have interfered with their capacity to enter into and maintain relationships. A third of the sample (32%) felt that many of their relationships with family and friends had become closer since diagnosis. Most studies of social support and HIV have been conducted on gay men which limit the generalizability of the findings. Nonetheless, there is a trend towards consolidating existing relationships in this group rather than broadening their social networks. This may stem from a fear of rejection, a decreasing support network as a consequence of deaths in the gay community, physical manifestations of illness that may interfere with social functioning, and apathy.

Communication and Disclosure within the Family

Foremost among the problems that people infected with HIV may face that may have implications for relationships, is information about the disease and the person's condition, and the dissemination thereof. A decision to inform others of the diagnosis carries the risk of a double disclosure; it may simultaneously reveal a previously hidden lifestyle. While stigma-related experiences or a fear of stigma are commonly discussed by people with HIV, we are only beginning to study patterns of disclosure of HIV status in families.

Although most relationships undergo some change where either or both spouses are infected with HIV, it is not possible to predict the nature and outcome of these changes (Dew, Ragni & Nimorwicz, 1991). It is difficult to determine whether the changes in some relationships are as a direct result of the disclosure of the diagnosis, or whether the disclosure highlighted or exacerbated an existing problem in the relationship. Some couples may become closer, others remain companions but cease sexual relations, while some relationships end abruptly or deteriorate over time. In spite of health prevention efforts of carers and counsellors, the disequilibrium that results where one partner is infected may result in sexual risk taking in order to restore balance in the relationship (Bor, Prior and Miller, 1990). Either or both partners may also experience increased alienation in the relationship as they adapt to and cope with HIV in different ways. A proportion of heterosexual and gay couples will seek counselling to deal with relationship problems (George, 1990; Myers, 1991).

The dynamics of relationships between parents and their children and disclosure of HIV infection to them is a more complex matter. Children may be either infected with HIV or affected by other family members who are themselves infected. Most children worldwide who have been diagnosed with HIV infection were infected perinatally and for this reason the mother and possibly other family members will also be infected. Parents face the difficult task of achieving some balance in the child's life between normal routines and the added demands placed on all spheres of life brought on by illness. Whether or not the child has been infected with HIV, there is a chance that children in the family will become orphans, which may lead to social and emotional deprivation.

Parents of an HIV infected child face the dilemma of 'if', 'how' and 'when' to tell their child his or her HIV status. Most research into this problem has been conducted with families in which the child was infected through contaminated treatment for haemophilia or through blood transfusions (Miller *et al.*, 1989; Tsiantis at al, 1990). In most of these cases, there is a greater chance that only the child in the family has been infected. The issue of disclosure to non-infected siblings in the family has been addressed in clinical practice (Bor, Miller & Goldman, 1992), but has not been the subject of research.

In a study by Courville and colleagues (1992), the majority of parents (80%) had not told their HIV-infected child the diagnosis even though their average age was ten years and presumably most children would be aware of health-related problems as a consequence of regular visits to the hospital. Some reasons parents gave for disclosure were: 'I knew it was the right time', 'We disclosed in response to our child's negative comments about AIDS' and 'There was unplanned disclosure in the emergency room'. The terminology used by parents when breaking the news to their child was varied: 'You have bad blood', 'You have something like AIDS', 'Santa Claus will come to take you away when you are asleep' and 'Take your medicines so you won't die'. The reasons given for not disclosing the diagnosis to children included: fear of the child disclosing to others, which may threaten parental confidentiality, fear that disclosure may exacerbate the disease process, and concern about the effect on family stability. The stage at which parents choose to disclose the diagnosis to a child, and how they do this, is an important topic since it yields insights into family dynamics and how each member comes to terms with the diagnosis and illness.

THE FAMILY'S RESPONSE TO ILLNESS

Most families have to endure a long period of uncertainty about the course of illness. This is because the latent period before overt clinical symptoms of HIV disease are diagnosed can last a decade or more. The anticipation of a loss through physical illness in the family can disturb the current functioning of each family member who may be immobilized by the fear or dread of facing the loss. The shift from an asymptomatic to a symptomatic phase of illness may reactivate stress in the family system. Shock, fear, isolation, guilt, blame, feelings of being overwhelmed and psychophysiological distress may all resurface (Leff & Walizer, 1992), although this is commonly tempered by a measure of relief as the course of illness becomes clearer and more certain. Family members may be called on to provide greater material and emotional support at this stage. Changes in family relationships may be quite marked at this point of transition, sometimes punctuated by emotional tension, fighting or withdrawal. This stems from anxiety over people's needs not being met or an excess of support, both of which may become destructive to relationships. Family members face a particular dilemma at the symptomatic phase of the disease. On the one hand there is a social expectation that they will offer hope and support to the member who is unwell, while at the same time they are faced with the reality that treatment and resources may be limited or ineffectual. This can lead to secrets in the family as some members, including the infected family member who is unwell, are protected from the gravity of the situation.

The family looks inward as the illness progresses and death becomes imminent, and rivalry may surface between family members as they struggle to redefine their relationship with the dying person. At this stage, the parents, siblings and where appropriate, the patient's partner, become the most important source of emotional support (Catania *et al.*, 1992). There may be arguments about approaches to care and decisions about advanced life support directives such as resuscitation (Lipman & Johnson, 1992). Friends and more distant relatives may seek to create some distance between themselves and the family by decreasing their contact and visits through fear or a difficulty in dealing with separation, loss and dying. Themes of blame and guilt may resurface and may serve to protect family members from the emotional pain relating to 'separation anxiety, existential aloneness, denial, sadness, disappointment, anger, resentment, exhaustion and desperation' (Rolland, 1990). The feelings may be both intense and ambivalent; there may be a desire to be closely and deeply connected with a family member and, at the same time, a need to escape the emotional pain and a longing to feel disconnected from the person and the problem. The dying person may rely on the family for emotional and practical support. In turn, the family turns to its own social network for support, both during the course of illness, and in the period of bereavement that may follow. As a consequence of some of the unique problems experienced by those affected by HIV disease, the interfaces may be disrupted between the individual and the family, and between the family and its social network.

THE IMPACT OF BEREAVEMENT ON SURVIVORS

Research in social psychiatry has demonstrated that the death of a partner, spouse or other relative can affect the psychological and physical health of survivors or others who are bereaved. These findings have important implications for those affected by

TABLE 9.3
Problems experienced by bereaved families

- isolation and stigma may persist
- fear of infection may persist for many months
- secrets surrounding the diagnosis may persist
- despair about the future
- emotional, social and financial loss (deprivation)

HIV as some of those who are bereaved may themselves be infected with HIV. Recent studies have sought to investigate whether bereavement has an adverse effect on the function of the immune system; whether survivors infected with HIV progress to AIDS more quickly than others who have not experienced a bereavement; and, whether social support buffers people infected with HIV from stress and the deleterious effects of adverse life events. Results of a recent study (Chesney *et al.*, 1992) suggest that the survivor's immune system is not adversely affected by an AIDS-related bereavement.

In parts of Africa which have been heavily affected by deaths resulting from AIDS, rituals associated with funeral arrangements and mourning have had to be abandoned. Financial and other demands on kinsmen and neighbours have become a significant burden as a result of multiple deaths (Ankrah, 1993). The survival of some clans in Africa could be threatened by a lack of availability of marriage partners for both young adults reaching maturity and those who have been widowed. A trend towards marrying very young women who are seemingly free from infection has also been noted.

THE IMPACT OF HIV DISEASE ON FAMILY STRUCTURE AND ROLES IN THE FAMILY

Changes in the structure of the family may become evident at different stages of illness. Normal developmental patterns are reversed in HIV disease. Children may die before their parents, leaving grandparents to look after themselves at a time

TABLE 9.2
Changes in the structure of the family

- increased widowhood
- increased orphanhood
- grandparents becoming carers
- children dying before their parents
- loss of productivity, financial ruin
- shift in roles
- children coming home to die at a stage when most have left home to establish themselves separately to their family
- parents deciding not to have children, in some cases

when they might look forward to increased support from their own children. Grandparents may have to take on the responsibilities of a parent once again and care for grandchildren orphaned by the loss of their parents. In other cases, young adults come home to die at a stage where children would be establishing themselves away from home. The disruption to some families may be compounded by their having to migrate. Refugees with HIV may become dislocated from a familiar and supportive environment which may exacerbate problems associated with coping and adjustment.

Where parents are both infected, there is an increased likelihood that their children will be orphaned. As the number of 'AIDS orphans' worldwide increases and the extended family becomes overburdened with orphans, an increasing number will have to be cared for in institutions rather than within the extended family (Hunter, 1991; Preble, 1990). Traditional views and attitudes towards sex, marriage and emotional bonds between spouses may result in sexual risk-taking in spite of health education messages (Larson, 1989). Termination of the mother's childbearing has profound implications not only for her nurturing role, but also for the family's relationship with the extended family and the community, and for future economic security (Ankrah, 1993). Even where targeted counselling is offered to couples where one or both partners is infected with HIV, there may be an overriding desire to have a child (Dublin, Rosenberg & Goedert, 1992; Goldman, Miller & Lee, 1992). There may also be periods where people lapse into unsafe sexual practices (Kelly, Lawrence & Brasfield, 1991) as a means of revitalizing or redressing the balance in a sexual relationship in which one partner is infected.

Illness almost always places a financial burden on families. This results from the direct costs of care and treatment and the disruption caused by loss of productivity. Where ill health interferes with the family breadwinner's mobility and employment, income may need to be replaced by other family members. In some cases, the role of the breadwinner cannot be substituted or replaced by others either because they are too ill themselves to work or they are fully committed to caring for other family members who may be unwell. This scenario is now all too common in parts of sub-Saharan Africa (Ankrah, 1993).

PROVIDING PSYCHOLOGICAL SUPPORT TO FAMILIES AFFECTED BY HIV DISEASE

An understanding of the impact of HIV disease on the family needs to be translated into supportive and therapeutic actions with individual family members and the family system as a whole. Approaches to family counselling are derived from systems theory and address relationships, recursiveness, context, developmental themes and belief systems (Bor, Miller & Goldman, 1992; Miller & Bor, 1988; Walker, 1991). Counselling about the family and relationships can be conducted with an individual, a couple or indeed, the family. Counselling is not dependent on everyone being present at a session since ideas about the family and relationships can be addressed with an individual. Some of these ideas can be addressed as follows:

1. Introduce the idea of 'the family' by talking to the individual about his or her family. Discuss relationships, changes in them and obstacles to change.
2. Take a family history. Draw up a family tree with the client and discuss each person's view of relationships (McGoldrick & Gerson, 1985) in the past, in the present, an anticipates them being in the future. The client or each person present at the session can then be asked to consider how he or she considers other family members would view these same relationships.
3. Enquire about definitions of the family. Ask about who is seen to be in or outside the family. If important people are not spoken about, ask how they fit into the description of the family.
4. Obtain a clearer view of boundaries and alliances in the family by asking who has been told about the diagnosis, what they have been told and from whom secrets have been kept. Ask about what this may mean for different relationships that some people know while others may not.
5. Discuss how each person has been told the diagnosis and what it means for their relationships with other family members. If no-one has been told, explore themes of secrecy in the family, fears about telling and what effect it may have on relationships if others were to know the diagnosis.
6. Talk about the future and each person's hopes and fears for the future. Ask about how the person with HIV sees their role or influence on the family throughout the course of illness, and any legacies thereafter.
7. Enquire about past experience of loss in the family and explore how this affects family members in relation to HIV.
8. Ask what issues or problems might be facing the family if HIV were not a problem.
9. Ask about support: who supports whom; how support is offered; what support is needed; and, how the family finds support for itself.
10. Some hints for conducting counselling sessions. (a) When sitting with the family, ensure that everyone's views are heard and that each person has an equal amount of time to put their views forward. (b) Adopt a curious and non-oppositional stance. Avoid prescribing how people should conduct their relationships. (c) Help to understand how beliefs or ideas may have come about and what they may mean for the future. (d) Address both the painful aspects of coping with HIV disease and address the competencies and strengths of family members. (e) Convey hope and encouragement without denying the reality of pain and suffering.

CONCLUSION

In most societies, health and illness are at one level a private, individual matter, while at another, they have implications for relationships and social functioning. As with all illnesses, HIV disease affects the entire family system. Disruption in families affected by HIV may take many forms as relationships and tasks undergo change. While each family has to process and adjust to these changes in its own way, we do not as yet have a clear view as to how culture, ethnicity or religion mediates this process, although the implications of HIV disease for an individual are inextricably linked to the social context where prevention, infection, illness, treatment and care occur. Beliefs about the illness and the meanings surrounding the route of infection are both important in psychotherapeutic work with these families. By studying the impact of HIV disease on the family, we come to understand, in part, the social context of HIV disease. As the focus for care in the 1990's for those affected by HIV disease shifts from the individual to the family, we can anticipate a concomitant change in the focus of psychosocial research.

REFERENCES

Ankrah, M. (1993) The imapct of HIV/AIDS on the family and other significant relationships. *AIDS Care*, **5**, 5–22.

Atkins, R., Amenta, M. (1991) Family adaptation to AIDS: a comparative study. *Hospice Journal*, **8**, 71–83.

Barnett, T., Blaikie, P. (1992) *AIDS in Africa*. London: Belhaven Press.

Beckett, A., Rutan, J. (1990) Treating persons with ARC and AIDS in group psychotherapy. *International Group Psychotherapy*, **40**, 19–29.

Blendon, R., Donelan, K. (1988) Discrimination against people with AIDS: the public's perspective. *New England Journal of Medicine*, **319**, 1022–1026.

Bor, R., Miller, R., Goldman, E. (1992) Theory and Practice of HIV Counselling: A Systemic Approach. London: Cassell.

Bor, R., Miller, R., Goldman, E., Kernoff, P. (1989) The impact of AIDS/HIV on the family. *Practice*, **1**, 49–65.

Bor, R., Miller, R., Salt, H. (1989) Secrecy-related problems in AIDS management. *Journal of the Royal College of Physicians*, **23**, 264–267.

Bor, R., Prior, N., Miller, R. (1990) Complementarity in relationships of couples affected by HIV. *Counselling Psychology Quarterly*, **3**, 217–220.

Catania, J., Turner, H., Kyung-Hee, C., Coates, T. (1992) Coping with death anxiety: help-seeking and social support among gay men with various HIV diagnoses. *AIDS*, **6**, 999–1005.

Coates, J., Graham, L., Boeglin, D., Tielker, S. (1990) The effects of AIDS on the family system. Families in Society: *Journal of Contemporary Human Services*, April, 195–201.

Chesney, M., Folkman, S., Cooke, M., Bocellari, A., Coates, T., Collette, L. (1992) Effect of partner death on CD4 levels in HIV positive and HIV negative caregiving men. *Abstracts of the VIIIth International Conference on AIDS*. Amsterdam.

Courville, T., Blum, S., Gunchin, L., Brunell, P., Isreale, V., Wittek, A., Srugo, I., Mekjian, M., Adams, J. (1992) Disclosure versus non-disclosure of HIV/AIDS diagnosis to children with transfusion associated HIV-1 infection. *Abstracts of the VIIIth International Conference on AIDS*, Amsterdam.

Dew, M., Ragni, M., Nimorwicz, P. (1991) Correlates of psychiatric distress among the wives of hemophilic men with and without HIV infection. *American Journal of Psychiatry*, **148**, 1016-1022.

Donlou, J., Wolcott, D., Gottlieb, M., Landsverk, J. (1985) Psychosocial aspects of AIDS and AIDS-related complex: a pilot study. *Journal of Psychosocial Oncology*, **3**, 39–55.

Dublin, S., Rosenberg, P., Goedert, J. (1992) Patterns and predictors of high-risk sexual behaviour in female partners of HIV-infected men with haemophilia. *AIDS*, **6**, 475–482.

Frierson, R., Lippmann, S., Johnson, J. (1987) AIDS: psychological stresses on the family. *Psychosomatics*, **28**, 65–68.

Gambe, R., Getzel, G. (1989) Group work with gay men with AIDS. *Social Casework*, **70**, 172–179.

Geis, S., Fuller, R., Rush, J. (1986) Lovers of AIDS victims: psychosocial stresses and counselling needs. *Death Studies*, **10**, 43–53.

George, H. (1990) Sexual and relationship problems among people affected by AIDS: three case studies. *Counselling Psychology Quarterly*, **3**, 389–399.

Gibb, D., Duggan, C., Lwin, R. (1991) The family and HIV. *Genitourinary Medicine*, **67**, 363–366.

Goldman, E., Miller, R., Lee, C. (1992) Counselling HIV positive haemophilic men who wish to have children. *British Medical Journal*, **304**, 829–830.

Hart, G., Fitzpatrick, R., McClean, J., Dawson, J., Boulton, M. (1990) Gay men, social support and HIV disease: a study of social integration in the gay community. *AIDS Care*, **2**, 163–170.

Hunter, S. (1991) Orphans as a window on the AIDS epidemic in sub-Saharan Africa: initial results and implications of a study in Uganda. *Social Science and Medicine*, **31**, 681–690.

Kaisch, K., Anton-Culver, H. (1989) Psychological and social consequences of HIV exposure. *Psychology and Health*, **3**, 63–75.

Kayongo-Male, D., Onyango, P. (1984) The Sociology of the African Family. London: Longman.

Kelly, J., Lawrence, J., Brasfield, T. (1991) Predictors of vulnerability to AIDS risk behaviour relapse. *Journal of Consulting and Clinical Psychology*, **59**, 163–166.

King, M. (1990) Psychological aspects of HIV infection and AIDS: what have we learned? *British Journal of Psychiatry*, **156**, 151-156.

Larson, A. (1989) Social context of HIV transmission in Africa: historical and cultural bases of East and Central African sexual relations. *Reviews of Infectious Diseases*, **11**, 716–731.

Leff, P., Walizer, E. (1992) The uncommon wisdom of parents at the moment of diagnosis. *Family Systems Medicine*, **10**, 147–168.

Levine, C. (1990) AIDS and changing concepts of the family. *The Milbank Quarterly*, **68**, 33–58.

Lipman, M., Johnson, M. (1992) Resuscitation and HIV. *Genitourinary Medicine*, **68**, 151–153.

Lipp, J. (1991) Living with HIV and AIDS. *Dulwich Centre Newsletter*, **2**, 7–16.

Lovejoy, N. (1989) AIDS: impact on the gay man's homosexual and heterosexual families. *Marriage and Family Review*, **14**, 285–316.

Martin, D. (1989) HIV infection and the gay community: counseling and clinical issues. *Journal of Counseling and Development*, **68**, 67–72.

McCann, K., Wadsworth, E. (1992) The role of informal carers in supporting gay men who have HIV related illness: what do they do and what are their needs? *AIDS Care*, **4**, 25–34.

McGoldrick, M., Gerson, R. (1985) *Genograms in Family Assessment*. New York: W. W. Norton.

McGrath, J. Ankrah, M. Shumann, D., Nkumbi, S., Lubega, M. (1993) AIDS and the urban family: its impact in Kampala, Uganda. *AIDS Care*, **5**, 57–72.

Miller, R., Bor, R. (1988) *AIDS: A Guide to Clinical Counselling*. London: Science Press.

Miller, R., Goldman, E., Bor, R., Kernoff, P. (1989) AIDS and children: some of the issues in haemophilia care and how to address them. *AIDS Care*, **1**, 51–57.

Murphy, P., Perry, K. (1988) Hidden grievers. *Death Studies*, **12**, 451–462.

Myers, M. (1991) Couples therapy with HIV-infected men. *Psychiatric Annals*, **21**, 466–470.

Namir, S., Wolcott, D., Fawzy, F., Alumbaugh, M. (1987) Coping with AIDS: psychological and health implications. *Journal of Applied Social Psychology*, **17**, 309–328.

Ostrow, D., Monjan, A., Joseph, J., Van Raden, M., Fox, R., Lawrence, K., Dudley, J., Phair, J. (1989) HIV-related symptoms and psychological functioning in a cohort of homosexual men. *American Journal of Psychiatry*, **146**, 737–742.

Powell-Cope, G., Brown, M. (1992) Going public as an AIDS family caregiver. *Social Science and Medicine*, **34**, 571–580.

Preble, E. (1990) Impact of HIV/AIDS on African children. *Social Science and Medicine*, **31**, 671–680.

Reidy, M., Taggart, M., Asselin, L. (1991) Psychosocial needs expressed by the natural caregivers of HIV infected children. *AIDS Care*, **3**, 331–343.

Rolland, J. (1987) Chronic illness and the lifecycle: a conceptual framework. *Family Process*, **26**, 203–221.

Rolland, J. (1990) Anticipatory loss: a family systems developmental framework. *Family Process*, **29**, 229–244.

Sealey, J., Kajura, E., Bachengana, C., Okongo, M., Wagner, U., Mulder, D. (1993) The extended family and support for people with AIDS in a rural population in south west Uganda: a safety net with holes? *AIDS Care*, **5**, 121–126.

Tsiantis, J., Anastasopoulos, D., Meyer, M., Paniz, D., Ladis, V., Platokouki, N., Aroni, S., Kattamis, C. (1990) A multi-level intervention approach for care of HIV-positive haemophiliac and thalassaemic patients and their families. *AIDS Care*, **2**, 253–266.

Ussher, J. (1991) Family and couples therapy with gay and lesbian clients: acknowledging the forgotten minority. *Journal of Family Therapy*, **13**, 131–205.

Walker, G. (1991) In the Midst of Winter. New York: W.W. Norton.

Zich, J., Temoshok, L. (1987) Perceptions of social support in men with AIDS and ARC: relationships with distress and hardiness. *Journal of Applied Social Psychology*, **17**, 193–215.

10

Behavioural Bisexuality Among Men

PETER WEATHERBURN AND PETER DAVIES

SEXUAL ACTIVITY WITH BOTH MALES AND FEMALES

Prevalence and Implications

Whilst UK government funded bodies, such as the Health Education Authority (HEA) and international organisations such as the World Health Organization (WHO), have showed sporadic interest in the need for specific research on, and interventions targeted at men that have sex with both men and women, our understandings of this group have advanced little in the last ten years or so. This is especially surprising given that men who have sex with both men and women have long been seen as crucial to the pattern of sexual spread of HIV and the future incidence of HIV/AIDS (Winkelstein *et al.*, 1986; Bennett *et al.*, 1989; Boulton & Weatherburn, 1990; Ekstrand *et al.*, 1993). This widespread assumption is based on the belief that homosexual men and heterosexual men form two hermetic communities. With this view of the world the problem becomes the containment of infection within the former – glossed as a 'risk group' – and avoidance of spread in the latter – referred to as the 'general population', which, as many commentators implicitly continue to assume, would not otherwise be at any risk of HIV infection. From this (offensive and simplistic) analysis, the notion of 'bridge' groups or 'access points' emerge. The most popular of these is 'bisexual' men.

The essential problem with this model is that common to all those approaches which seek to understand the physical processes of sexual transmission by referring to social identities and labels. For, despite the fact that there are women and men who will affirm the identity 'bisexual', there are many more who, terming themselves gay or straight[1] will engage, regularly or infrequently in sex with partners of either gender. On the other hand, there are many of those who term themselves 'bisexual' who will, for significant periods, perhaps even for life, remain behaviourally monosexual. Hence, what is at issue is the specific pattern of sexual activity, particularly the prevalence of those acts most likely to be implicated in the sexual transmission of the HI virus: vaginal and anal intercourse (Padian *et al.*, 1987; Johnson & Laga, 1988).

In the context of the epidemiology of HIV/AIDS the self-avowed sexual identity of men who have sex with both men and women is of relatively little consequence. The often demonstrated, but widely disregarded fact that there is no straightforward relationship between self-proclaimed sexual identity and sexual behaviour (Fitzpatrick *et al.*, 1989; Boulton & Weatherburn, 1990; Weatherburn *et al.*, 1990) argues very strongly for ignoring sexual identity in an epidemiological study of the factors associated with HIV transmission. This does not mean that identity is wholly irrelevant but that it is behaviour that is the crucial (indeed the only true) determinant of HIV risk.

Failure to take seriously the distinction between behaviour and identity often leads to totally unhelpful conjecture such as:

> 'The present and future course of Acquired Immune Deficiency Syndrome (AIDS) will depend largely on the dynamics of sexual transmission of the Human Immunodeficiency Virus (HIV) in the general population. One growing source of concern is the potential transmission through bisexual contacts.'
> (Tielman, Carballo & Hendriks, 1991)

Whilst the book from which this extract originates proclaims itself to be the 'first effort to assess current knowledge on bisexuality and to explore the relevance of bisexuality in the AIDS epidemic' (Tielman, Carballo & Hendriks, 1991) it makes a most fundamental error by conflating social categories (bisexual) with behavioural patterns (sex between two persons). There can be no such thing as 'bisexual contact' (above), 'bisexual practices' (Tielman, Carballo & Hendriks, 1991) or 'bisexual sex' (Garcia Garcia *et al.*, 1991) unless three or more people are involved. If sexual contact between two persons really has to be categorised it has to be termed homosexual or heterosexual. Those who insist on identifying 'bisexuals' as a risk group must demonstrate, if their arguments are to be regarded as sound, that bisexual men and women behave differently with their contacts of either sex than those who are exclusively heterosexual or homosexual. This seems unlikely.

We are not arguing that the sexual behaviour of self-defined bisexuals is of no consequence. It has been shown that identification with gay community has an important effect on the pattern of risk behaviour of men having sex with men (Kippax *et al.*, 1992). If it could also be shown that bisexually identified individuals

---

[1] It is interesting that the presumed identify of the majority has no term to refer to it other than those which emerge as antonyms to labels applied to the minority (heterosexual from homosexual) or affirmed by that minority (straight from gay). Attempts to popularize terms such as 'glums' (as opposed to 'gays') or 'breeders' have not met with widespread acceptance.

had different patterns of behaviour than those who did not identify as such, then their identification as a group becomes important for epidemiology as well as health promotion.

WHO HAS SEX WITH BOTH MEN AND WOMEN?

Bisexual Men

Definitions of Bisexuality
The vast majority of studies of bisexuals has concentrated either on issues of identity and other broadly psychological factors such as coping, adjustment, motivation and personality; or have adopted anthropological and historical methods in an attempt to examine bisexuality in temporal or cultural contexts. Such studies (see Boulton & Weatherburn, 1990 for a review) usually define bisexuality in terms of self-proclaimed identity or, less commonly, in terms of affections, intentions or emotions. Hence such bisexuals may not necessarily currently engage in sexual behaviour with both males and females but may identify with the bisexual movement politically or because of feelings or future intentions. That is, persons who are attracted to, and/or intend to have sex with members of both genders at some point in the future may identify, and be identified as bisexual.

It has been argued that since the sexual revolution of the 1960's and early 1970's it has become increasingly easy to self-identify as bisexual. Indeed, in a few countries an entire bisexual commercial and social scene has developed. In the UK, no such scene exists and bisexuality remains unacknowledged either as a social category or an available social identity. Furthermore, bisexuality remains stigmatised by wider society and, to some extent within gay and lesbian culture (MacDonald, 1981; Wolf, 1987) and has been widely pathologised as a transitory or transitional state, a denial of homosexuality and even a myth (Ross, 1979; MacDonald, 1981). This, coupled with the lack of a straightforward and cohesive social or political structure, may make self-identification as bisexual both difficult and relatively unusual.

Alternatively, bisexuality may be defined solely in terms of sexual behaviour within a given time period. Given that sexual behaviour is the key determinant of HIV risk this seems a most appropriate means of defining bisexuality in this context. However, if we adopt such a definition we must bear in mind that this is not a social category: we are not discussing a set of persons who share a common set of preconceptions or lifestyle, but who share a broadly similar behavioural pattern.

Even admitting that a behavioural definition is the more appropriate does not exhaust the difficulties. Problems then arise over the time period involved. Thus, a person may be termed behaviourally bisexual if he has had sex with both genders during the course of his life. However, if the primary interest is in patterns of sexual behaviour as they effect HIV transmission this time period may be rather too long. In order to be of any true epidemiological use we have to use behavioural bisexuality to refer to sex with both genders in the last 5 years, or less. In fact much of the following discussion will use behavioural bisexuality to refer to sex with both genders during the last year. Not only is this time period easily short enough to have epidemiological significance, but apart from lifetime it is the period most commonly used in studies of sexual behaviour.

Henceforth, we will use to the term 'behavioural bisexual' to describe men who have sex with both men and women, within a given time period, and 'bisexual' to refer only to men that label themselves as such.

It is important to recognise that the question 'who counts as a bisexual ?' has no single answer. The population identified in different studies will differ: those interested in the dynamics of HIV transmission will be interested in the behavioural bisexuals. Those interested in identity formation and its impact on behaviour will focus on the self-identified. Other projects will identify other specific groups. Problems have arisen in the past over the choice of inappropriate groups for such studies – for example the assumption that patterns of behaviour of self-defined 'bisexuals' mirror and exhaust the pattern of all behavioural bisexuality.

The problem is magnified if cross-cultural comparisons are made. Within North American, Northern European urban, post-industrial culture in the wake of the sexual liberation movements of the 1960s and 1970s, a bisexual identity and community has in places emerged. In other parts of the world, other patterns are common. In Mediterranean societies, male behavioural bisexuality is treated quite differently. (Lancaster, 1988; Carrier, 1971; 1976; Young, 1973; Tapinc, 1992; Murray, 1992). The assumption that these different cultural manifestations emanate from an essential bisexual personality remains at best an unproven conjecture, at worst an example of Western scientific imperialism.

Patterns of Bisexuality

While behavioural bisexuality appears to occur in a large number of diverse contexts, it seems to lead to the formation of a bisexual identity in only a very small minority of cases (Blumstein & Schwartz, 1977). Indeed Boulton (1991) has argued that because of the dichotomous notions of sexuality in the West identity is more likely to reflect the individual's reference group or the subculture in which they are involved, especially where there is no public reference group or community available to validate or support a bisexual identity. Hence 'most of those who engage in bisexual behaviour remain as isolated individuals, having little contact with other bisexual men and being hidden within the homosexual community or the 'general population'' (Boulton, 1991).

Whilst skilfully evading the question of definition and its impact by reference to a number of extensive theoretical reviews (Paul, 1984; Hansen & Evans, 1985; Klein *et al.*, 1985; Zinik, 1985; Morrow, 1989) Ross (1991) proposed that there were eight major patterns of bisexuality which could be distinguished worldwide: defensive; Latin; ritual; married; secondary; equal interest in male and female partners; experimental and technical. Without even pausing to explain those categories whose meaning is not self evident, it is easy to see that whilst this ingenious taxonomy of bisexuality is fascinating and not without considerable surface validity, it tells us little of patterns of sexual behaviour. The only common factor between persons in any, or indeed all of these categories is that must, at some point in their lives have sex with both males and females.

Similarly, but far more specifically, Boulton *et al.*, (1989) have identified six distinct patterns of bisexuality: transitional (as part of the process of 'coming out' as gay); unique (almost exclusively homosexual or heterosexual with occasional deviations); serial (alternating patterns of exclusive hetero- and homosexuality); concurrent – straight (predominately heterosexual with some homosexual contacts); concurrent – gay (predominately homosexual with some heterosexual contacts); and, concurrent – contact magazines (large numbers of homosexual and heterosexual contacts).

Since these patterns have the distinct advantage of describing modes and types of sexual contact they are of considerable potential in understanding the sexual behaviour of men that have sex with both men and women. However, since they are based on a small sample (n = 35) of men recruited to a study of bisexuality their validity with regard to describing all men that have sex with both men and women is questionable.

Clearly then, however we define bisexuality it is not a unitary concept. It means various things to various people. As some commentators suggest there may indeed be types of bisexuals (Boulton, 1991). However, this may be fitting into artificial constructed typologies persons who, at best, know nothing of such categorization and, more probably would refuse to be pigeon-holed in such a way.

The Prevalence of Bisexuality

Judging the prevalence of bisexuality is difficult whichever of our earlier broad definitions is adopted. By assuming a widespread social stigma and/or legal constraints attached to such an identity, we recognise that although self-identified bisexuals clearly exist the prevalence of the identity may grossly underestimate the proportion of men (and women) that have sex with both men and women. However, we must acknowledge that where the stigma attached to homosexuality is greater than that attached to bisexuality, or where relatively little stigma exists, then we may find that the prevalence of bisexual identified men may overestimate the true rate of behavioural bisexuality. For example, Winkelstein *et al.* (1986) found that among a sample of over 1,000 single men in San Francisco, a city with its own independent bisexual social and commercial scene, while 16.3% of men self-identified as bisexual, only about half of these had had sex with a male and a female in the preceding year. In short, not only may behavioural bisexuals not necessarily identify as bisexual, but self-identified bisexuals may not necessarily currently engage in behavioural bisexuality.

As we have discussed it is possible to concentrate on those persons whose behavioural patterns identify them as bisexual even if their self-proclaimed identity does not. Whilst this would appear to be an appropriate means of moving debates forward, especially for those concerned with HIV related issues, it makes it especially difficult to judge the prevalence of behavioural bisexuality. Before we can make any estimate of prevalence we need to discuss rates of behavioural bisexuality among men who identify as gay or heterosexual, whilst recognising the stigma attached to bisexuality from both communities.

Gay Men

Most estimates of the size of the 'homosexual population' begin with Kinsey's finding that 4% of the men in his sample were exclusively homosexual in behaviour (1948). This figure is then adjusted (often on the flimsiest of pretexts) so that, for example Magee's (1966) book on the subject is entitled 'One in Twenty'. Most British commentators (for example, Schofield, 1965; West, 1968; 1977) take Kinsey's figures and refer to the conclusion of the Wolfenden committee (1957) that similar figures obtain in the UK. It is worth, therefore, reproducing Wolfenden's remarks

> '... some of our medical witnesses expressed the view that something very like (Kinsey's) figures would be established in this country if similar enquiries were made. The majority, while stating quite frankly that they really did not know, indicated that their impression was that his figures would be on the high side for Great Britain.' (para. 38)

Thus, the guesses of a group of medics, who freely admitted their ignorance established the received wisdom on the prevalence of homosexuality for more than a thirty years. With the advent of the UK's own national study of sexual attitudes and behaviour (Johnson *et al.*, 1992) it is likely that their figures will gain as much prominence in the years to come. They report 6.1% of men ever having any homosexual experience; 3.6% reporting ever having a homosexual partner (that is, a male partner with whom anal sex or oro-genital sex or other forms of genital contact had occurred); 1.4% reporting a partner in the past 5 years; and 1.1% in the last year.

Which of these two remarkable studies reflects the true picture of the proportion of men in the whole population which have ever, or are currently, homosexually active is likely to fuel heated debate for some considerable time. Whilst Kinsey's (1948) study has the advantage of a staggering depth and breadth of coverage its sampling frame is relatively weak and it may be both temporally and culturally specific. On the other hand, the methods adopted by the British study mean that the estimates will necessarily be underestimates of the true level (see below).

More importantly in this context, whatever the overall proportion of homosexually active males within the overall population, studies suggest that less than half of those persons who identify as gay or lesbian have been exclusively homosexual throughout their lifetimes (Weatherburn *et al.*, 1990; Fitzpatrick *et al.*, 1989; Bennett *et al.*, 1989). Furthermore, as table 10.1 demonstrates, studies also suggest that at least 10% of homosexually active men are behaviourally bisexual in any given year (Bell & Weinberg, 1978; DHSS, 1987; Ekstrand *et al.*, 1993) and some 5% are behaviourally bisexual in as short a time period as a month (McManus & McEvoy, 1987; Fitzpatrick *et al.*, 1989; Weatherburn *et al.*, 1990).

In our cohort study of 930 homosexually active males (Weatherburn *et al.*, 1990; Weatherburn et al., 1992; Davies *et al.*, 1993), recruited predominantly from those who lay claim to a gay identity and consider themselves attracted exclusively or primarily to men, we found that not only had 61% engaged in sexual behaviour with a female during the course of their lifetime but that in the last year 9.3% have had sex with both men and women and 2.5% had sex only with women. These figures tie in fairly closely with the Kinsey ratings reported by the cohort, in which

TABLE 10.1
Rates of 'bisexuality' in studies of homosexually active men

McManus & McEvoy (1987) UK: 1,292 homosexually active males responding to postal questionnaire	Reported current female partner	5%
DHSS (1987) UK: 3 sets of gay or venues (n = 298, 284, 251)	Female partner in last year	27% 32% 29%
Fitzpatrick et al. (1989) UK: 356 men who had sex with a man in last 5 years	Female partner in: Last month Last year Lifetime	 4% 10% 58%
Bennett et al. (1989) Australia: 176 homosexually active males recruited from venues attracting 'closeted' homosexuals	Female partner in: Last 6 months Lifetime	 31% 82%
Weatherburn et al. (1990) UK: 930 homosexually active males	Female partner in: Last month Last year Lifetime	 5.4% 11.7% 60.6%
Humphreys (1970) USA: 100 men who engaged in sex with men in public toilets	Married to and living with female partner	54%
Bell & Weinberg (1978) USA: 685 men with same sex preference	Female partner in last year: White homosexual males Black homosexual males	 14% 22%
Ekstrand et al (1993) USA: probability sample of 1,034 single men who had sex with a man in last two years	Self identified as bisexual Self identified as bisexual and female partner in last 2 years	13.5% 10.4%

just over 90% identified themselves as either predominantly or exclusively homosexual. However, if our primary interest in behavioural bisexuality amongst gay or bisexual identified population is in risk behaviours, we must note that in the year before interview, only 54% of men who had a female partner had engaged in anal intercourse with a male and vaginal intercourse with a female.

Similarly, Fitzpatrick *et al.* (1989) found that 52% of the homosexually active men they interviewed had ever had a female partner, 10% had done so in the preceding year and 9% thought of themselves as bisexual. However, a third of those that thought of themselves as bisexual had not had a female partner in the previous year, whilst almost half of those men that did report a female partner in that time-frame, described themselves as gay.

While, conflicting methodologies have given rise to divergent figures on the prevalence of behavioural bisexuality among gay identified men it is clear that something in the region of half of all men that identify as gay have had sex with a female at some point in their lives. Given that typologies of patterns of bisexuality (Ross, 1991) recognise that many men pass through periods of 'experimentation' prior to sexual identity and sexual object choice becoming more fixed, this is not particularly surprising but it does emphasize what Blumstein & Schwartz (1977) called the discontinuous nature of many men's sexual histories.

More importantly, the studies outlined in table 10.1 emphasize that at least 10% of homosexually active men also have sex with female partners in any given year. Since one year is easily as short enough a time period to have epidemiological significance in terms of HIV transmission, this suggests that at least 1 in 10 of homosexually active and possibly gay identified males are behaviourally bisexual. What exact proportion of this population also identify as bisexual it is impossible to say, but it appears that at least half of them do not. Whilst doubts over the exact proportion of homosexually active males in the population render any further conjecture unwise it seems relatively clear then, that a significant proportion of gay identified men are behaviourally bisexual.

Heterosexuals

General population surveys invariably collect data on the overall proportion of men in the sample that report ever having sex with a man, or having sex with both men and women. Unfortunately methodological incompatibilities (such as exact questions or time frames used) make comparison of these data difficult, and these problems are compounded by factors such as the failure to collect data relating to sexual identity and details of sexual practices, and by cultural and temporal differences.

As we can see from table 10.2 the estimated rate of lifetime behavioural bisexuality in the general population varies between 1.5% (Foreman & Chilvers, 1989) and 46% (Kinsey *et al.*, 1948). While some of this variance must clearly arise from sampling and design differences this amounts to massive variation in potential rates. While some, if not most of these estimates include homosexually active men that self-identify as gay or bisexual (Johnson *et al.*, 1992; ACSF, 1992; Sundet *et al.*, 1988; Ross, 1988) failure to report on sexual identity makes it difficult to judge exactly what effect such variables would have on estimates of the rate of behavioural bisexuality.

In fact the only studies that report such issues in sufficient detail to make any estimate of the proportion of heterosexual men that have engaged in sexual activity with both men and women are Kinsey *et al.* (1948); and Lever *et al.* (1989). Taking

TABLE 10.2
Rates of 'bisexuality' or homosexual experience in general population surveys

Foreman & Chilvers (1989) UK: 480 white men aged 15–49 years	Ever had 'homosexual intercourse' and had female partners	1.5%
Sundet *et al.* (1988) Norway: random sample of about 6,300 men and women	Men who ever had partners of both sexes	2.9%
Johnson *et al.* (1992) UK: 18,876 men and women from random household survey*	Ever had 'homosexual partner'	3.6%
	Ever had homosexual experience	6.1%
ACSF (1992) France: 9.928 men from random househould survey*	Ever had male partner	4.1%
	Ever had both male and female partners	3.2%
Ross (1988) Australia: geographically stratified sample of 2601 persons over 21 years old	Currently married men with male partner in last year	4.2%
	Previously married men with a male partner in the last year	6.4%
Lever *et al.* (1989) USA: 62,352 men answering Playboy readers' survey	Adult homosexual and heterosexual experiences	120%
	Adult homo- and heterosexual experiences and identified as bisexual	3.4%
Kinsey *et al.* (1948) USA: about 5300 men in convenience sample	Overt homosexual experience to orgasm after adolescence, but not exclusively homosexual	33.0%
	Neither exclusively homosexual or exclusively heterosexual	46.0%

Kinsey *et al.* (1948) first we must recognise that the study has proved seminal for two main reasons. First, it revealed that the incidence of homosexual behaviour was much greater than had hitherto been supposed. Secondly, it suggested that men could be arranged along a continuum of sexual response, moving from those who are completely heterosexual in their behaviour, to whom he gave a 'score' of 0, through varying degrees of mixed heterosexual-homosexual response, to those who are completely homosexual, to whom he gave a 'score' of 6. It is not clear whether a seven-point scale is preferable to one with any other number of grades in dividing up this continuum, and indeed, Kinsey specifically refers to gradations within each of the categories (p. 647), but the labelling has entered into the realm of common knowledge. Kinsey writes pungently:

> 'Males do not represent two discrete populations, heterosexual and homosexual. The world is not divided into sheep and goats. Not all things are black nor all things white ... Only the human mind invents categories and tries to force facts into separated pigeonholes. The living world is a continuum in each and every one of its aspects. The sooner we learn this concerning human sexual behaviour, the sooner we shall reach a sound understanding of the realities of sex'.

In fact, although nearly 50 years have passed since the bulk of this data was collected it is worth reiterating at length Kinsey's summative generalisations (p. 650–1) on the incidence of homosexual behaviour. He records that in the white male population as covered by his study:

37% of the total male population has at least some overt homosexual experience to the point of orgasm between adolescence and old age.
30% have at least incidental homosexual experience or reactions over a three year period between the ages of 16 and 55.
25% has more than incidental homosexual experience or reactions for at least three years between the ages of 16 and 55.
18% have at least as much of the homosexual as the heterosexual in sexual their histories.
13% has more of the homosexual than the heterosexual for at least three years between the ages of 16 and 55.
10% are more or less exclusively homosexual for at least three years between the ages of 16 and 55.
8% are exclusively homosexual for at least 3 years between the ages of 16 and 55.
4% are exclusively homosexual after the onset of adolescence.

If we subtract Kinsey's (1948) figure of 4% exclusively homosexual from his 37% of the total male population which has overt homosexual experience to the point of orgasm between adolescence and old age, then we find that 33% of males are behaviourally bisexual over their lifetimes. Alternatively, if we exclude 'to the point of orgasm' Kinsey *et al.*, (1948) report that, through the course of their lives 50% of men are exclusively heterosexual, 4% are exclusively homosexual and 46% are behaviourally bisexual.

Recent national surveys of sexual behaviour in both the UK (Johnson *et al.*, 1992) and France (ACSF, 1992) have suggested that Kinsey's figures on the prevalence of homosexual activity are overestimates. The difference is said to emerge from the fact that Kinsey was collecting his data during the War years when homosexual activity was particularly prevalent. Alternatively, it is possible that these national studies underestimate the prevalence of homosexually active men because of factors such as political and moral sensitivity dictating question style and content; fear around confidentiality and anonymity where participation is not on a volunteer only basis; and where a massive number of interviewers is necessary. While factors such as these are not necessarily specific to massive random household surveys, they serve as exemplars of problems that are especially important in studies of this scale. While such studies are necessary to assess broad parameters of sexual behaviour their sheer scale necessitates simple coverage of some very complex issues.

Turning to Lever *et al.*'s (1989) study of 80,324 readers of Playboy magazine we find that 86.7% of their male sample are exclusively heterosexual; 1.3% are exclusively homosexual; 11.1% are predominantly heterosexual; and 0.9% are predominately homosexual. If we sum the later two categories we find that 12% of the male readers of soft-porn are behaviourally bisexual. Of these 7,484 behaviourally bisexual males 28.2% define themselves as bisexual and 69.9% define themselves as heterosexual. Of course there are problems with extrapolating from a readers' survey of a heterosexually orientated soft-porn magazine to the wider population but, one could reasonably argue, these problems should serve to underestimate the reported rate of homosexual activity, rather than exaggerate it.

Clearly then these data confirm that a significant proportion of heterosexually identified men in the entire population are behaviourally bisexual, at least at some point in their lives. While exact rates have, thus far, proved impossible to quantify it seems fair to assert that the figure lies somewhere in the region of 5–15%. If forced, the authors' best guess would be closer to Lever *et al.*'s (1989) figure of 12% than Johnson *et al.*'s (1992) 6.1%, whilst recognizing that this is significantly lower than Kinsey *et al.* (1948) would predict. Based on the fact that about one fifth of gay identified men that are behaviourally bisexual in their lifetimes are also behaviourally bisexual in any given year, then we can also estimate that about 1–2% of heterosexually identified men are behaviourally bisexual in any given year.

While all these data definitely confirm is that exact estimates of the rate of behavioural bisexuality are very difficult to obtain, they do indicate that, irrespective of self-proclaimed sexual identity, a significant proportion of all men are behaviourally bisexual. They also indicate that homosexual activity is not only not confined to men that identify as gay or bisexual, but that the assumption that it is likely to be dangerously misleading.

CONCLUSION

Perhaps the most important implication of all the above is the simple recognition that sexual identity neither precludes nor prescribes any sexual activity or practice. There is no straightforward relationship between sexual identity and sexual behaviour. Not only do a significant proportion of gay men have sex with females partners, but there is substantial evidence to suggest that some proportion of heterosexually identified men have sex with male partners. In the majority of these cases the behavioural bisexuality of these men does not appear to lead to a bisexual identity.

Two agendas emerge from this conclusion. First, it is appropriate to extend epidemiological studies and those involved with parameterisation to include the large proportion of behaviourally bisexual men and women who do not identify as bisexual. While this is not a simple undertaking, neither is it impossible, as other studies of difficult to define and socially invisible groups have shown. Secondly, studies of and interventions in bisexual communities need to be move beyond parameterisation and identify the ways in which such communities have an impact on HIV preventative behaviour. It may, indeed, be appropriate in some circumstances actively to encourage the formation of groups of this kind.

These agenda are appropriate – indeed urgent – for many Western countries. As HIV prevention programmes emerge in other cultures, however, it is equally important for us not to attempt to impose our very different cultural traditions or understandings of 'bisexuality'. What is appropriate in London, Paris or San Francisco will not necessarily be appropriate in Rio de Janiro or Mexico City.

REFERENCES

ACSF Investigators, (1992) AIDS and Sexual Behaviour in France. *Nature*, **360**, 407–409.

Bell, A.P., & Weinberg, M.S., (1978) Homosexualities: A Study of Diversity Among Men and Women; New York,Simon and Schuster.

Bennett, G., Chapman, S., & Bray, F. (1989) A potential source for the transmission of the human immunodeficiency virus into the heterosexual population: bisexual men who frequent 'beats'. *Medical Journal of Australia,* **151**, 314–318

Blumstein, P., Schwartz, P. (1977) Bisexuality in Men; *Urban Life*, **5**, 339–358

Boulton, M., Schramm Evans, Z., Fitzpatrick, R., Hart, G. (1989) Bisexual Men: Identity and Behaviour in Sexual Encounters. Paper presented at the twenty first Annual Conference of the Medical Sociology Group, Manchester, England.

Boulton, M., Weatherburn, P. (1990) Literature Review on Bisexuality and HIV transmission. Report commissioned by the Social and Behavioural Research Unit, Global Programme on AIDS, World Health Organization, July 1990.

Boulton, M., (1991) Review of the Literature on Bisexuality and HIV Transmission. In Tielman R.A.P, Carballo M., Hendriks A.C., (eds) Bisexuality and HIV/AIDS: A Global Perspective, New York, Prometheus Books, pp. 187–209.

Carrier, J.M., (1971) Participants in Urban Mexican Male Homosexual Encounters; *Archives of Sexual Behaviour*, 1(4), 279–291.

Carrier, J.M., (1976) Cultural Factors Affecting Urban Mexican Male Homosexual Behaviour; *Archives of Sexual Behaviour*, 5(2), 103–124.

Davies, P.M., Hickson, F.C.I., Weatherburn, P., Hunt, A.J. (1993) Gay Men, Sex and AIDS. London, Falmer Press.

DHSS (Department of Health and Social Security) AIDS: Monitoring response to the Public Health Education Campaign, February 1986 – February 1987, London, HMSO.

Ekstrand, M.L., Coates, T.J., Guydish, J.R., Hauck, W.W., Collette, M.S., Hulley, S.B. (1992) Bisexual Men are Not a Common Vector for Spreading HIV Infection to Women: The San Francisco Men's Health Study, *American Journal of Public Health*, (under review).

Fitzpatrick, R., Hart, G., Boulton, M., McLean, J., Dawson, J. (1989) Heterosexual sexual behaviour in a sample of homosexually active males. *Genito-Urinary Medicine*, **65**, 259–262.

Foreman, D., Chilvers, C. (1989) Sexual Behaviour of Young and Middle-Aged Men in England and Wales. *British Medical Journal*, **298**, 1137–1142.

Garcia Garcia, M. de L., Valdespino, J., Izazola, J., Palacios, M., Sepulveda, J., (1991) Bisexuality in Mexico: Current Perspectives in Tielman R.A.P, Carballo M., Hendriks A.C., (eds) Bisexuality and HIV/AIDS: A Global Perspective, New York, Prometheus Books, pp. 41–58.

Hansen, C.E., Evans, A. (1985) Bisexuality Reconsidered: An Idea in Pursuit of a Definition. *Journal of Homosexuality,* 11(1&2), 1–6.

Humphreys, L. (1970) Tearoom Trade: Impersonal Sex in Public Places Chicago, Aldine.

Johnson, A.M., Laga, M. (1988) Heterosexual transmission of HIV. *AIDS,* 2(suppl 1), S49-S56.

Johnson, A.M., Wadsworth, J., Wellings, K., Bradshaw, S., Field, J. (1992) Sexual Lifestyles and HIV Risk. *Nature,* 360, 410–412.

Kinsey, A.C., Pomeroy, W.B., Martin, C.E. (1948) Sexual Behaviour in the Human Male. Philadelphia, W.B. Saunders.

Kippax, S., Dowsett, G.W., Davis, M., Rodden, P., Crawford, J. (1992) Sustaining Safe Sex or Relapse: Gay Men's Response to HIV; paper presented at the VIIIth International Conference on AIDS, Amsterdam, TuD 0545.

Klein, F., Sepekoff, B., Wolf, T.J. (1985) Sexual Orientation: A Multi-Variable Dynamic Process. *Journal of Homosexuality,* 11(1&2), 35–49.

Lancaster, R.N., (1988) Subject Honour and Object Shame: The Construction of Male Homosexuality and Stigma in Nicaragua; *Ethnology,* 27(2), 111–125.

Lever, J., Roger, W., Carson, S.P., Hertz, R., Kanouse, D. Behavioural Patterns of Bisexual Men in the US in 1982. VIIth International Conference on AIDS, Montreal, Canada, 1989, Abstract TDP 18.

MacDonald, A., (1986) Bisexuality: some comments on research and theory. *Journal of Homosexuality,* 6, 21–36.

Magee, B. (1966) One in Twenty. London, Secker and Warburg.

McManus, T.J., McEvoy, M. (1987) Some Aspects of Male Homosexual Beaviour in the UK: a Preliminary Study. *British Journal of Sexual Medicine,* April.

Morrow, G.D., (1989) Bisexuality: An Exploratory Review. *Annals of Sex Research,* 2, 283–306.

Murray, S.O. (1992) The 'Underdevelopment' of Modern/Gay Homosexuality in Meso-America; in Plummer, K. (ed): Modern Homosexualities: Fragments of a Gay and Lesbian Experience; Routledge, London, pp. 29–38.

Padian, N., Marquis, L., Francis, D., *et al.* (1987) Male to female transmission of human immunodeficiency virus. *Journal of the American Medical Association,* 258, 788–791

Paul, J.P. (1984) The Bisexual Identity: An Idea Without Social Recognition. *Journal of Homosexuality,* 9, 45–63.

Ross, M.W. (1979) Bisexuality: Fact or Fallacy? *British Journal of Sexual Medicine,* (Feb): 49–50.

Ross, M.W. (1988) Prevalence of Risk Factors for HIV Infection in the Australian Population. *The Medical Journal of Australia,* 149, 362–365.

Ross, M.W. (1991) A Taxonomy of Global Behaviour, in Tielman R.A.P, Carballo M., Hendriks A.C., (eds) Bisexuality and HIV/AIDS: A Global Perspective, New York, Prometheus Books.

Schofield, M. (1965) Sociological Aspects of Homosexuality: A Comparative Study of Three Types of Homosexual. London, Longman.

Sundet, J., Kvalem, I., Magnus, P., Baakketeig, L. (1988) Prevalence of risk-prone sexual behaviour in the general population of Norway. In Fleming *et al.* (eds) 'The Global Impact of AIDS' New York, Allen R Liss.

Tapinc, H. (1992) Masculinity, Femininity and Turkish Male Homosexuality in Plummer, K. (ed): Modern Homosexualities: Fragments of a Gay and Lesbian Experience; Routledge, London, pp. 39–52.

Tielman, R.A.P., Carballo, M., Hendriks, A.C., (eds) (1991) Bisexuality and HIV/AIDS: A Global Perspective, New York, Prometheus Books.

Weatherburn, P., Davies, P.M., Hunt, A.J., Coxon, A.P.M., McManus, T.J. (1990) Heterosexual Behaviour in a Large Cohort of Homosexually Active Men in England and Wales *AIDS Care,* 2(4), 319–324

Weatherburn, P., Hunt, A.J., Hickson, F.C.I., Davies, P.M. (1992) The Sexual Lifestyles of Gay and Bisexual Men in England and Wales. London, HMSO.

West, D.J. (1968) Homosexuality. Harmondsworth, Penguin.

West, D.J. (1977) Homosexuality Reconsidered. Harmondsworth, Penguin.

Winkelstein, W., Wiley, J.A., Padian, N., Levy, J. (1986) Potential for transmission of AIDS-associated retrovirus from bisexual men in San Francisco to their female sexual contacts. *Journal of the American Medical Association,* **256**, 901

Wolf, T.J. (1987) Group Counselling for Bisexual Men. *Journal for Specialists in Group Work,* (Nov): 162–165.

Wolfenden, J. (1957) Report of the Committee on Homosexual Offences and Prostitution, London, HMSO Cmnd 247.

Young, A. (1973) Gay Gringo in Brazil, in The Gay Liberation Book; Ramparts Press, San Francisco, pp. 60–67.

Zinik, G. (1985) Identity Conflict or Adaptive Flexibility? Bisexuality Reconsidered. *Journal of Homosexuality,* 11(1&2), 7–19.

11

Prisons: Heterosexuals in a Risk Environment

PAUL J. TURNBULL AND GERRY V. STIMSON

HIV infection and AIDS in prisons are part of the same epidemic that is being experienced outside of prisons. Far from being isolated communities, prisons in most countries are characterised by a continual flow of people from, and then back into, the community. The prevalence of HIV and AIDS, and the behaviours that risk transmission might therefore be expected to reflect the problems in the wider society. Prisons, however, have a greater concentration of those who may have been exposed to HIV. Implicit to some behaviours with a risk of HIV infection is an element of illegal activity, which can often lead to imprisonment.

As in the community the problem of HIV and AIDS in prisons has a significant heterosexual dimension. Within prisons there are heterosexuals with HIV and behaviours occur among heterosexuals with a risk of HIV transmission. Unlike in the community, though, transmission through heterosexual sex is unlikely within prison and is rarely a behavioural risk issue. Most custodial establishments are single sex institutions or the sexes are segregated. The heterosexual dimension of HIV and AIDS in prison is not immediately obvious, but on further analysis the nature of prison populations, the prevalence of HIV, and the injecting and sexual behaviours that occur within prisons have many implications for heterosexuals within and outside prisons.

Prisons have an additional burden. Prisons do not contain a representative section of the population: they contain disproportionate numbers of younger, more sexually active people who, through their pre-existing sexual and drug using behaviour, are at higher risk of HIV infection (NACRO Briefing, 1990; Farrell and Strang, 1991). Many people who engage in activities which might have a high risk of HIV infection - such as drug injecting and prostitution - are at a greater risk of imprisonment.

Furthermore, prisons draw people from wide geographic areas and diverse cultural backgrounds, and disproportionately represent those with poor social resources – such as the homeless and the poor – and have become repositories for the mentally ill. It has been clearly described in the literature that these people will suffer further deprivation in terms of HIV. Prisons may therefore concentrate people with higher levels of HIV infection and behavioural risk (Brewer and Derrickson, 1992).

Prisons are environments in which some individuals engage in HIV risk behaviours which they would otherwise not do outside. Prisons displace individuals from their usual environments, practices and behaviours, and sexual and drug taking behaviour can alter as a result. For example, some ostensibly heterosexual men may have sex with men in prison since they may desire sexual pleasure. So prisons not only contain a disproportionate number of people with pre-existing risk exposure, but they may also be conducive to novel behaviours for those with no pre-existing risk behaviours.

This population is then placed in conditions which are less than adequate. Many prisons are over-crowded with poor sanitation, and prison medical services are poorly developed and staffed. Prisoners have no access to self-care resources, nor a choice in the medical treatment they receive. Furthermore, these conditions influence the provision of appropriate HIV prevention policies, and humane care for those symptomatic with HIV infection and AIDS. The majority of prisoners do not have access to the resources for HIV prevention (e.g. condoms or cleaning materials, such as bleach for injecting equipment).

These factors all occur within a context of confinement, where institutional needs often take priority over those of the individual (Sim, 1990). Marginalisation, stigmatisation, and unnecessary confinement exacerbate conditions for those at high risk of HIV infection, those with HIV disease, and those needing care and treatment (Harding *et al.*, 1990; Turnbull *et al.*, 1991). Methods of prevention and treatment not only have institutional limitations but, in many countries, face political objections.

Why do these issues that occur within the closed environment of a custodial institution have any relationship to heterosexual AIDS? Exposure to HIV in the prison environment will be translated to people outside as interaction between those who have engaged in risk behaviours in prison and the wider heterosexual community is inevitable. Injecting drug users play a pivotal role in this process (Brewer and Derrickson, 1992). As will be shown, many injecting drug users experience imprisonment, during which many are exposed to the risk of HIV infection (Dolan *et al.*, 1989; Covell *et al.*, 1992). The majority of injecting drug users have heterosexual sexual relationships and, on their release from custody, will resume this pattern of behaviour (Turnbull *et al.*, 1991). Most male injecting drug users have non-injecting female sexual partners (Donoghoe, 1992; Rhodes *et al.* (forthcoming)).

Prisons, therefore, concentrate people at higher risk from diverse geographical areas, who then mix in a setting conducive to high risk behaviour but with few prevention resources. The prison environment is one in which many may be exposed to HIV, some for the first time, who then return to the community.

PRISONS AND HIV: THE INTERNATIONAL CONTEXT

Since the isolation and identification of HIV in 1984, the virus has been found among populations held in prisons. The realisation that these populations would experience disproportionate levels of HIV infection came quickly with a number of studies finding higher than average HIV prevalence across a broad range of prisoners.

Levels of HIV infection in prisons vary widely and tend to reflect levels in the communities from which prisoners are drawn. In the United States the percentage of HIV positives among 9,000 male and female prisoners tested in Iowa between 1986 and 1989 was 0.2%, and 3.4% among 15,000 male prisoners tested in Georgia between 1988 and 1989 (Hammett & Moini, 1990). Much higher rates were found in New York State, where in 1990 it was estimated that 17 to 20%, or approximately 9,000 of the State's 54,000 inmates, were HIV positive. More than 800 had developed symptoms of AIDS (PAAC Notes, 1990).

Harding has estimated the overall prevalence of HIV infection in European prisons to be in excess of 10% (Harding, 1987), but again the prevalence rate varies greatly between, and within, countries. In England and Wales, prisoners known by the Prison Medical Service to be HIV positive (about 60 at any one time) are acknowledged to be only a small proportion of actual cases. In research we conducted in England in 1990–91, an attempt was made to estimate actual levels of HIV infection by interviewing and anonymously testing 452 ex-prisoners within three months of their release. The highest rates of HIV infection were found among those who had injected drugs before imprisonment – 15.5% of women injectors and 7.7% of men. HIV infection was also identified in non-injecting women and in heterosexual non-injecting men (Turnbull *et al.*, 1991).

In France, testing of 500 consecutive entries to one prison found a prevalence of 13%. In 1989 in Les Baumettes prison, Marseille, which has 5,000 admissions per year and 2,000 prisoners at any one time, there were 266 prisoners with HIV infection, including 29 with AIDS and 134 with an AIDS-related complex (Gestaut, 1992).

Screening of more than 30,000 Italian prisoners found 17% to be HIV positive in 1986. Another study in Italy found 36% of drug injectors in prison to be HIV positive, and a rate of 8% for prisoners with no known risk factors (Heilpern & Eggar, 1989).

However, in other European countries, much lower rates have been found. In Belgium an HIV prevalence rate of 1% was found, in Luxembourg 2%, in Cyprus 0% and in Portugal 0.1% (Harding *et al.*, 1990). In a recent study of a Scottish prison an HIV prevalence rate of 4.5% was documented (Bird *et al.*, 1992).

The available information on HIV prevalence shows that in Western European countries injecting drug users are the critical link in transmission within prisons, and ultimately to the heterosexual community. To assess the risk of transmission and the implications of this for the heterosexual community, an understanding of the composition of the prison population and risk behaviours while incarcerated is essential.

PRISON POPULATIONS

The nature and size of prison populations vary greatly. Conditions in which prisoners are accommodated and the arrangement of penal systems are equally diverse. Within countries there may be a mix of young offenders' institutions, holding jails, local jails, and prisons for different categories of prisoner. In England prisons range in size from the smallest which holds less than 100 inmates, to the largest such as Wandsworth and Wormwood Scrubs which might each hold up to 1,500 prisoners (HM Prison Service, 1990).

At any one time, prisons in England and Wales hold around 45,000 remand and sentenced prisoners. But prison populations are not static and in England and Wales the total throughput of prisoners is around 150,000 each year, many of whom are moved from prison to prison.

Prison over-crowding is a particular problem in some countries, though again conditions vary greatly. In the Netherlands and Germany, for example, cells hold a single occupant and integral sanitation is provided. At the other extreme, prisons can be run as a compound or camp system where numerous inmates share large dormitories. In England and Wales many prisoners share cells designed for one occupant: in 1990 nearly 12,000 prisoners did so. Over 40% of prisoners have no access to night sanitation (HM Prison Service, 1990).

Approximately one million people are confined in prisons and jails in the United States. Since 1980, the prison populations of federal prisons in 18 states have doubled in size, while, in the same period, California and New Jersey had three-fold increases (PAAC Notes, 1990).

DRUG INJECTORS IN THE PRISON SYSTEM

Most prisons contain high numbers of drug users and injectors, the majority of whom are heterosexuals. This includes those sentenced for drug offences and others who have been sentenced for illegal activities conducted to finance their drug use.

In New York, 24% of men and 30% of women arrestees reported that they had injected drugs at some time (PAAC Notes, 1990). In England, 11% of men and 23% of women had been dependent on drugs in the six months before imprisonment, and 7% and 15% respectively had injected drugs in the six months preceding imprisonment (Maden *et al.*, 1990 (a),(b)) . It can therefore be estimated that, overall, 7.5% of the prison population in England and Wales, around 3,400 people, had injected prior to imprisonment (Turnbull *et al.*, 1992).

Higher numbers of injectors are reported among Scottish prison populations. In a study in Saughton Prison, Edinburgh, 35% of all inmates interviewed said that they had injected drugs before imprisonment (Dye and Isaacs, 1991).

These data allow a tentative estimate to be made of the prevalence of HIV infection among drug injectors in prison. It might be estimated, using data on the prevalence of injecting before imprisonment and sero-prevalence data on recently released injectors, that there are around 285 drug injectors in prison with HIV infection in England and Wales at any time (Turnbull *et al.*, 1992). Rates of HIV infection may be higher in Scottish prisons.

HIV infection in prisons is thus inextricably linked to drug use. Drug use and drug injecting increases the risk of imprisonment. The majority of problem drug injectors will have been in custody at some time. Research in England has found that between 61% and 76% have been incarcerated (Donoghoe *et al.*, 1990; Stimson *et al.*, 1988; Dolan *et al.*, 1990). Drug injecting also increases the risk of HIV infection. Putting the two together may indicate that the prison population will contain a higher concentration of HIV infection than there is in the community as a whole. In order to understand the dynamics of heterosexual spread and the role of the prison population in the heterosexual transmission of HIV, this group's HIV risk behaviour while in prison is therefore of special significance and requires careful consideration.

HIV RISK BEHAVIOUR WITHIN PRISONS

Drug injecting and sexual behaviour occur within prisons, even though both are often proscribed activities. This, combined with denial that these behaviours occur and the stigma attached to these behaviours, has meant that information on these behaviours within prison has been difficult to collect and is scarce. Much more is known about drug use and drug injecting in prison than about sexual behaviour.

Prisons are not closed systems. A large variety of people have access to prisons, including prisoners' visitors, those providing services in prison, prison staff, and suppliers of the wide range of items consumed within prisons each day, for example food and other materials. Drugs are smuggled into prison institutions through the above routes and others and are used chiefly by those who used drugs before imprisonment.

A wide range of UK evidence suggests that between 25–30% of people who inject drugs before imprisonment manage to continue to do so whilst they are in prison (Stimson *et al.*, 1988; Dolan *et al.*, 1990; Turnbull *et al.*, 1991; Covell *et al.*, 1992). In Scotland, it is reported that 8% of a random sample of *all* prisoners had injected in prison at some time (Power, 1991). Drugs are injected with syringes brought in from outside or stolen from the prison hospital, or with improvised injecting equipment made from makeshift materials.

The restricted supply of syringes in prison means that injecting equipment is normally shared (Stimson *et al.*, 1988; Dolan *et al.*, 1990; Turnbull *et al.*, 1991; Covell *et al.*, 1992). One needle may be passed between many groups of prisoners in different parts of a prison, often being exchanged for drugs. For those who continue to inject in prison, their risk of exposure to HIV infection is undoubtedly increased.

Less is known about sexual behaviour in prison. Levels of sexual activity vary by country and by institution, with high levels of sexual behaviour being reported in American institutions and low levels in prisons in Scotland. Studies conducted in England and Wales have found that the majority of men who engaged in sexual activity while incarcerated had unprotected oral or anal sexual intercourse with other men. The men involved in sexual activity with other men will not be exclusively homosexual or bisexual; some are heterosexual men with no previous history of homosexual contact.

The extent of coerced or non-consensual sexual activity within prisons is believed to be widely under-reported (Heilpern & Eggar, 1989). Research from the United States has estimated various levels of sexual assault at 1% to 2.9% of prisoners (Heilpern & Eggar, 1989). In a study conducted in England and Wales of 29 men reporting sexual activity in prison, eight of those mentioned being pressurized into having sex (Turnbull *et al.*, 1991).

Thus far it would appear that the risk of HIV transmission is present in prison but only exceptionally on a scale and in such circumstances as to propel HIV infection. There are only a few studies which have mapped trends in sero-conversion within custodial settings. The limited amount of data available suggests low HIV transmission rates. In the United States, the Federal Bureau of Prisons reported data based on 98,000 time interval tests, which showed only 14 sero-conversions, all of which occurred within the first six months of confinement. In a study of sero-conversion within Maryland prisons, in a population of 422, there were 29 who were infected with HIV at incarceration and two who sero-converted while in prison.

However, there are exceptional circumstances. The major outbreak of HIV infection among drug injectors in Thailand, rising from 0 to 40% within the space of a few months, probably first occurred within the Thai prison system. It was only identified when prisoners were subsequently released, due to an amnesty, and when many of the drug users recently released from prison were tested for HIV at methadone clinics. Though these conditions were unusual, and not entirely a comparable situation, they clearly demonstrate the potential spread of HIV within a custodial setting.

RISK IN THE COMMUNITY AND IN PRISON

Comparing the risk of HIV transmission within prisons with that outside is difficult. Nevertheless, it is the key to assessing the role of prisons in the spread of heterosexual AIDS. While injecting diminishes in prison, those who continue to inject are much more likely to share syringes. Injectors who have adopted safe injecting practices in the community (by not sharing used injecting equipment or by cleaning used equipment effectively) are unlikely to have these alternatives available to them in prison. For those who continue to inject and share in prisons the patterns of social mixing are different: those in custody are effectively sharing outside of their usual social network. Prisoners are drawn from large geographical areas and there is considerable movement of prisoners between prisons. The multiple use of syringes by drug injectors within prison may mean that they are effectively sharing with more people inside than outside and are exposed to many different networks of sharers.

The occurrence of sexual intercourse is again less frequent in prison, but when it does occur it is of higher risk, due to the unavailability of condoms. Those sexually active in prison may be engaging in a novel type and pattern of behaviour with a network of partners from diverse geographical locations. Such people may be exposed to HIV for the first time while in prison.

The fact that the vast majority of prisoners are eventually released into the community means that any exposure to HIV in the prison setting may be transmitted to people outside. Conversely, the risk of HIV transmission in prison will inevitably increase as the prevalence of HIV among those entering custodial institutions increases. This in turn augments the risk of HIV transmission to those linked to the released prisoner population through risky sexual activity and or injecting behaviour. On their release, injectors, who have been exposed to HIV in prison, return to previous sharing networks and to their sexual partners, many of whom do not themselves inject drugs (Donoghoe, 1992; Rhodes *et al.*, forthcoming). Similarly, men who had sex with men in prison may return to previous (heterosexual) sexual partners. These scenarios suggests the link between the potential transmission of HIV infection in prisons to the heterosexual population outside.

THE PRISON RESPONSE

In epidemiological terms, the heterosexual aspects of HIV infection and AIDS in prisons in England and Wales are still predominantly problems of prevention rather than the care and treatment of people with HIV disease.

This is not to underestimate the challenge to providers of care and treatment for people with HIV disease within prison. Prisons internationally are backwaters of health care. Many American prisons have no formal arrangements for medical care, and some only call on outside help when needed. A few have no medical facility whatsoever. In England and Wales there are only 104 full-time Medical Officers in prisons, supplemented by 300 National Health Service (NHS) doctors working part-time. Over half of prisons are served entirely by part-time NHS doctors. Many prisons worldwide use irregular prison staff to provide nursing care.

Prisons have often failed to keep pace with developments in AIDS treatment in the community. One study in New York found that the median time from diagnosis to death was 159 days for prisoners with AIDS who had a history of drug injecting, compared to 318 days for non-prisoners with similar drug histories. A quarter of AIDS cases within New York prisons were not diagnosed until autopsy (PAAC Notes, 1990).

In the immediate future, the main heterosexual risk is connected with drug injecting. However, the scale of HIV prevention activities for drug injectors in prison is currently minimal. There is a movement towards a public health model of HIV prevention within many countries; however, this model has not yet been adapted by prisons. This lack of foresight may have significant consequences for the spread of heterosexual AIDS.

There are many alternatives to tackle the problem of HIV transmission within prison, some of which can be addressed before people reach prison. For example, prison does not effectively prevent continued drug injection. Many drug injectors carry on injecting in prison and return to drug injecting on release (Turnbull *et al.*,

1991; Dolan *et al.*, 1990). Prison cannot be seen as providing a short or longer term solution to individuals' drug problems. Consideration therefore has to be given to the diversion of drug injectors from custody and the provision of suitable alternative help and treatment in the community. This is an issue for all involved in law enforcement and the criminal justice system. The rising number of injectors in prisons throughout the world should force a major revision of the place of the criminal justice system in the management of the drug user (Brewer, 1991).

There are many disincentives to prisoners to reveal their pre-prison risk behaviour or HIV status if known. In many prisons worldwide, testing, where it takes place, is conducted more in the interests of staff than of prisoners, and may serve as a basis for segregation, and consequently encourages marginalisation and stigmatisation.

This discrimination against drug injectors, men who have sex with men and HIV positive people within prison, discourages them from seeking education, testing and treatment. This curtails efforts to prevent new HIV infection and to treat persons living with HIV disease.

The occurrence of unprotected sexual intercourse in prison means that consideration must be given to this in any HIV prevention strategy. Providing condoms and education on their use would be one way to help to reduce the risk of sexual transmission. The provision of condoms within prisons is a difficult and contentious issue, however, and in England and Wales this does not occur. Nevertheless, many prison systems in Europe make condoms available. In a recent survey of 32 prison systems in 17 European countries, 22 reported that condoms were available to prisoners (Harding & Schaller, 1992).

In Britain, prisoners are unlikely to be offered treatment for their drug problems of a standard and quality of that which is available in the community. Indeed there is every incentive to drug users not to disclose their drug use because of the discrimination and marginalisation they may suffer. This position has to be reversed, and this can only be achieved by providing access to acceptable drug treatment on demand, delivered in a supportive and non-coercive manner. Treatment for problem drug use should be expanded and made more 'user-friendly'.

It is only recently that methadone detoxification has been introduced into many prisons in England and Wales. While this is a step in the right direction this treatment option will be insufficient: methadone maintenance should also be made available as it is in the community. In a variety of settings methadone maintenance has been shown to reduce the risk of HIV infection through lessening injecting and syringe sharing, and it has been suggested it would be feasible and practical to include this as a treatment option within prisons (Ball *et al.*, 1988; Serraino *et al.*, 1989).

The sharing of needles and syringes is a complex issue. For a number of reasons it is unlikely that sterile injecting equipment will be made available in UK prisons, as they are in the community, through syringe exchange and distribution schemes. Some prisons have offered information on syringe cleaning in general literature on HIV and AIDS, and bleach is made available to disinfect used syringes in prisons in San Francisco and in Melbourne. The provision of cleaning agents, such as bleach, to disinfect needles and syringes, with ease of access, confidentiality and instructions on use appears to be an acceptable compromise, and is an effective measure which must be given high priority.

Prison provides an opportunity to educate and inform a population that other initiatives may have missed. The freeflow of people into and out of prisons, and the movement of individuals from communities back to their partners, provides a suitable population for HIV education. HIV and AIDS education should be a priority for all prisons: programmes can target risk behaviours that occur in prison and in the community. Education needs to be provided for both prisoners and staff, and should provide explicit and clear advice about resources available within the prison setting (and the community) for HIV prevention.

However, prisoners may distrust the provision of advice, help and treatment by prison authorities. This indicates the need for outside organisations, including the broader health care system and agencies specifically involved in AIDS and drug use, to be brought into prison to provide such services.

The initiatives outlined above will not come about through goodwill alone. Prisons are vastly under-resourced and have many competing priorities. HIV and AIDS is but one issue in the daily round of prison life; overcrowding, poor sanitation, boredom and security are all competing interests. But the potential for the spread of HIV within prisons and the wider community must not be understated.

It is necessary to ensure that strategies for HIV prevention, for care and treatment, and for dealing with drug use, are codified with clear and itemised details of service and quality standards. This means bringing HIV and AIDS, and drugs, within the sphere of competence of prison scrutineers, whether these are national prison bodies or external visitors.

PRISONS AND PUBLIC HEALTH

HIV and AIDS provide us with a 'diagnosis' of disabling and disabled institutions. They bring into sharp relief the inadequacies of our health, welfare and penal systems. It is difficult to graft HIV and AIDS prevention and care services onto a prison health care system that cannot yet provide decent basic welfare and health services. However, the health and welfare of the prison population is inextricably linked with the health and welfare of the population as a whole.

Prisons could serve as an exceptional place to achieve public health objectives in the prevention of HIV infection. HIV serves to highlight serious shortfalls in prison health care and appropriate AIDS policies, and developing appropriate HIV and AIDS policies is linked with an improvement in prison health care. Traditionally, many prisons' medical care systems have been solely oriented towards treatment, and have not easily adopted a public health perspective, yet it is vitally important that this approach becomes part of prison medical practice. Failure to do so may have major consequences for the spread of HIV and for those within and outside of prisons.

ACKNOWLEDGEMENT

The authors wish to acknowledge AVERT for the support they have given to this work.

REFERENCES

Ball, J.C., Myers, C.P., Friedman, S.R. (1988) Reducing the risk of AIDS through methadone maintenance treatment. *Journal of Health and Social Behaviour*, **29**, 214–226.

Bird, A.G., Gore, S.M., Jolliffe, D.W., Burns, S.M. Anonymous HIV surveillance in Saughton Prison, Edinburgh. *AIDS, 6*, 623–628.

Brewer, T.F. (1991) HIV in prisons: the pragmatic approach. *AIDS, 5*, 897.

Brewer, T.F., Derrickson, J. (1992) AIDS in prison: a review of epidemiology and preventive policy. *AIDS, 6*, 623–628.

Covell, R.G., Frischer, M., Taylor, A., Goldberg, S.G., Mckeganey, N., Bloor, M. Prison experience of injecting drug users in Glasgow. Forthcoming in *Drug and Alcohol Dependence.*

Dolan, K.A., Donoghoe, M.C., Stimson, G.V. (1990) Drug injecting and syringe sharing in custody and the community: an exploratory survey of HIV risk behaviour. *The Howard Journal of Criminal Justice, 29*(3), 177–186.

Donoghoe. M.C. (1992) Sex, HIV and the injecting drug user. *British Journal of Addiction, 87*, 405–416.

Donoghoe, M.C., Dolan, K.A., Stimson, G.V. (1990) National Syringe Exchange Monitoring Study. Interim Report. The Centre for Research on Drugs and Health Behaviour, Charing Cross and Westminster Medical School.

Dye, S., Isaacs, C. (1991) Intravenous drug misuse among inmates: implications for spread of HIV. *British Medical Journal, 302*, 1507.

Farrell, M., Strang, J. (1991) Drugs, HIV, and prisons. *British Medical Journal, 302*, 1477–1478.

Gastaut, J.A., Durrand, D.W., Jussy, R. (1992) Health Care for HIV positive patients at the 'Baumettes' prison, Marseille, France. VIII International Conference on AIDS, Amsterdam, July 1992; PoD 5057- D396

Hammet, T., Moini, S. (1990) HIV/AIDS in U.S. prisons and jails: epidemiology, policy and programmes. Presented at the HIV/AIDS and Prisons Conference November 1990 Melbourne, Australia.

Harding, T. (1987) AIDS in Prison. *The Lancet*, 1260–1263.

Harding, T., Manghi, R., Sanchez, G. (1990) HIV/AIDS and Prisons: a survey covering 54 prison systems in 45 countries. *Report commissioned by the World Health Organisation Global Programme on AIDS*, Geneva.

Harding, T., Schaller, G. (1992) HIV/AIDS and Prisons: Updating and Policy Review. *Report for the World Health Organisation Global Programme on AIDS*, Geneva.

Heilpern, H., Egger, S. (1989) AIDS in Australian prisons. Issues and Policy Options. *Report commissioned by Department of Community Services and Health,* Canberra.

HM Prison Service Report on the work of the Prison Services April 1989 – March 1990.

NACRO Briefing. (1990) Imprisonment in England and Wales: some facts and figures.

Maden, A., Swinton, M., Gunn, J. (1990a) Drug dependence in prison. *British Medical Journal,* **302**, 880.

Maden, A., Swinton, M., Gunn, J. (1990b) Women in prison and use of illicit drugs before arrest. *British Medical Journal,* **301**, 1133.

PAAC Notes, News Journal of the Physicians Association for AIDS Care (1990). *National Commission on AIDS releases report on HIV disease in correctional facilities.* 3(1), 16–21.

Power, K.G., Markova, I., Rowlands, A., McKee, K.J., Anslow, P.J., Kilfedder, C. (1992) Intravenous drug use and HIV transmission amongst inmates in Scottish prisons. *British Journal of Addiction* 87, 35–45.

Rhodes, T.J., Donoghoe, M.C., Hunter, G.M., Stimson, G.V. (Forthcoming *British Journal of Addiction*).

Serraino, D., Franchesschi, C. (1989) Methadone maintenance programmes and AIDS. *Lancet,* 30, 22.

Sim, J. (1990) Medical power in prisons. Milton Keynes: Open University Press.

Stimson, G.V., Alldritt, L.J., Dolan, K.A., Donoghoe, M.C., Lart, R.A. (1988) Injecting Equipment Exchange Schemes: *Final Report. Monitoring Research Group, Goldsmiths' College,* London.

Turnbull, P.J., Dolan, K.A., Stimson, G.V. (1991) Prisons, HIV and AIDS: Risks and Experiences in Custodial Care. Horsham: AVERT.

Turnbull, P.J., Stimson, G.V., Dolan, K.A. (1992) Prevalence of HIV infection among ex-prisoners in England. *British Medical Journal,* 304, 90–91.

12

HIV Testing, Counselling and Behaviour change

LORRAINE SHERR AND SUSAN QUINN

HIV infection continues unabated. From the first awareness of the epidemic the crucial role of behaviour change for prevention of initial infection and subsequent limitation of virus spread was acknowledged. Early in the 1980s a test was available to examine the presence of antibody for HIV. The HIV antibody test has been an invaluable tool in the management of the epidemic worldwide. The test, however has strengths and limitations. As an antibody test it only registers presence of antibody after a period of anything up to 12 weeks. It also gives no further information such as mode of infection, time of infection, disease state, virus concentration, presence or absence of opportunistic infections or prognosis.

The test itself, though fairly simple to implement, carries a high emotional consequence (Perry, 1990) and from the initiation of the test there has been a concerted effort to ensure optimum procedure in test handling. This has included, in the main, a careful examination of HIV factors for the individual potentially facing HIV testing, thorough pre and post test counselling and discreet handling of results. Such handling allows not only for psychological preparation for the test and outcome, but also allows an opportunity for intervention in individual risk behaviour which may need adjustment irrespective of whether the person being counselled proceeds to be tested or not, or whether the test is positive or negative. Such pre and post test counselling has prompted widespread international training of counsellors.

Pre and post test counselling (Green & McCreaner, 1989) are time consuming and costly procedures. They have been justified not only on the criteria of quality of

This chapter was drawn from a study funded by the AIDS Unit, Department of Health UK to the British Psychological Society AIDS/HIV Special Interest group on. The authors gratefully acknowledge the assistance of the DOH and members of the BPS AIDS/HIV Special Interest group.

care, but on a variety of other dimensions. As testing for HIV carries a high emotional cost, such counselling has been put forward as 'preventive medicine' to ameliorate, prevent or prepare clients for intense emotional reactions. Furthermore it has been argued that behaviour change is a necessary component of HIV disease management. Although behaviour change is often not explicit in testing procedure, there is a need to examine the extent to which such counselling has been effective in behaviour change, and whether this is true of all groups, particularly heterosexuals, in this context.

The literature has revealed that such an examination is highly complicated and many questions remain unanswered. The seemingly straightforward question 'does counselling for sexual behaviour change work?' is complex and may well prove unhelpful. Instead the empirical questions should be concerned with the ways in which such intervention can be shown to work; on whom, under which circumstances, in which setting, under which conditions and for how long. There should also be an understanding of the limitations of such interventions, when they are frustrated, why they do not reach a desired outcome and how this may be remedied.

Broad groups of the population have been the subject of HIV testing – many such groups drawn from heterosexual subsamples in different countries. Ideally such testing has been carried out in the presence of pre and post test counselling. This chapter sets out to examine the links between such HIV testing, counselling and behaviour change. Such an analysis will provide a comprehensive insight into the potential role of HIV testing and counselling in HIV containment and the implications and pitfalls of such procedures. This raises a number of questions:

1. What is involved in HIV testing?
2. What do the studies show on testing and its ramifications?
3. Are there systematic differences between groups?
4. To what extent has behaviour change been monitored?
5. Which behaviours are under review?
6. What are the methodological problems with the studies, particularly concerning behavioural and outcome measures?
7. How do the findings compare between heterosexual and gay groups.
8. Are there differences between short and long term outcomes?
9. What are the implications for counsellors?

HETEROSEXUALS

'Heterosexuals' is a term which covers a wide array of individuals. This definition may include their sexuality which in some studies is presumed rather established, but also relates to other categories such as life circumstances (pregnancy, prostitution, prostitute clients, haemophilia, haemophiliac spouses, drug users, drug user partners sexual or sharing) place of abode (general population, urban or rural dwellers), age (adolescents, children, infants) or other factors (blood bank attenders). Testing, counselling and data exist for many of these categories. Of note is a consistent male/female difference where the lower rates of HIV are recorded in females yet the highest levels of testing are prevalent among females. Behaviour change is often noted more in females than males.

COUNSELLING

There are two definitions widely used around HIV work to explain counselling. The British Association for Counselling has developed the following definition, generally endorsed by the Bond report (Bond, 1992).

> "Counselling is the skilled and principled use of relationships which develop self knowledge, emotional acceptance and growth, and personal resources. The overall aim is to live more fully and satisfyingly. Counselling may be concerned with addressing and resolving specific problems, making decisions, coping with crises, working through feelings and inner conflict, or improving relationships with others. The counsellor's role is to facilitate the client's work in ways that respect the client's values, personal resources and capacity for self determination."

The World Health Organization (WHO) Global Programme on AIDS (GPA) provides a definition of HIV counselling (Carballo & Miller, 1989) as follows:

> "HIV counselling is an ongoing dialogue and relationship between the client or patient and counsellor with the aims of preventing HIV transmission and providing psychosocial support to those affected, directly or indirectly, by HIV. In order to achieve these aims, counselling seeks to encourage and enhance self-determination, to boost self confidence, improve family and community relationships and quality of life". Prevention counselling comprises five steps:
> - Examine the lifestyle of the individual or group of individuals and work with them to understand the risks.
> - Identify the meanings such behaviour has for them.
> - Identify and define the potential for behavioural change.
> - Work with the individual to achieve and sustain appropriate and chosen changes in behaviour.
> - Provide a supportive and trusting counsellor and client relationship.

Pre and post HIV test counselling only form a part of the total counselling input to HIV and AIDS care, but often mark the initial contact point.

The components of counselling need specific clarity if different studies are to be compared and contrasted and if outcome data from one area is to be generalised to another area. The very central notions 'counselling' and 'behaviour change' are problematic and therein lies the key to some of the grave difficulties in interpreting this body of research. 'Counselling' has been used as a catch all phrase for a multitude of interventions. It has ranged from unskilled counsellors using scripted dialogue on single occasions, to highly skilled counsellors using in depth intervention on multiple occasions. The extent to which these terms cover the same commodity must come under question and render the studies incapable of comparison. There is also considerable variation as to what is implied by counselling. It is sometimes pre and post test, it is sometimes post test only (and then sometimes only for those who are positive). It is sometimes in depth with lengthy follow up, whereas at others it is short, cursory and not by trained counsellors. Video, information packs, group discussion and face to face interviews have all been reported under the 'counselling' umbrella. A lack of consistency makes comparability low. It includes situations where testing is voluntary or compulsory, planned or unplanned.

WHO DOES THE COUNSELLING

There is great variation on the training of individuals carrying out counselling, and the time and intensity of the counselling sessions (Wilkins *et al.*, 1989). Bor *et al.* (1992) estimate that counselling can take ten minutes and can be carried out by medical staff. Sherr *et al.* (1992) found that non mental health trained health care workers responded well to short training but were unable to shift their personal deeply held myths. Sherr *et al.* (1992) found that General Practitioners felt uncertain about counselling skills and desired training. Furthermore, the less proficient they were with such skills the more likely they were to refer their patients on to hospital care. Meadows *et al.* (1990) in a study of HIV pre test counselling and testing in pregnancy, found that individual personality factors of the midwives accounted for HIV testing uptake more so than client variation or risk factors.

Numerous programmes on counsellor training have been described yet few relate such training to client outcomes such as test uptake, emotional adjustment or simple satisfaction and knowledge gain.

There is some dialogue as to which profession should undertake the counselling (Timmis *et al.*, 1991; Bor *et al.*, 1991; Brown Peterside *et al.*, 1991; Leukefeld *et al.*, 1990; Gillespie *et al.*, 1991; King *et al.*, 1989; Holman *et al.*, 1988; Bor Miller & Salt, 1991; Naji, 1989). It can be done by counselling experts (such as psychologists, social workers or psychiatrists), by health care workers, particularly trained to do the counselling (such as nurses, midwives, doctors) or by lay people also specifically trained. Clearly the higher skilled counsellors are more costly and economic factors are often key elements in deciding protocols. Cockroft (1989) noted that counselling will increasingly become the role of occupational health professionals. At times written information is substituted for counselling. Sherr & Hedge (1990) examined the counselling effects of leaflets to address ante natal needs and found that they had some specific limitations and were best used as adjuncts to counselling rather than substitutes.

BEHAVIOUR CHANGE

'Behaviour change' can refer to total change, partial change, or any change. Some workers look at one off changes, and other, more sophisticated research designs look at change and fluctuation over time. Outcome variables for behaviour change have included several sexual behaviours (such as insertive anal/vaginal sex), prophylactic behaviours (such as the use of condoms), decision making behaviours (such as the decision to terminate or continue a pregnancy) or reproductive behaviours (such as subsequent pregnancies). Some of these behaviours are difficult to equate with each other. Confusion can be further compounded by a lack of systematic timing and monitoring of counselling input in the studies. Some refer to pre HIV test counselling only, others to pre and post test counselling and others only at post test work. Subjects are often blurred, with some studies reporting on the HIV positive, some on the HIV negative and others on both.

Not surprisingly there is a wide variety of findings. In some cases behaviour change is attained, in others it is not. In some cases this is maintained at long term follow up, in others it is not. For some individuals behaviour fluctuates, so that at one follow up point they may be having risk exposure and at a subsequent follow up they may not. Some women terminate their pregnancies, others do not. Some couples split up, others do not. Some people adopt condoms regularly, sporadically or never. The data is at best ambiguous and at worst confusing. Meta studies (Higgins, 1991; Carael, 1991) which have tried to make sense of the data run the risks of comparing studies which are not comparable, of giving equal weighting to badly designed small studies and large prospective cohort studies. In such efforts to simplify the complex, they run the risk of providing biased and inaccurate outcome data.

An analysis of the research also runs the risk of negating a procedure on the grounds of limited outcome when the procedure never set out to address such outcomes in the first place. There is little empirical evidence in the psychological literature that one off interventions have immediate, dramatic and long lasting consequences.

As most of these studies are carried out in the real world as opposed to the laboratory, it would be seen as unethical to either deny a client counselling or to isolate a client from the many other inputs which may intervene between the counselling and behaviour change (such as peer pressure, social norm adjustment, health education, general public information, dialogue with a high status individual such as a doctor or information seeking).

CAN ONE OFF SESSIONS CHANGE BEHAVIOUR?

There is very little general evidence that one off interventions can effect lasting behavioural change. Yet there is certainly anecdotal evidence that this is possible. Different counselling strategies may be more or less effective. There has been little outcome research on this topic. The interventions tried to date include groups (Kelly & Lawrence, 1990; Hedge & Glover, 1990), couples (Usher, 1990), individuals (Ostrow, 1991), mass media (Sherr, 1987) and peer support (Valdiserra *et al.*, 1990).

WHO ARE THE SUBJECTS?

Cross study comparisons are often difficult because subjects are blurred, with the HIV positive and negative appearing in many studies. Risk categorisation is often a theme where groups are divided on a number of indices including risk behaviour (such as gay men, drug users, haemophiliacs), other evidence of sexual behaviour (such as STD attenders, sex workers) those who are part of screening programmes for another reason (such as pregnant women and clinic attenders) those already identified at risk (such as discordant couples) or others simply isolated on the basis of their gender, age or place of residence (such as women, adolescents, inner city dwellers).

THE LINKS BETWEEN HIV COUNSELLING, TESTING AND BEHAVIOUR CHANGE

Testing alone rarely motivates total behavioural change (Miller and Pinching, 1989). The majority of the studies come from gay men revealing that wide ranging behaviour change is possible in the short term. The heterosexual studies are varied.

Heterosexuals

Heterosexuals are generally an under researched group. Work that is to hand often applies to a variety of different cultural settings and it is unclear to what extent data from one such centre can be generalised to another.

Muller *et al*. (1992) reported on a study in Kampala where anonymous counselling and testing were offered. Counselling was provided by 'professional health workers with a 4 week HIV training course'. In total 12,204 clients were tested. No refusal rates were reported. Behavioural intentions stated prior to test results and after test results were examined. No differences were found between those found to be positive and those found to be negative. No data was given on behavioural intentions prior to counselling and testing. 200 clients returned for a follow up visit; 2 (1%) who were initially negative had seroconverted (both urban women), 67% reported that they had maintained sexual relationships within their relationships since the first test result and 19% now used condoms. 25% reported sexual abstinence since the first test result, 6% reported casual sexual contacts; using condoms in 3% of cases. This is in sharp contrast to the pre-test rate of 25% casual sex.

Mhalu *et al*. (1989) studied 605 subjects including 347 women and 258 men from Tanzania. They received counselling for one year and were supplied with condoms. Results showed an increased condom use and lowered the number of partners.

Samuel *et al*. (1991) examined changes in sexual behaviour of 209 heterosexual men enrolled in a prospective study. Few details were given on any counselling input but HIV testing was carried out and on follow up number of partners decreased. Only one seroconversion occurred during the study.

Discordant Couples

There is a growing literature on discordant couples (see chapter 5). They provide an interesting insight into behaviour change issues in the presence of a known HIV positive partner. Yet few address the fact that subjects are usually identified after a period of ignorance, during which unsafe behaviour has usually taken place. Sero conversion has systematically not occurred for these subjects. Few studies compare or control their data against concordant couples. Yet it is in this area that the greatest and most consistent long term changes in behaviour have been monitored after HIV testing and counselling.

Muller *et al.* (1992) looked at 86 couples in Uganda. 61 tested HIV negative and 21 were discordant for HIV (6 men and 15 women) and 4 couples had both partners positive. The most common differences in response to a positive test result were to separate (51%), to stay together (25%), to stay together but not to have sex (9%) and to use condoms regularly (6%). After discordant test results the most common difference was the intention to separate (77%), to stay together and not have sex (6%) and to stay together and practice safe sex (6%).

Johnson *et al.* (1990) studied 110 couples where heterosexual contact was the only risk factor (UK). 69% of the male partners were IDUs and 25% of the female sexual partners were HIV + ve. In the HIV negative group, marked decreases in the frequency of intercourse was noted as was more condom use. Yet half the group still practiced unprotected intercourse. The level and continuity of counselling was not made clear.

Kamenga *et al.* (1991) studied 149 subjects in Zaire. The risk group comprised discordant couples who received post test counselling and intensive home-based follow-up at one and 18 months. No pre-test counselling was reported, rather 'notification of serostatus' and subsequent counselling. Condom uptake increased from 5% to 70.7% at 18 month follow up. 18 couples experienced extensive stress, which was ameliorated by counselling.

Peterson *et al.* (1989) studied 54 Couples in San Francisco to increase safer sex among the 43 discordant couples in the sample. Follow-up was every six months and resulted in a reduction of anal intercourse and less intercourse generally for thirty of the 43 couples.

Drug Users

A number of studies in drug users are available. However subgroups are rarely differentiated. Those in treatment may differ systematically from those not motivated for such treatment or rejected from programmes. Multiple risks may be present and behavioural outcomes are often focussed at needle sharing behaviour rather than at sexual behaviour. Some studies do examine both factors and find that it is often easier for individuals to adjust their personal behaviour compared to their interpersonal behaviour.

It is challenging to know whether pre test counselling alone reduces risk behaviour (Des Jarlais & Friedman, 1987; Power *et al.*, 1988), and how to deal with those intoxicated with drugs or alcohol during pre test counselling. Many studies report behaviour change after intervention for this group. For example, Celsyn (1991) assessed counselling in a random design study where drug users were either exposed to AIDS education only, AIDS education and counselling and testing and a waiting list control. After a four month follow up there was an increase in condom use and needle hygiene for both the intervention groups, but no difference between the groups. Yet in Italy, Gregis (1991) found among 462 HIV positive male idus only 57% abstained from sharing while 8.4% shared frequently. With regard to sexual behaviour 53% always used condoms with negative partner while 20% used them rarely or never.

It is unclear which component of counselling or testing accounts for the behaviour change. Gibson (1991) examined the impact of brief counselling on 300 IDUs in California who randomly received brochures or brief counselling. Counselling led to a significant decrease in unprotected sex, sustained after a year. Needle sharing was reduced in both groups. Martin *et al.* (1990) studied 189 IDUs who received multiple input (audio/video presentation plus pre post test counselling). Syringe sharing decreased from 35% to 12% in 6 months. Sexual behaviour proved more resistant to change. Condom use in at risk situations increased from 49% to 70%.

Few workers examine the negative effects of intervention. Trapido *et al.* (1990) studied female partners of drug users who were exposed to a counselling programme targeted at the reduction of high risk behaviours. They found 50% changed positively, 10% changed negatively and 40% recorded no change. Some subjects decline testing after counselling (Sonnex *et al.*, 1989) mostly as a result of a sense of inability to cope with the results. This inability is reflected in some subjects failing to return for results (21% in Edinburgh; Brettle *et al.*, 1988 – 30% USA: CDC 1986).

Sasse *et al.* (1988) studied drug users in Italy. 428 HIV + ves were compared with 688 HIV-ves and 92 untested. 74% of those + ve had modified their use compared to 53% of HIV negatives and 54% untested. Sexual behaviour modifications were also noted. They do not discuss counselling in detail but caution that, despite change, it was lower in those testing negative which may be as a result of a false sense of security.

Des Jarlais (1989) examined behaviour change in drug users and the long term ability to maintain such change. Of 317 subjects reporting behaviour change, 203 (64%) maintained the changes while 36% did not. Nicolsi *et al.* (1991) looked at risk behaviours in 933 IDUs with follow up of 460 subjects. 30% stopped injecting but no improvement in sexual behaviour was noted.

Adolescents

There are few good prospective studies focussing on adolescents generally and testing, counselling and behaviour change specifically. This marks not only a gap in the research, but means that knowledge is limited and the ability to generalise to this population is also limited. The studies that do exist show rapid gains in knowledge but severe limitations in behaviour change. They also raise some of the problems which teenagers have where their choices are limited and they are abused or unable to negotiate sex.

Kipke *et al.* (1990) raised a number of queries with regard to counselling adolescents. They suggest there is a need for several counselling sessions, but given no indication of how long these should be, how close together they should occur and who should do the counselling. They conclude that the minimum is one pre and one post test session.

Hingson *et al.* (1989) surveyed American teenagers to examine transmission, changes in knowledge and behaviour. The study was based on Massachusetts State wide surveys carried out between 1986 and 1988 on 16 to 19 year olds. They reported an increased knowledge of the virus over the 2 years from 52%–82%. Alcohol and drug misuse declined. Among sexually active teenagers, changes in behaviour was reported from 16% – 34%. Mass media and school education increased knowledge but there was a need for more personal forms of counselling. The teenagers who saw GPs were more likely to use condoms. However of 80% who saw a GP in the last year, only 13% were counselled about AIDS. Thus the GPs were not the ideal source of counselling support.

Griffin Scott & Hastings (1991) showed a miss-match between young people's knowledge and their behaviour. They knew how AIDS was transmitted and the methods of reducing the risk, but did not put this knowledge into practice. These workers concluded that there was a need to promote the confidence and skills to practice safer sex by educating the young from 12 years upwards. This was confirmed by Ammon (1991).

Futterman *et al.* (1990) looked at 15 HIV + ve adolescents tested prior to the study. Sexual abuse was reported in 9 of the 15 and survival sex in 7 of the 15. (This is an important factor in 'choice' in risk behaviours. When an individual is forced or has no choice, all the counselling and testing may be ineffective or irrelevant). All the female subjects continued minimal or no condom use after HIV diagnosis. After HIV status known, 33% of males were abstinent, 33% increased condom use and 33% continued high risk sex. Counselling was reported as 'inadequate' as were referrals for this group.

Women

Studies purely on women are few and far between. Data for women usually is monitored within couples, or within other groups such as pregnant women, sex workers, haemophiliacs or drug users. Thus the variables which are studied are often confounded. Although there is a body of data, it is often submerged under other subheadings, rather than the study of women *per se*. A few studies do exist and others, where specific data on the woman has been gathered, will be summarised.

Sherr & Strong (1991) found that HIV testing did not differentiate sexual behaviours of women (N = 153). Trapido *et al.* (1990) studied the impact of a programme targeting the reduction of high risk behaviours in the partners of drug users. Although many changed to avoid risk, some maintained risk exposure and some were resilient to change. Barbour *et al.* (1989) studied 17 family planning clinic attenders who took up the offer of HIV counselling and information. One in four proceeded to HIV testing. Beavor (1993) studied 46 women and described the HIV counselling they had received around testing. Those who were not counselled did not consider the possibility of a positive result and suffered greater levels of psychological distress when this occurred.

Lindan *et al.* (1990) studied 1,469 women prospectively who were given an educational video plus a group discussion HIV counselling and free condoms prior to HIV testing (no refusals given). Prior to the study 9% had tried condoms and 3%

had reduced the number of partners. At six months follow up 34% claimed safer sex, 21% were using condoms, 16% were using spermicides, 2% had fewer partners. The test itself and the video were rated as the most important factor in behaviour change.

Pregnancy

Pregnant women are the group who have perhaps been subjected to the most HIV testing world wide. The only equal sized group is probably blood donors, but they are often anonymous. Despite a large number of such studies (Sherr, 1991) pre and post test counselling is rarely mentioned, carried out, described or evaluated. Most of the studies look at testing, serostatus and termination of pregnancy as outcome measures with few looking at sexual behaviour or behavioural change. The lack of counselling in these settings may be an issue for urgent consideration. Counselling is usually measured in terms of numbers of women who agree to subsequent HIV testing. Although termination of pregnancy is an option for many women, the majority do not consider a termination and when they do this is rarely associated with their HIV status (Selwyn, 1989). On follow up women who had previously terminated a pregnancy in the presence of HIV are highly likely to have had a subsequent pregnancy (Sunderland, 1992).

Sexual behaviour change in pregnant women may well be an issue for research and intervention. Van de Pere (1991) showed that pregnant women who contract HIV during pregnancy have a heightened vertical transmission rate. No studies have given data of condom use during pregnancy, on the serostatus and sexual behaviour of male partners or long term behaviour change. The studies on HIV testing in this group generally include notions of satisfaction, acceptability of the test, uptake of the test and subsequent outcomes.

Meadows *et al.* (1991) studied 98 ante natal attenders and found that counselling was carried out by the midwife at the booking appointment. Only one third were satisfied. Stevens *et al.* (1989) found that the anxiety generated from HIV testing was significantly higher than anxiety recorded for other ante natal tests and the reassurance generated from test results significantly lower. Meadows *et al.* (1990) showed great variation in test uptake after counselling which relied on the midwife more than the client or the risk behaviours. In a follow up (Meadows & Catalan, 1991) they examined the counselling and found midwives did not appear to be offering accurate pre test counselling in many cases. Those in risk groups were neither counselled nor tested. Much misinformation, especially among ethnic minorities was noted.

Temmerman *et al.* (1990) examined the impact of a single session of post partum counselling on HIV infected women on their subsequent reproductive behaviour. 1,507 mothers enrolled in the study and 94 HIV positive women were identified who were compared with a control group of consecutive subsequent deliveries. Subjects were interviewed at two weeks and one year. Condom use was low for both despite counselling. An educational programme did increase the level of general knowledge but failed to support the hypothesis of a positive effect on attitudes around testing and an increase in desire for voluntary testing.

Blood Donors

In most Western countries blood donors are screened for HIV. Due to the sheer volume of this group, few receive face to face counseling. In the UK for example, written information is the norm, plus attempts to exclude individuals who may be at risk or to donate their blood for research purposes only. Sociological studies have described some of the emotional trauma of individuals identified as HIV positive through such screening, and would point to a need for constant attention to this group. Very few studies examine behaviour change in this group and little data is to hand on the role of HIV testing, counselling and behaviour change for blood donors in general.

Los *et al*. (1989) studied 500–600 blood donors in the Netherlands. They were randomly allocated to groups receiving information leaflets with the overall finding that there was poor uptake and reading of such leaflets.

Lefrere *et al*. (1992) interviewed 74 HIV positive blood donors in France who were not counselled. On post test counselling it was found that they all reported risk factors and had donated their blood in order to ascertain serostatus.

Haemophilia

Much of the heterosexual data comes from groups who are doubly affected by haemophilia and HIV. Such couples have been studied to examine sexual behaviour, transmission rates and psychological burden over time. Psychological stress was high for these clients (Parish and Mandl, 1991, Klimes *et al*., 1992). Behaviour change was monitored with this group (Dublin *et al*., 1992), but was not maintained over time for all couples. Few studies give details of the nature and extent of counselling. Many of these clients were tested for HIV infection very early on in the epidemic and pre test counselling was not studied systematically.

Sex Workers

Sex workers have been studied internationally and may be a rich source of data on heterosexual couples. Yet the studies must be viewed in context as sex for money plays a different role in the West (Ward and Day, 1990; McKegeney, 1992), Africa (Wilson, 1993; Ngugi, 1991) and Asia (Swadiwuldhipong *et al*., 1990). It is most common for female sex workers to be studied, and less common for male sex workers or the male partners of female sex workers to be approached.

Most studies show that despite counselling and testing, few give up their sex work (Manaloto, 1990), but many take up condom use (Swaddiwudhipong *et al*., 1990; Ngugi, 1988, 1991); especially if these are provided free of charge.

Children

There are very few reports in this group in that no clear behaviour change has been identified, and it is rare, almost non existent for any report to discuss any pre or post test counselling with children. This does not mean that children are not tested, indeed many are. Permission, if it is sought, often is focussed on one or both parents.

Children are usually too young to understand and there are few clear guidelines about what counselling children should (or do) receive, from whom, at what age and about disclosure. This area marks a serious deficit in the literature, as children may go on to grow up and become sexually active. There is some literature on haemophiliac children (Miller and Goldman, 1989) and other review articles of children generally (Gibb & Duggan, 1992; Melvin & Sherr, 1993), but almost no relevant empirical studies.

STD Attenders

Sexually transmitted diseases (STDs) are both co-factors for HIV infection and disease progression. They may also mark risk factors which are equally associated with STDs and HIV infection.

Counselling often affects test uptake (Burgess *et al.*, 1992; Erickson *et al.*, 1990), especially among those with high risks for HIV. Yet some studies report the lowest uptake among the groups with the highest seroprevalence (McDonald *et al.*, 1990). Counselling has resulted in some changes such as decreases in numbers of partners (Hooykas, 1991) although this was not associated with changes in sexual behaviours practiced with them.

Zenilman *et al.* (1992) examined the effectiveness of HIV testing and post test counselling on subsequent behaviour in STD attenders in Baltimore. Comparisons were made between 868 + ve patients and 1104 −ve patients in terms of STDs for 23 months after testing. 71% of the positives returned for their result (and then received post test counselling) compared to 63% HIV negatives who returned. High levels of repeated STDs (indicators of possible risk) were reported for both groups, higher in the HIV negatives.

Meta Studies

A number of meta-studies have been carried out which attempt to analyse the whole issue of HIV testing, counselling and behaviour change (Higgins, 1991; Carael *et al.*, 1991; Landis *et al.*, 1992; Des Jarlais *et al.*, 1990).

These have shown that there is evidence of behaviour change, but it is unclear to what extent the behaviour changes and what are the crucial factors prompting such change. Few studies exist which isolate HIV testing from counselling. Some of the better studies (Higgins, 1991) examine the literature according to groups (gay men, intravenous drug users, pregnant women, heterosexuals) with some variation in findings.

Des Jarlais (1990) concluded that an analysis of studies using hard data have shown much more AIDS risk reduction than would have been expected from the lay images of drug users as individuals with self destructive motivations.

WHEN BEHAVIOUR CHANGE DOES NOT OCCUR?

There is much debate about the concept 'relapse'. This is somewhat of a red herring where workers are so concerned with the correct terminology that they fail to grasp the real issue which is specifically the ability to bring about a behaviour change in the first instance and to continue with this behaviour change in the long term. The majority of studies where behaviour change is shown are themselves short term studies. A few longer term studies are now emerging with a much more complex picture.

Numerous studies have documented consistent groups who do not alter their behaviour in the longer term (Routy *et al.*, 1990, n = 20; McKusker, 1992; Sherr *et al.*, 1992).

PAYING LIP SERVICE TO COUNSELLING

Many studies state they have carried out counselling but this is not according to the definitions of true decision making and informed consent situations. For example those where the outcome of the test may entail exclusion from employment, insurance etc. or those where testing is compulsory for admission (such as the military) St Louis *et al.* (1991).

Counselling may also ensure consent to testing which is often missing (Henry *et al.*, 1991). Counselling may be carried out by primary health carers, and there may be an element of coercion. For example Lindsay *et al.* (1991) examined 'routine voluntary prenatal HIV counselling and testing'. They 'encouraged testing'. 4,731 women registered for ante natal care and 4,574 (97%) consented to HIV testing. More acceptors than rejectors thought the counselling session helpful.

THE PSYCHOLOGICAL EFFECT OF HIV TESTING

The wide literature endorses that there is more to HIV counselling than behaviour change. All tests are associated with negative emotional consequences (Marteau, 1989). There is clear evidence that there is a psychological cost to HIV testing which needs to be described (Perry, 1990; Salt *et al.*, 1989; Miller, 1988). This includes anxiety, depression, suicidal ideation and phobic anxiety states in those who are AIDS anxious but HIV negative. Essentially any counselling and testing protocol, whatever its aim, must take this into account when planning policy and procedure. This is probably why testing without counselling is seen in informed circles as unethical, and is thus a factor in the majority of counselling – testing – behaviour change studies. Random allocation and true clinical design is difficult if not impossible as withholding counselling in any group must be deemed as unethical. Many individuals who are HIV positive report retrospectively that they did not know the test was being carried out and were dissatisfied with the procedure (McCann and Wadsworth, 1991; Mansson, 1990).

THOSE WHO DECLINE TESTING

Behaviour change has rarely been studied in those who decline testing. This would be one way of determining if counselling on its own or in conjunction with testing contributed to behaviour change. Yet those who decline testing after counselling may differ systematically from those who proceed.

CONCLUSIONS

Behaviour change has been monitored, to varying degrees, in many studies often despite the fact that it was not the main goal of some studies. The modes and mechanisms of such change are poorly understood. The link between counselling testing and behaviour change has not been proven to be causative, and many other variables may intervene. It is unclear which component (or which group of components) is responsible for behaviour change when it occurs – the counselling, the testing, the two in combination, the outcome – or it could be closely related to factors which triggered the individual to come forward to seek testing in the first instance.

Behaviour change is not unitary. It includes a variety of sexual behaviour changes (reduction in number of partners, reduction in casual partners, adjustment of type of sexual behaviours utilised, notably anal intercourse,increase in condom usage); drug behaviour changes (decreases in sharing of needles/syringes, increase of bleach use to clean out equipment). Yet these may fluctuate according to circumstance and time for any given individual. The literature reveals that in some instances behaviour change is attained, in others it is not.

Meta studies which have tried to make sense of the data run the risk of comparing studies which are not comparable, or giving equal weighting to badly designed studies with low subject numbers to large prospective cohort studies. In such efforts to simplify the complex, they run the risk of providing biased and inaccurate outcome data. Detailed analysis shows that some behaviours are easier to alter than others. Established high risk behaviours may be easier to avoid than the initiation of newer lower risk behaviours (McKusick *et al.*, 1985). It may be easier for individuals to initiate new behaviours than to maintain these over time (Ostrow, 1990). Some behaviours are particularly difficult to adopt and others have simply not been evaluated over time. The conclusions can be summarised in table 1 below.

The challenge then is whether to abandon pre-test counselling or whether to encourage HIV testing. From the studies surveyed it is clear that the situation is complex, that single counselling sessions will have limited and possible short term effects (more likely affording transient rather than permanent risk reduction) and that factors such as the skill of the counsellor and the content of the counselling session have been underinvestigated. The only way directly to answer some of these questions is to mount clearly defined research which will, unavoidably, suffer from the problems of clinically applied work where design con straints are present due to ethical considerations. The studies do show, quite clearly, that the lack of counselling is perceived as a bad thing in retrospective views and that the psychological cost of testing generally, and HIV seropositivity specifically is high. Counselling is the only preventive tool available and this role of counselling must be acknowledged in any programme, but the costs would increase if testing became more widespread.

TABLE 12.1

- Behaviour change is rarely total

- Salience is a key factor

- Single person behaviour (e.g. needle sharing) are easier to influence than interpersonal behaviours (such as sex)

- Behaviour change for some groups are more difficult (namely some groups of women, those who are sexually abused, those who are uninfected)

- There is clear confusion in the literature between
    i) behaviours to prevent transmission
    ii) behaviours to prevent infection
These are the same behaviour changes, but (i) refers to the behaviour of those already infected, and (ii) refers to the behaviour of those currently uninfected. There is another level of distinction between those who are currently uninfected but indulging in risk behaviours with someone known to be infected, compared to those carrying out behaviours with individuals of unknown infection status or those known to be infection free

- Behaviour change is a complex notion and many theories do not address or measure it fully

- Behaviour change is a marker and not an end point in HIV infection

- Few studies document fully or explain when behaviour change does not occur

- Behaviour change is often studied out of social context

REFERENCES

Ammon, A. (1991) Can adolescents transfer their knowledge about AIDS into their Partnership Relations?

Barbour, R., Macintyre, S., McIlwaine, G., Wilson, E. (1989) Uptake of AIDS counselling and testing at a Scottish family planning clinic *BJ of Family Planning* 15(2), 61–62

Beavor, A. (1993) *AIDS Care* 5(2) (in press).

Bond, T. (1992) HIV Counselling Second Edition. British Association for Counselling, Department of Health Joint Project, Daniels Publishing

Bor, R., Miller, R., Johnson, M. (1991) A testing time for doctors counselling patients before an HIV test. *BMJ*, **303**, 905–7.

Bor, R., Miller, R., Salt, H. (1991) Uptake of HIV Testing following counselling *Sexual and Marital Therapy Journal*, 6(1), 25–28.

Brown-Peterside, P., Sibbald, B., Freeling, P. (1991) Aids: Knowledge, skills and attitudes among vocational trainees and their trainers.' *British Journal General Practitioners*. 41(351), 401–5.

Burgess, M., Taylor, S., McManus, T.J. (1992) HIV Screening in an STD Clinic, VIII Int Conf on AIDS Amsterdam

Carael, M., Cleland, J., Adeokun, L. (1991) Overview and selected findings of sexual behaviour surveys *AIDS* 5, (suppl l), 565–74

Carballo, M., Miller, D. (1989) HIV Counslling Problems and Opportunities Defining the New Agenda for the 1990s *AIDS Care* 1(2).

CDC (1986) Centres for Disease Control

Cockroft, A. (1989) AIDS/HIV counselling in occupational health. *AIDS Care*, 1(1).

Day, S., Ward, H. (1990) The Praed Street Project: A Cohort of Prostitute women in London, in M. Plant (ed.) AIDS Drugs and Prostitution in London, Tavistock

Des Jarlais, D., Friedman, S. (1988) HIV infection among persons who inject illicit drugs: problems and prospects, *Journal of AIDS* 1, 267–273

Des Jarlais, D.C., Tross, S., Abdul Quader, A., Kouzi, A., Friedman, S.R. (1989) IDU and maintenance of behaviour change Int Conf *AIDS* 5, June, abstract THD06

Des Jarlais, D., Friedman, S., Casriel, C. (1990) Target groups for preventing AIDS among IDU: The hard data studies *Jnl of Consulting and CLinical Psychology* 58(l), 50–56

Dublin, S., Rosenberg, P., Goedert, J. (1992) Patterns and predictors of high risk sexual behaviour in female partners of HIV infected men with Haemophilia *AIDS* 6, 475–82

Erickson, B., Wasserheit, J., Rompalo, A., Brathwaite, W., Glasser, D., Hook, E. (1990) Routine voluntary HIV screening in STD clinic clients, characterization of infected clients. *Sex Transm Dis* 17(4), Oct-Dec, 194–99

Futterman, D., Hein, K., Kipke, M., Reulback, W., Clare, G., Nelson, J., Orane, A., Gayle, H. (1990) HIV + adolescents HIV testing experiences and changes in risk related sexual and drug use behaviour. Int Conf *AIDS* Abs SC 663

Gibb, D., Duggan, C. (1992) AIDS and Children, Editorial *G U Medicine*.

Gibson (1991) Abstract International AIDS Conference

Gillespie, P., Bateman, J. (1991) The Role of General Practitioners in the Prevention and Management of HIV/AIDS. *Druglink*

Green, J., McCreaner, A. (1989) Counselling in AIDS and HIV Infection, Blackwell Scientific Publications, Oxford

Gregis (1991) Abstract International AIDS Conference

Griffin Scott, Hastings (1991) Making safer sex easier – lessons from an anti AIDS initiative. *Journal Inst of Health Ed* 29(3).

Henry, K., Maki, M., Willenbring, K., Campbell, S. (1991) The impact of experience with AIDS on HIV testing and counselling practices a study of US infectious disease teaching hospitals and Minnesota hospitals. *AIDS Educ Prev* 3(4), 313–21

Hedge, B., Glover, L. (1990) Group intervention with HIV seropositive patients and their partners *AIDS Care* 2(2), 147–54

Higgins, D.L., Galavotti, C., O'Reilly, K.R., Schnell, D.J., Moore, M., Rugg, D.L., Johnson, R. (1991) Evidence for the effects of HIV Antibody Counselling and Testing on Risk Behaviours. *JAMA* 266(17), 2419–2429.

Hingson, R., Strunin, L., Berlin, B., Meeren, T. (1989) Beliefs about AIDS use of alcohol drugs and unprotected sex among Massachusetts adolescents. Alcohol Epidemiology Symposium ICCA Netherlands.

Holman, S., Minkof, H., Hoegsberg, H., Beller, B., Goldstein, G. (1988) – A model programme for routinely offered HIV anti-body testing in pregnancy. Presented at the 4th International Conference on AIDS in Stockholm Sweden.

Hooykas, C., Van der Linden, M., Van Doornum, G., van der Velde, F., van der Pligt, J., Coutinho, R. (1991) Limited changes in sexual behaviour of heterosexual men and women with multiple partners in The Netherlands *AIDS Care* 3(l), 21–30

Johnson, A., Mclean, K., Davidson, S., Petherick, A., Shergold, C., Brettle, R. (1990) Sexual behaviour change in a prospecive study of heterosexual partners of HIV infected men. *Int Conf AIDS* 6(2), 1990 20–23 June abstract FC 652

Kamenga, M., Ryder, R., Jingu, M., *et al.* (1991) Evidence of marked sexual behaviour change associated with low HIV-1 seroconversion in 149 married couples with discordant HIV 1 serostatus experience at an HIV counselling centre in Zaire *AIDS* 5(1), 61–67

King, M.B. (1989) Psychological and social problems in HIV infection. *British Medical Journal* 299, 713–17

Kipke, M., Futterman, D., Hein, K. (1990) HIV infection and AIDS during Adolescence *Medical CLinics of North America* 74(5).

Kelly, & Lawrence (1990) The impact of community based groups. *AIDS Care* 2(l), 25–36.

Klimes, I., Catalan, J., Garrod, A., Day, A., Bond, A., Rizza, C. (1992) Partner of Men with HIV infection and Haemophilia. *AIDS Care* 4(l), 149–57

Landis, S.E., Schoenbach, V., Weber, D., Mittal, M., Krishan, B., Lewis, K., Koch, G. (1992) Results of a randomized trial of partner notification in cases of HIV infection in North Carolina. *N Engl J Med* 326(2), 101–6

Lefrere, J., Eighouzzi, M., Paquex, F., Dalla, N., Nubel, L. (1992) Interviews with anti HIV positive individuals detected through the systematic screening of blood donations – consequences on predonation medical interview, *Vox Sanguinis* 62(1), 25–28

Leukefeld, C. AIDS Counselling and Testing U.S. Public Health Service, National Institute of Drug Abuse, Rockville.

Lindan, C., Allen, S., Nsengumuremyi, F., Black, D., Schwalbe, J., Levy, J., Hulley, S. (1990) HIV testing and education: promote safer sex among urban women in Rwanda Int Conf AIDS Abs SC 669

Lindsay, M., Adefris, W., Peterson, H., Williams, H., Johnson, J., Klein, L. (1991) Determinants of acceptance of routine voluntary HIV testing in an inner city prenatal population. *Obstet Gynecol* 78(4), 678–80

Mansson, S.A. (1990) Psychosocial Aspects of HIV Testing: the Swedish Case. (1990) *AIDS Care* 2(l), 5–16

Martin, G.S., Serpelloni, G., Galvan, U., Rizzetto, A., Gomma, G., Morgante, S., Rezza, G. (1990) Behavioural change in injecting drug users: – Evaluation of an HIV/AIDS Education Programme. *Aids Care* 2(3), 275–279.

McKegeney, N., Barnard, M. (1992) Selling sex female street prostitution and HIV risk behaviour in Glasgow, *AIDS Care* 4(4), 395

McDonald, A., Whyte, B., Jacogs, D., Philpot, C., Bradford, D. *et al.* (1990) Voluntary HIV antibody testing among STD clinical patients: a pilot study. *The Med Jnl of Aust* 153, 12–14

Meadows, J., Jenkinson, S., Catalan, J., Gazzard, B. (1990) Uptake rates. *AIDS Care* 2(3)

Meadows, J., Catalan, J. (1991) Who consents to HIV antibody testing and why? Paper presented at the London Conference of the British Psychological Society, City University.

Melvin, D., Sherr, L. (1993) The Child in The Family. *AIDS Care* 5(1),

Mhalu, F., Hirji, K., Ijumba, P. (1991) A cross sectional study of a programme for HIV infection control among public house workers *Journal of AIDS* 4(3), 290–6

McCann, K., Wadsworth, E. (1991) The experience of having a positive HIV antibody test. *AIDS Care* 3(l), 43–53.

McCusker, J., Stoddard, A., McDonald, M., Zapka, J., Mayer, K. (1992) Maintenance of behaviour change in a cohort of homosexually active men *AIDS* 6, 861–68

Miller, D., Acton, T., Hedge, B. (1988) The worried well: their identification and management. *Journal of the Royal College of Physicians* 22(3), 158–65

Miller, D., Pinching, A. (1989) HIV tests and counselling current issues *J AIDS* **suppl** l(3), 3187–93

Miller, R., Goldman, E., Bor, R., Kernoff, P. (1989) AIDS and Children; some of the Issues in Haemophilia care. *AIDS Care* 1(1)

Muller, O., Barugahare, L., Schwartlander, B., Byaruhanga, E., Kataaha, P., Kyeyune, D., Heckmann, W., Ankrah, M. (1992) HIV prevalence attitudes and behaviour in clients of a confidential HIV testing and counselling centre in Uganda. *AIDS* 6, 869–874

Naji, S., Russell, T., Foy, C.J.W., Gallagher, M., Rhodes, T.J., Moore, M.P. (1989) HIV Infection and Scottish General Practice: Workload and current practice. *J. Royal College of General Practitioners.* 39, 234–238.

Ngugi, E., Plummer, F., Simonsen, J. *et al.* (1988) Prevention of transmission of HIV in Africa: Effectiveness of condom promotion and health education among prostitutes *Lancet* 2, 887–90

Nicolsi, A., Molinari, S., Musicco, M., Saracco, A., Ziliani, N., Lazzarin, A. (1991) Positive modification of injecting behaviour among intravenous heroin users from Milan and northern Italy 87–89 *Br Jnl of Addiction* 86(1), 91–102

Ostrow, D. (1992) Paper presented at the International AIDS Conference, Amsterdam

Perry, S., Jacobsberg, L., Fishman, B. (1990) Suicidal Ideation and HIV testing *JAMA* 2, 263(5), 679–82

Peterson, H., Padian, N., Glass, S., Moreno, A., Ajaniku, I., Wofsy, C. (1989) Behaviour modification in couples enrolled in a study of heterosexual transmission. *Int AIDS Conf Abstract* pg 115 no TAP 100

Power, R., Hartnoll, R., Daviaud, E. (1988) Drug injecting AIDS and Risk Behaviour Potential for Change and Intervention Strategies, *British Journal of Addiction* 83, 649–54

Samuel, M., Guydish, J., Ekstrand, M., Coates, T., Winkelstein, W. (1991) Changes in sexual practices over 5 years of follow up among heterosexual men in San Francisco, *J Acquir Immune Defic Synd,* 4 (9), 896–900

Salt, H., Miller, R., Perry, Bor, R. (1989) Paradoxical interventions in counselling for people with an intractable AIDS-worry. *AIDS Care* 1(1), 39.

Sasse, H., Salmaso, S., Conti, S., Rezza, G. (1988) Significance of HIV antibody testing as a preventive measure in IDUs, *AIDS* 2(5), 402–403

Sherr, L. (1987) Summary Evaluation of the UK Health Education Camapign on AIDS, *Psychology and Health*

Sherr, L. (1991) HIV and AIDS in mothers and babies, Blackwell Scientific Publications, Oxford.

Sherr, L., Strong, C., Goldmeier, D. (1990) *Counselling Psychology Quarterly.* 3(4), 343–352.

Sherr, L., Davey, T., Strong, C. (1991). Counselling implications of anxiety and depression in AIDS and HIV infection: A pilot study. *Counselling Psychology Quarterly* 4(1), 27–35.

Sherr, L., Hedge, B. (1990) The Impact and Use of Written Leaflets as a Counselling Alternative in Mass Ante Natal Screening. *AIDS Care* 2(3).

Sherr, L., Victor, C., Jeffries, S. (1992) AIDS Patient Care

Sherr, L., Strong C. (1992) Safe sex and women. *Genito Urinary Medicine* 68, 1.

Sonnex, C., Petherick, A., Hart, G.J., Adler, M.W. (1989) An appraisal of HIV antibody test counselling of IDUs. *AIDS Care* 1(3), 307

St Louis, M., Conway, G., Hayman, C., Miller, C., Petersen, L., Dondero, T. (1991) HIV infection in disadvantaged adolescents *JAMA* 266(17)

Sunderland, A., Minkoff, H., Handte, J., Moroso, G., Landesman, S. (1992) The impact of HIV serostatus on reproductive decisions of women. *Obs and Gyne* 79(6), 1027–31

Swaddiwudhipong, W., Nguntra, P., Chaovakiratipong, C., Koonchote, S., Lerdlukanavonge, P., Chandoun, C. (1990) *Southeast Asian Jnl of Trop Med and Public Health* 21(3), 453–7

Temmerman, M., Moses, S., Kiragu, D., Fusallah, S., Wamola, I.A., Piot, P. (1990) Impact of single session post partum counselling on HIV infected women on their subsequent reproductive behaviour. *AIDS Care* 2(3)

Timmis, C. (1991) Counselling patients before an HIV test. *BMJ.* 303, Letter

Ussher, J.M. (1990) Cognitive behavioural couples therapy with gay men referred for counselling in an AIDs Setting: A pilot setting. *AIDS Care* 2(1), 43.

Valdiserra, R., Lyter, D., Leviton, L., Callahan, C., Kingsley, L. (1990) Preventing HIV infection in gay and bisexual men – experimental evaluation of attitude change from two risk reduction interventions. *AIDS Int and Prevent.* 2(2), 95–108

Van De Pere, P., Simonson, A., Msellati, P. (1991) Postnatal Transmission of HIV type 1 from mother to infant: a prospective cohort study in Kigali Rwanda. *New England Journal of Medicine* 91, 325, 593–8

Ward, J., Day, S., Donegan, C., Harris, J. (1990) HIV risk behaviour and STD incidence in London prostitutes VI Int Conf on AIDS San Francisco ABST FC 738

Wilkins, H.A., Alonso, P., Baldeh, S., Cham, M.K., Corrah, T., Hughes, A., Jalteh, K.O., Keita, K., Oelman B., Pickering, H. (1989) Knowledge of AIDS, use of condoms and results of counselling subjects with asymptomatic HIV2 infection in the Gambia. *AIDS Care* 1(3), 247–256

Zenilman, J., Erickson, B., Fox, R., Rechart, C., Hook, E. (1992) Effect of HIV post test counselling on STD incidence *JAMA* 2617(6), 843–5

13

Psychological Needs and Services for Heterosexuals with HIV Infection

DONNA L. LAMPING AND ITESH SACHDEV

"I can deal with my own poor health but losing my husband and watching him die is and will be the worst thing I'll ever experience in my life. I'm not angry about getting HIV. I get angry with other people being ill. My heart goes out to them. What will it take to stop this infection? Education isn't getting across enough..." (34-year-old woman, infected with HIV through heterosexual contact)

"I think that being a straight female that much more emphasis needs to be put on at least this part of the population. Straight males as well. I find it very sad and frustrating when I hear my friends say they didn't practice 'safer sex' or they did at first but after the first few times they stopped...People just aren't aware that it can be the person next door..." (31-year-old woman, infected with HIV through heterosexual contact)

"We're dealing with a population that is increasingly diverse. When I first started my job I had only gay men as patients. Now I have wives of infected individuals, children, i.v. drug users, and so on. I'm becoming more aware of the breadth of this problem and the challenge of dealing with mental health with such a broad population." (HIV caregiver)

The voices of heterosexuals with HIV infection and their caregivers speak powerfully about the psychological impact of the disease and the concomitant need for services to address HIV-related mental health problems. Women, persons who have been exposed to HIV infection through blood and blood products, injection drug users, and heterosexual men who have contracted HIV through sexual activity with an infected partner, represent a diverse group whose distinctive needs have not typically been addressed by health care services traditionally oriented to gay men in the West.

The purpose of this chapter is to contribute to an understanding of psychological needs and services for heterosexuals with HIV infection. Data from a recently completed large-scale national survey of HIV-related mental health needs and services in Canada (Lamping, Sewitch, Clark, & Ryan, 1990a, 1990b; Lamping, Hamel, & Di Meco, 1990) are analyzed first, to identify the specific psychological needs of heterosexuals with HIV infection; and second, to assess services related to the mental health needs of this population. A brief review of the literature is presented on the psychological impact of HIV on various groups of heterosexuals, including women, haemophiliacs, and injection drug users, followed by a description of the national survey on which the data presented in this chapter are based, and presentation and discussion of results pertinent to psychological needs and services for heterosexuals with HIV infection in Canada.

PSYCHOLOGICAL IMPACT OF HIV INFECTION IN HETEROSEXUALS

The literature on the psychological impact of HIV infection has focused primarily on the psychosocial and neuropsychological consequences of HIV infection in the gay male community, and to a lesser extent in injection drug users (see review by Lamping & Sewitch, 1990). However, as the number of persons with HIV infection increases in other groups, the literature has begun to consider the unique psychological problems of persons in specific groups. This section reviews issues related to the psychological impact of HIV infection in women, haemophiliacs, and injection drug users.

Women
Much of the literature on the psychological consequences of HIV infection in gay males is equally relevant to women with HIV infection (Hays & Lyles, 1986; James, 1988). However, there are a number of specific issues to consider (Cochran & Mays, 1989; Ickovics & Rodin, 1992; Shaw & Paleo, 1986). First, the fact that women often become infected with HIV through sexual contact with an infected male partner can lead to unique emotional reactions, including a feeling of betrayal, anger, and inadequacy (Buckingham & Rehm, 1987; Evans, 1987). Second, the usual problems regarding disclosure of HIV infection are compounded by the fact that disclosure of HIV infection in women implies disclosure about her male partner's sexual or drug-related behaviour (Buckingham & Rehm, 1987). Third, the role disruptions experienced by women with HIV infection are particularly problematic, given the traditional role expectations of women in relation to responsibilities to family and children (Buckingham & Rehm, 1987; Saint-Jarre, 1989; Shaw & Paleo, 1986; Wofsy, 1987; Zuckerman & Gordon, 1988). Fourth, the sense of isolation may be even more profound in women with HIV infection who, unlike gay men, may lack a supportive network (Rickert, 1989; Saint-Jarre, 1989; Wofsy, 1987) and for whom special services, information and understanding are either unavailable or difficult to find (Battle, 1986; Buckingham & Rehm, 1987; Maire, 1988; Wofsy, 1987). Fifth, the fact that the course of HIV infection is different in women than in men presents a unique set of problems (Ickovics & Rodin, 1992; Mantell, Shinke, & Akabas, 1988; Zuckerman & Gordon, 1988).

Finally, there are a host of fertility and reproductive-related issues that create special psychosocial problems for women with HIV infection (Maire, 1988; Mantell *et al.*, 1988; Minkoff, 1987; Sachs, Tuomala, & Frigoletto, 1987).

Haemophiliacs
Haemophiliacs with HIV infection experience with double psychological burden of having a chronic illness in addition to HIV infection. Little is known about the psychological impact of HIV infection in haemophiliacs, as they are few reports in the literature about those who are actually infected. Haemophiliacs and their families report a high level of distress about AIDS risk which tends to decrease over time but which continues to interfere with daily activities (Agle, Gluck, & Pierce, 1987). Parents report greater distress about AIDS risk than either haemophiliacs or partners, which may lead to overprotective child-rearing practices (Agle *et al.*, 1987). Clinical reports suggest problems similar to those experienced in other HIV infected groups, although a high degree of denial in haemophiliacs and their families has been suggested (Veroust & Ferragu, 1988). Although the literature in this area is sparse, the special problems related to HIV infection and mental health in haemophiliacs are beginning to be studied (e.g. Naji, Wilkie, Markova, Forbes, & Watson, 1986).

Injection Drug Users
The psychological consequences of HIV infection in injection drug users may be more devastating than in any other high risk group (Caputo, 1985). In general, injection drug users have a greater number of psychological problems than non-drug users, and fewer psychosocial resources to cope with the stresses of HIV infection (Batki, Sorensen, Faltz, & Madover, 1988). Added to the psychosocial stresses common to HIV infection in general, injection drug users are faced with a unique set of psychosocial issues which increase mental health risk.

First, drug use is associated with a number of behaviours that may compromise the psychosocial resources of the individual in coping with HIV infection. Many injection drug users are known to have pre-existing personality disorders and psychiatric complications (Caputo, 1985; Flavin & Frances, 1987; Ginzburg, 1984). Injection drug users engage in socially sanctioned behaviours such as needle sharing, that are known to increase HIV-risk (Des Jarlais, Wish, *et al.*, 1987; Friedman, Des Jarlais, & Sotheran, 1986; Selwyn, Feiner, Cox, Lipshutz, & Cohen, 1987) in addition to having highly reinforcing consequences (Black, Dolan, & DeFord, 1986; Des Jarlais, Friedman, & Strug, 1986; Mulleady, 1987).

Second, because the minimal social reinforcement inherent in drug use is the only available source of support, injection drug users with HIV infection are extremely socially isolated. Unlike gay males, injection drug users have little sense of community, no organized advocacy, and are particularly hard to reach (Caputo, 1985; Ginzburg, 1984; Greif & Price, 1988; Velimirovic, 1987). Drug use is known to be associated with high rates of criminality and unemployment, which intensifies social problems and social isolation (Ginzburg, 1984). In addition, many injection drug users are from less advantaged social groups and experience additional HIV-related problems because of their minority group status (Peterson &

Marin, 1988). Women injection drug users who are infected with HIV share not only the problems common to men in this group, but also the unique problems of non-drug using women with HIV infection (Mondanaro, 1987; Mulleady, 1987).

Third, the combined effect of HIV infection and drug use has serious neuropsychological consequences. Findings from one study suggest a 40% prevalence of psychological dysfunction in injection drug users with AIDS, with greatest difficulty in basic cognitive functioning (Jordan, Grallo, Mashberg, Gordon, & Kapila, 1987). Results from another study of HIV seropositive injection drug users showed evidence of impaired neuropsychological function even in the absence of symptoms (Silberstein *et al.*, 1987).

NATIONAL SURVEY OF HIV-RELATED MENTAL HEALTH NEEDS AND SERVICES IN CANADA

To address issues related to the mental health of Canadians with HIV infection, the Federal Centre for AIDS established a Working Group on HIV Infection and Mental Health in December 1988. The task of the Working Group, which was comprised of health care professionals across Canada representing a broad range of specialities relevant to mental health, was to recommend ways to solve problems and improve mental health services available to those affected by HIV (Health and Welfare Canada, 1992).

As part of this task, a collaborative research team comprised of university researchers and commuity-based health care professionals, conducted a national survey of HIV-related mental health needs and services in 1,262 persons affected by HIV infection in Canada. Details of the study methods and results are described elsewhere (Lamping, Sewitch, Clark, & Ryan, 1990a, 1990b; Lamping, Hamel, & Di Meco, 1990). Briefly, three separate questionnaires were developed to assess HIV-related mental health needs and services in persons with HIV infection, caregivers, and family members/significant others. These were distributed through 124 key HIV-related service providers in five general categories of service provider agencies, including primary health care facilities, community health clinics, social service agencies, community-based organizations, and private practice doctors. Service providers from 51 institutions and agencies in four major cities (Halifax, Montreal, Toronto, and Vancouver) and in 24 community-based groups across Canada participated in the study.

Preliminary versions of the three self-administered questionnaires were pretested in a sample of 52 respondents from seven cities across Canada (Lamping, Sewitch, Clark, & Ryan, 1990b). Final versions of the questionnaires were then developed on the basis of results obtained from the pretest. The questionnaires were similar in format and content, and consisted of three parts: background information about demographic, illness, and treatment-related characteristics; a scale to measure HIV-related psychological distress (HIV Impact Scale-HIVIS; Hamel, 1992; Lamping & Hamel, 1991) and four questions about perceived health status, happiness, and life satisfaction used in large-scale national household surveys in Canada (General Social Survey; Statistics Canada, 1987; Canada Health Survey;

Health and Welfare Canada and Statistics Canada, 1981); and questions about mental health services (e.g. awareness, use, need, barriers, etc.).

A total of 1,747 questionnaires were distributed to service providers. Of these, 1,262 were returned indicating a return rate of 72.2% for the entire sample. Respondents included 581 persons with HIV infection, 459 caregivers, and 222 family members/significant others. Of these, 1,023 (81%) completed questionnaires in English and 239 (19%) in French. The sample included 142 respondents from Halifax, 303 from Montreal, 349 from Toronto, 258 from Vancouver, and 210 from Canadian AIDS Society community-based groups.

The demographic and illness-related characteristics of the sample of 581 persons with HIV infection who participated in the national survey correspond closely to the 3,771 adults with AIDS in the Canadian population (Federal Centre for AIDS, 1990). The distribution of males and females in the sample is equivalent to the Canadian population of persons with AIDS (94% and 6% respectively). The age distributions are also similar. The percentages of persons with HIV infection in the sample by age, compared to the Canadian population of persons with AIDS are: 21% and 20% for under 29 years, 46% and 44% for 30–39 years, 27% and 25% for 40–49 years, and 7% and 11% for 50 years and over. The distribution of risk factors in the sample is also consistent with that of the Canadian population of persons with AIDS. Corresponding percentages in the national survey sample, compared to the Canadian population of persons with AIDS, are: 72% and 79% for homosexual/bisexual activity only, 3% and 1% for injection drug use only, 3% and 3% for both homosexual/bisexual activity and injection drug use, 6% and 5% for recipient of blood/blood products, 6% and 7% for heterosexual activity, and 9% and 5% for unknown/no identified risk factors.

Characteristics of Respondents

First, the background characteristics of the sample of heterosexual men and women were compared to gay men, and then differences within the heterosexual sample were examined by comparing heterosexual men and women.

Heterosexual Men and Women vs. Gay Men

The sample of 581 persons with HIV infection who participated in the national survey included 121 heterosexuals (85 men, 36 women) and 457 gay men. Three respondents who were unable to be classified by sex or sexual preference due to missing data were excluded from further analysis. Table 13.1 presents background data on demographic, illness, and treatment-related characteristics of the subsamples of heterosexual men and women compared to gay men. Heterosexual men and women were comparable to gay men in the sample in terms of work status, living status, source of income, diagnosis, taking AZT/ddI, and perceived physical health, but were younger ($p = .01$), more likely to be French speaking ($p = .0005$) and Black ($p = .04$), less well-educated ($p = .0004$). There were expected differences in the distributions of the two groups in terms of risk factors ($p = .00001$); heterosexuals were from various risk groups, including injection drug use, recipient of blood/blood products, and heterosexual activity, whereas the majority of gay

Table 13.1
Demographic, Illness, and Treatment-Related Characteristics of Heterosexual Men and
Women and Gay Men

| | Heterosexuals | | Gay men |
	Men (N = 85)	Women (N = 36)	(N = 457)
Age (years) Mean (SD)	35.88 (9.64)	30.81 (7.79)**	36.68 (7.33)*
Range	20–74	17–55	18–59
Language			
English	62 (73)	26 (72)	396 (87)
French	23 (27)	10 (28)	61 (13)***
Education			
High school or less	33 (39)	23 (64)	133 (29)
At least some university/college	52 (61)	13 (36)*	324 (71)
Work Status			
Working	40 (48)	14 (40)	211 (47)
Not working	44 (52)	21 (60)	242 (53)
Ethnicity			
Asian	2 (2)	0 (0)	5 (1)
Black	4 (5)	3 (8)	6 (1)
Latin American	1 (1)	0 (0)	6 (1)
Native American	0 (0)	0 (0)	10 (2)
White	74 (89)	31 (86)	398 (88)
Other	0 (0)	1 (3)	8 (2)
None	2 (2)	1 (3)	22 (5)*
Living status			
Living alone	26 (31)	11 (31)	175 (39)
Living with others	58 (69)	25 (69)	279 (62)
Source of Income			
Employment	38 (45)	15 (43)	204 (45)
Welfare/social assistance	21 (25)	14 (40)	100 (22)
Other (e.g. disability/ pension, unemployment, private)	25 (30)	6 (17)	149 (33)
Diagnosis			
HIV Asymptomatic	24 (29)	7 (20)	76 (17)
HIV Symptomatic	23 (28)	13 (37)	148 (33)
AIDS	36 (43)	15 (43)	222 (49)

Table 13.1
Demographic, Illness, and Treatment-Related Characteristics of Heterosexual Men and
Women and Gay Men

	Heterosexuals		Gay men
	Men (N = 85)	Women (N = 36)	(N = 457)
Risk Group			
Homosexual/bisexual activity (only)	0 (0)	0 (0)	419 (92)
Injection drug use (only)	14 (17)	6 (17)	0 (0)
Both homosexual/bisexual activity and injection drug use	0 (0)	0 (0)	23 (5)
Recipient of blood/blood products	33 (39)	3 (8)	0 (0)
Heterosexual activity	10 (12)	22 (61)	0 (0)
Other or unknown	28 (33)	5 (14)***	15 (3)***
Currently on AZT/ddI			
Yes	56 (67)	15 (42)	312 (68)
No	28 (33)	21 (58)*	145 (32)
Perceived physical health (1 = Poor, 4 = Excellent)			
Mean (SD)	2.32 (1.00)	2.39 (0.93)	2.33 (0.97)

*** $p < .001$
** $p < .01$
* $p < .05$

Note. Statistical comparisons are between gay men vs. heterosexual men and women and between heterosexual men and heterosexual women.

men were in the homosexual/bisexual activity risk group with a small percentage in the combined homosexual/bisexual activity and injection drug use group.

Heterosexual Men vs. Women
Within the HIV-infected heterosexual subsample, women were comparable to men in terms of language, work status, ethnicity, living status, source of income, diagnosis, and perceived physical health, but were younger, less well-educated, and less likely to be taking AZT or ddI. The distributions of men and women across risk groups were quite different ($p = .000001$). Although there was a similar distribution of heterosexual men and women in the injection drug user risk group, the proportion of women who contracted HIV through heterosexual activity with an HIV-infected partner was five times higher than among heterosexual men. The proportions of men who contracted HIV through blood/blood products and through either a combination of risk factors or unknown sources (*Other* category) were higher than in women.

Summary
Although there are differences in background characteristics between the sample of heterosexuals (including men and women) and gay men, the majority of differences between the two groups are due to differences between men and women rather than to differences between heterosexuals and gay men. That is, although heterosexual men and women as a group are younger and less well-educated than gay men, these group differences are due mainly to heterosexual women being generally younger and less well-educated than either heterosexual or gay men. Another major difference between heterosexual men and women is the fact that women in the sample are most likely to have contracted HIV through heterosexual activity with an HIV-infected partner rather than through blood/blood products or a combination of risk factors. In this sense, heterosexual women are similar to gay men in having contracted HIV through sexual behaviour rather than through other non-sexual behaviour.

Measurement of Psychological Needs and Services

Psychological needs and services were measured using a combination of scales developed for the national survey as well as standard survey questions used in previous research.

Measurement of Psychological Needs
HIV-related psychological distress was measured using the HIV Impact Scale (HIVIS; Lamping & Hamel, 1991), a 40-item scale which assesses the distress associated with problems commonly experienced by persons with HIV infection. The HIVIS was developed on the basis of a comprehensive review of the literature on HIV infection and mental health (Lamping & Sewitch, 1990) and through expert opinion and key informant interviews. For each item, respondents indicate *How much have you been bothered by this problem during the past month?* using a 5-point Likert scale (1 = *Not at all*, 5 = *A lot*). The HIVIS yields a total mental health distress score (HIVIS Total) by averaging the responses over all questions, as well as scores on the five conceptually derived subscales described above. Total HIVIS scores and subscale scores ranged from 1 to 5. The reliability and validity of the HIVIS have been demonstrated (Hamel, 1992; Lamping & Hamel, 1991), showing strong internal consistency (.94, .92, .89) and good test-retest reliability (.71, .60), as well as good convergent validity with the Profile of Mood States (.78, .75, .68), the SF-36 mental health scale (-.81) and the Brief Symptom Inventory (.62), and good discriminant validity with the SF-36 physical health subscale (-.06) and perceived physical health (-.05). The HIVIS was included as part of the questionnaire distributed to persons with HIV infection in the national survey.

Four questions were also included to measure perceived health status and life satisfaction based on items used in two large-scale national household surveys (General Social Survey; Statistics Canada, 1987; Canada Health Survey; Health and Welfare Canada and Statistics Canada, 1981). Included were questions about perceived physical and psychological health, happiness, and life satisfaction. Respondents gave self-ratings on each of the four dimensions on 4- or 5-point Likert scales, based on reference group instructions of ratings in comparison with persons of the same age.

Measurement of Mental Health Services

Awareness, use, and need for 20 HIV-related services broadly defined as being related to mental health were assessed. For each service, respondents indicated first, whether they were aware of the service, and second, whether they had used the service. To assess need, respondents then identified the three services from the list that they felt were most needed. This section also included other service-related questions, e.g. barriers to service use, frequency of use of different service providers, prior use of mental health services, and whether the respondent must travel or had to move to obtain services.

Psychological Needs

Psychological needs between heterosexual men and women and gay men were compared. Then, in order to determine whether any observed differences in psychological needs between heterosexuals and gay men may have been due to gender differences between the two groups, psychological needs between heterosexual men and women were compared.

Differences between groups were examined in three ways. First, the set of psychological problems rated as most distressing by each group were compared. Items on the HIVIS scale which scored > 2.70 were included among the most distressing problems, and these were ranked to form a list of most distressing problems. Second, the question of whether there were specific problems which were more or less distressing for one group compared to the other was asked. To do so, *t*-tests were used to compare mean scores between groups on each of the 40 HIVIS items. Finally, differences in psychological health, happiness and life satisfaction were examined using *t*-tests on mean scores for items measured by the national survey questions.

Heterosexual Men and Women vs. Gay Men

Table 13.2 presents the most distressing problems for heterosexual men and women compared to gay men. For both heterosexuals and gay men, *not being able to realize life goals* and *feeling uncertain about the future* are the two most distressing problems. Other problems which are among the most distressing to both groups include *feeling depressed, fear of loss of mental abilities or dementia, feeling anxious, getting sick or sicker, concern about not being able to care for myself, feeling helpless, financial difficulties,* and *feeling angry.* However, there are a number of concerns which appear in the list of most distressing problems for heterosexual men and women but not for gay men: *concern about confidentiality, feeling anger or frustration at the health care system, feeling lonely, being discriminated against, and feeling isolated.*

When mean scores were compared on each of the 40 HIVIS items between heterosexual men and women and gay men, differences were found between the two

Table 13.2
Most Distressing Problems

Heterosexual Men and Women	Gay Men	Heterosexual Men	Heterosexual Women
Not being able to realize life goals (3.35)	Feeling uncertain about the future (3.31)	Not being able to realize life goals/Feeling uncertain about the future (3.24)	Not being able to realize life goals (3.61)
Feeling uncertain about the future (3.29)	Not being able to realize life goals (3.22)	Fear about loss of mental abilities or dementia (3.00)	Feeling angry (3.53)
Feeling depressed (3.00)	Fear of loss of mental abilities or dementia (2.98)	Feeling anger or frustration at the health care system/Concern about confidentiality (2.88)	Feeling depressed/Feeling uncertain about the future (3.39)
Feeling angry (3.04)	Feeling anxious (2.88)	Feeling helpless/Getting sick or sicker/Feeling depressed/Feeling angry (2.84)	Feeling helpless/Feeling isolated/Financial difficulties (3.19)
Fear of loss of mental abilities or dementia (2.97)	Feeling depressed (2.85)	Feeling anxious (2.81)	Feeling lonely (3.17)
Feeling helpless (2.95)	Getting sick or sicker (2.83)	Concern about not being able to care for myself (2.80)	Telling others (3.08)
Concern about confidentiality (2.88)	Concern about not being able to care for myself (2.79)	Side effects of HIV medication (2.79)	Fear of dying (2.97)
Feeling anger or frustration at the health care system (2.87)	Feeling helpless (2.77)		Problems in my sexual life/Feeling less physically attractive (2.94)
Feeling lonely/Financial difficulties (2.83)	Financial difficulties (2.75)		Fear about loss of mental abilities or dementia (2.89)
Feeling anxious (2.81)	Feeling angry (2.71)		Concern about confidentiality (2.86)
Getting sick or sicker/Concern about not being able to care for myself (2.79)			Feeling anger or frustration at the health care system (2.83)
Being discriminated against (2.78)			Feeling anxious (2.81)
Feeling isolated (2.71)			Concern about not being able to care for myself (2.75)

Note. Mean scores for HIVIS items are indicated in brackets (possible range 1–5). Table includes all HIVIS items with scores > 2.70.

groups on seven scales. Heterosexuals reported higher distress than gay men on *not knowing where to go for help* ($p = .001$), *concern about confidentiality* ($p = .002$), *being discriminated against* ($p = .01$), *feeling angry* ($p = .02$), *rejection by others close to me, e.g. family or friends* ($p = .02$), and *telling others, e.g. who to tell, what to tell* ($p = .04$) and lower distress on *grief due to loss of friends to AIDS* ($p = .007$).

Finally, heterosexual men and women reported less happiness ($p = .03$), less life satisfaction ($p = .03$), and marginally lower perceived psychological health ($p = .06$) than gay men.

For both heterosexual men and women and gay men, uncertainties about the future and being unable to realize life goals, as well as concerns about increasing physical disability, financial difficulties and negative mood states are major sources of distress. However, the picture that emerges is one of increased psychological risk among heterosexual men and women as a group compared to gay men. Although heterosexuals as a group do not experience the high distress associated with losing friends to AIDS that gay men do, they are more distressed by a number of problems having to do with factors related to what would generally be interpreted as stigmatization. Heterosexuals as a group experience more discrimination and rejection, are more distressed by issues having to do with concerns about confidentiality and telling others, and are angrier, unhappier, and less satisfied with life than gay men. The extent to which these differences may be due to differences between men and women is considered in the next section.

Heterosexual Men vs. Women
Table 13.2 also presents the most distressing problems for men in the heterosexual sample compared to women. For both men and women, *not being able to realize life goals* is the most distressing problem. Other problems which are among the most distressing to both groups include *feeling uncertain about the future, feeling angry, feeling depressed, fear of loss of mental abilities or dementia, feeling anxious, concern about confidentiality, feeling helpless, feeling anger or frustration at the health care system, feeling anxious*, and *concern about not being able to care for myself*. There are two problems which appear in the list of most distressing problems for men but not for women: *getting sick or sicker* and *side effects of HIV medication*; and other problems which appear in the list of most distressing problems for women but not for men: *financial difficulties, feeling isolated, feeling lonely, telling others, fear of dying, feeling less physically attractive*, and *problems in my sexual life*.

In comparing mean scores between heterosexual men and women on each of the 40 HIVIS items, differences were found between the two groups on seven scales. Women reported higher distress than men on *being discriminated against* ($p = .02$), *feeling isolated* ($p = .02$), *feeling angry* ($p = .02$), *feeling depressed* ($p = .02$), *fear of dying* ($p = .03$), *rejection by others close to me, e.g. family or friends* ($p = .05$), and *self-blame, guilt* ($p = .05$).

Finally, women reported less life satisfaction ($p = .05$) and lower perceived psychological health ($p = .05$) than men.

For both heterosexual men and women, uncertainties about the future and not being able to realize life goals, concerns about increasing physical disability and confidentiality, negative mood states, and anger and frustration at the health care system are major sources of distress. However, there are several differences in distress between men and women. Whereas men are more concerned about the physical consequences of the disease, such as getting sick or sicker and side effects of medication, women are more distressed by the psychological consequences of HIV infection, such as feeling lonely, isolated, fearful of dying, and less satisfied with life, as well as by the effects of HIV on sexuality, in terms of feeling less physically attractive and more distressed by sexual problems. Women are also more distressed by financial difficulties. Clearly, women with HIV infection are at greater psychological risk than heterosexual men.

The differences between heterosexual men and women suggest that the initial differences found between heterosexuals as a group and gay men are largely due, again, to differences between women and both heterosexual and gay men. It could be argued that the differences in psychological distress between men and women may be due to the fact that women in the sample are younger and less well-educated. However, the fact that psychological distress as measured by HIVIS total scores is only weakly related to both age ($r = -.13$) and education ($r = .15$) suggests that the differences in distress between men and women are not due to differences in age or education. Accumulating evidence suggests a psychological profile for women with HIV infection which puts them at increased mental health risk compared to either heterosexual or gay men.

Mental Health Services

Mental health services between heterosexual men and women and gay men were compared, followed by comparisons between heterosexual men and women. Differences in awareness, use and need between groups were examined using Chi-square tests. First the proportions in each group who were aware of and had used services were compared. Then the proportions in each group who rated a service as being among the three most needed were compared. Finally, groups were compared in terms of other service-related questions, e.g. barriers to service use, frequency of use of different service providers, prior use of mental health services, and whether the respondent must travel or had to move to obtain services.

Heterosexual Men and Women vs. Gay Men

Table 13.3 shows the percentages of awareness, use and need for services for heterosexual men and women compared to gay men. In terms of awareness of services, heterosexual men and women as a group are clearly less aware than gay men. Of the 20 services which were assessed, heterosexuals were significantly less aware than gay men of 17 of the 20 services. There were no differences in awareness between heterosexuals and gay men for only three services: *child care, temporary lodging while receiving care,* and *foster care.*

Despite differences in awareness, there were few differences in the use of services between heterosexuals as a group and gay men. Service use was similar in the two groups for 16 of the 20 services. Heterosexuals, however, were less likely to use *information* ($p = .0005$) and *dental services* ($p = .02$) and more likely to use *child care* ($p = .01$) and *foster care* ($p = .01$) than gay men.

Table 13.3
Awareness, Use, and Need for Services: Heterosexuals vs. Gay Men

Services	% Aware of Services		% Used Services		% Need (% Ranked in Top 3)	
	Heterosexuals	Gay Men	Heterosexuals	Gay Men	Heterosexuals	Gay Men
Adequate information	72	86**	60	76***	36	34
Peer counselling	70	87***	43	45	29	35
Professional counselling	66	80**	35	43	29	33
Alcohol or drug treatment	52	70***	8	8	8	5
Stress management	44	56*	12	16	18	17
Recreational/social activities	45	65***	12	19	5	9
Telephone hotline	57	79***	20	16	3	5
Nutritional counselling	54	65*	23	21	11	13
HIV pre- and post-test counselling	53	71***	25	24	7	11
Alternative treatments	42	63***	22	27	17	19
Financial assistance	64	78**	45	41	49	44
Housing	33	48**	10	6	13	12
Child care	21	24	2	0*	4	1
Homemaker/homecare services	31	56***	7	9	8	7
Temporary lodging while receiving care	22	30	3	1	4	2
Hospice/palliative care	35	57***	2	2	1	5*
Foster care	20	21	4	.4*	3	2
Adequate medical care	56	72***	44	45	36	41
Visiting nurse	37	52**	7	9	2	5
Dental services	48	64**	21	32*	8	11

***$p < .001$
**$p < .01$
*$p < .05$

Need for services for heterosexuals as a group compared to gay men were then examined. The only service for which need differed between the groups was *hospice/palliative care* (p = .03). Heterosexuals expressed lower need for this service than did gay men. The first two columns of Table 13.4 show the ranking of services according to need for both groups. These rankings are based on information provided in Table 13.3 about the proportions of respondents who rated the service as being among the three most needed. The five most needed services are identical for each group and include *financial assistance, adequate medical care, peer and professional counselling*, and *adequate information*. The five least needed services are also similar between the two groups and included *foster care, hospice/palliative care, temporary lodging while receiving care, telephone hotline* and *visiting nurse*.

Table 13.5 presents comparisons between heterosexual men and women and gay men on other service-related issues. Heterosexuals were more likely to report *fear of what others might think* (p = .03) as being a barrier to service use, were more likely to have to travel from the city or town in which they live to obtain services (p = .005), and were more frequent users of hospital in-patient services (p = .01). Gay men were more frequent users of AIDS community-based groups (p = .004) and family doctor (p = .0001).

Again, the picture that emerges is one of increased isolation and stigmatization in heterosexual men and women compared to gay men with HIV infection. As a group, heterosexual men and women are much less aware of services, are more likely to report fear of what others might think as a barrier to service use, are more likely to have to travel to another town or city than the one in which they live to obtain services, and are more likely to seek services on a hospital in-patient basis rather than their family doctor. Despite these differences, use and need for services is highly similar between the two groups. That is, lower awareness of services among heterosexuals is not associated with lower use of services. The extent to which the observed differences between heterosexuals as a group and gay men may be due to differences between men and women is considered in the next section.

Heterosexual Men vs. Women

Table 13.6 shows the percentages of awareness, use and need for services for heterosexual men and women. There were no differences in awareness of services between men and women except for *homemaker services* of which women were more aware (p = .03). Therefore, the lower awareness of services in heterosexuals as a group compared to gay men is not attributable to gender differences. Differences in awareness between heterosexuals and gay men may more likely be a function of the more extensive network and support systems in many gay communities.

Despite similarities in awareness, there were several differences in the use of services between men and women. Women were more likely than men to have used *telephone hotline* (p = .004), *housing* (p = .02), *child care* (p = .03) and *professional counselling* (p = .05) and less likely to have used nutritional counselling (p = .04).

Need for services for men compared to women were then examined. Women were more likely to rate *child care* (p = .002) and men were more likely to rate *HIV pre-and post-test counselling* (p = .01) as among the three most needed services. The last two columns of Table 13.4 show the ranking of services according to need for

Table 13.4

Services Ranked According to Need

Heterosexual Men and Women	Gay Men	Heterosexual Men	Heterosexual Women
Financial assistance	Financial assistance	Financial assistance	Financial assistance
Adequate medical care/Adequate information	Adequate medical care	Adequate medical care/Adequate information	Peer counselling/Professional counselling
Peer counselling/Professional counselling	Peer counselling	Peer counselling/Professional counselling	Adequate information/Adequate medical care
Stress management	Adequate information	Alternative treatments	Stress management
Alternative treatments	Professional counselling	Stress management	Alternative treatments/Housing
Housing	Alternative treatments	Housing/Nutritional counselling	Alcohol or drug treatment/Child care
Nutritional counselling	Stress management	HIV pre- and post-test counselling/Dental services	Nutritional counselling/Homemaker services
Alcohol or drug treatment/Homemaker services/Dental services	Nutritional counselling	Homemaker services	Temporary lodging while receiving care
HIV pre- and post-test counselling	Housing	Alcohol or drug treatment	Recreational/social activites
Recreational/social activities	Dental services/HIV pre- and post-test counselling	Recreational/social activities	Telephone hotline/Foster care/Dental services
Child care/Temporary lodging while receiving care	Recreational/social activities	Telephone hotline/Temporary lodging while receiving care/Foster care/Visiting nurse	HIV pre- and post-test counselling/Hospice/palliative care/Visiting nurse
Telephone hotline/Foster care	Homemaker services	Hospice/palliative care	
Visiting nurse	Alcohol or drug treatment/Telephone hotline/Hospice care/Visiting nurse	Child care	
Hospice/palliative care	Temporary lodging while receiving care/Foster care		
	Child care		

Table 13.5
Other Service-Related Issues

Service-Related Issues	Heterosexuals % Yes	Gay Men % Yes	Heterosexual Men % Yes	Heterosexual Women % Yes
Barriers				
Didn't know where to go to get services	22	19	20	26
Location of services too far/too inconvenient	14	9	14	14
Lack of transportation	16	10	16	14
Possible loss of confidentiality	30	23	29	34
Fear of what others might think	27	18**	24	34
Had to wait too long to get services	14	13	10	23
Didn't feel welcome where services offered	10	10	8	14
Couldn't afford services	16	14	13	23
Agency not open when I needed help	9	6	8	11
Services not available in my language	3	1	4	0
Didn't feel well enough	10	13	9	14
Has used mental health services before	21	30	17	31
Must travel to obtain services	26	12***	26	26
Had to move to obtain services	12	8	10	17
Frequency of use of different service providers (1 = Never, 5 = Always)	Mean (SD)	Mean (SD)	Mean (SD)	Mean (SD)
Hospital in-patient services	1.80 (1.20)	1.48 (0.99)**	1.73 (1.19)	1.94 (1.24)
Hospital out-patient services	2.64 (1.42)	2.78 (1.47)	2.79 (1.50)	2.31 (1.19)
AIDS community-based groups	1.90 (1.32)	2.33 (1.48)*	1.77 (1.24)	2.22 (1.46)
Other community-based groups	1.43 (0.94)	1.41 (0.96)	1.43 (0.97)	1.46 (0.92)
Family doctor	2.60 (1.48)	3.15 (1.39)***	2.54 (1.55)	2.75 (1.32)
Church groups	1.21 (0.71)	1.32 (0.85)	1.19 (0.71)	1.25 (0.73)
Community health clinic	1.33 (0.86)	1.24 (0.75)	1.29 (0.81)	1.44 (1.00)

*** $p < .001$ ** $p < .01$ * $p < .05$

Table 13.6
Awareness, Use, and Need for Services: Heterosexual Men vs. Women

Services	% Aware of Services		% Used Services		% Need (% Ranked in Top 3)	
	Men	Women	Men	Women	Men	Women
Adequate information	75	66	63	51	37	31
Peer counselling	71	66	38	54	24	40
Professional counselling	64	71	29	49*	24	40
Alcohol or drug treatment	52	51	9	6	7	11
Stress management	43	46	10	17	16	23
Recreational/social acitivities	40	51	15	6	5	3
Telephone hotline	56	60	13	37**	3	3
Nutritional counselling	54	54	28	11*	12	9
HIV pre- and post-test counselling	53	54	24	29	11	0*
Alternative treatments	39	49	20	26	19	14
Financial assistance	60	74	46	43	47	54
Housing	29	43	5	20*	12	14
Child care	16	31	0	6*	0	11**
Homemaker/homecare services	25	46*	5	11	8	9
Temporary lodging while receiving care	21	23	4	0	3	6
Hospice/palliative care	31	43	1	3	1	0
Foster care	16	29	3	6	3	3
Adequate medical care	55	57	46	40	37	31
Visiting nurse	34	46	6	9	3	0
Dental services	48	49	23	17	11	3

** p < .01   * p < .05

both groups. These rankings are based on information provided in Table 13.6 about the proportions of respondents who rated the service as being among the three most needed. The five most needed services are identical for each group and include *financial assistance, adequate medical care, peer and professional counselling,* and *adequate information.* The five least needed services are also similar between the two groups and include *foster care, hospice/palliative care, telephone hotline,* and *visiting nurse.* For women, *dental services* and *HIV pre- and post test counselling* were lower in the list of needed services than for men, whereas for men *temporary lodging while receiving care* and *child care* were lower in the list of needed services than for women.

Table 13.5 presents comparisons between heterosexual men and women on other service-related issues. There were no differences between men and women on any service-related issues, including barriers to service use, frequency of use of different service providers, prior use of mental health services, or whether the respondent must travel or had to move to obtain services.

In general, heterosexual men and women are equally aware of services and similar in terms of need for services. There are differences between men and women in the use of services in the expected direction: women are higher users of housing, child care, and professional counselling. Interestingly, women are three times more likely to use telephone hotline services. The finding of women's preference for an anonymous information service is consistent with previous results which suggest greater stigmatization in this group. Despite these differences, however, the general picture is that of similar awareness and need for men and women. In the case of mental health services then, the differences in awareness and other service-related questions between heterosexuals as a group and gay men, reported in the previous section, cannot be attributed to gender differences.

Despite the fact that few overall differences emerged in these analyses between heterosexual men and women, examination of the pattern of results between all three groups, i.e. heterosexual men and women and gay men, reveals an interesting picture of differences in mental health services in which gender differences figure prominently. This is particularly true in the area of barriers to service use, in which case qualitative analyses of table 13.5 show that the percentage of respondents reporting a particular factor as a barrier is highest for women on 8 of the 11 barriers compared to heterosexual and gay men. Qualitative comparisons also indicate that compared to both groups of men, women are more likely to have had to move to obtain services, use hospital in-patient and community health clinics more frequently and hospital out-patient clinics less frequently than either group of men. Women use family doctor services and AIDS community-based groups more frequently than heterosexual men, but not as frequently as gay men.

IMPLICATIONS REGARDING PSYCHOLOGICAL NEEDS AND SERVICES FOR HETEROSEXUALS WITH HIV INFECTION

Two major findings relevant to psychological needs and services for heterosexuals emerge from these analyses. First, there is no unitary view of the psychological impact and mental health service needs of heterosexuals with HIV infection. That is, it may not be useful to ask questions about the psychological impact of HIV infection on heterosexuals as a group. Rather, such questions can only be considered in the context of specific subgroups of heterosexuals with HIV infection defined, most importantly, in terms of gender and also according to risk factor group. Evidence from the analyses of data obtained in the national survey show a differential psychological impact of HIV on women compared to men, suggesting that gender is a major factor to be considered when assessing psychological needs and services for heterosexuals with HIV infection. Although we were unable to evaluate differences between subgroups of heterosexuals defined on the basis of risk factors, due to relatively small numbers in several risk groups, evidence from several studies reviewed in this chapter indicate that risk factor status is also a major determinant of psychological needs and services. Future research with HIV-infected heterosexuals, with larger subgroups of male and female injection drug users and haemophiliacs, would permit an evaluation of the differential effects of gender and risk factor status on psychological needs and services.

Second, results from these analyses point clearly to the greater mental health risk in women with HIV infection compared to men. In terms of psychological needs, women experience significant distress due to isolation, discrimination, and rejection, and are more likely to have feelings of self-blame, guilt, fear, depression and anger. In addition, HIV infection has an even greater impact on women's sexuality than on men's, and is associated with more distressing financial problems. Compared to heterosexual and gay men, women experience more barriers to service use and are more likely to use services which permit greater anonymity, such as telephone hotlines. Women's increased psychological risk and isolation may be due to a combination of the stigmatizing effects of HIV together with the general disadvantaged status of women. In this sense, women are in a double social minority position which makes them even more vulnerable to the stigmatizing effects of HIV infection than men.

Despite the increasing number of women with HIV infection (Guinan & Hardy, 1987a, 1987b; James, 1988; Mantell *et al.*, 1988; Mays & Cochran, 1988; Zuckerman & Gordon, 1988), little attention has been given to the special psychosocial problems and mental health needs of women (Buckingham & Rehm, 1987; Cochran & Mays, 1989; James, 1988; Mantell *et al.*, 1988). This may be largely due to the fact that HIV infection is typically perceived as a gay disease (Adams, 1986). Moreover, because attention has focused primarily on women who are injection drug users, the needs of other women with HIV infection have largely been ignored (Mantell *et al.*, 1988). However, there are several reasons why it is important that the psychosocial needs of women with HIV infection be considered separately from men.

First, the increasing size of the population of HIV-infected women implies a probable increase in the need for mental health services for these women. Second, the fact that a large number of women with HIV infection are from the least advantaged groups in society, e.g. poor, urban, ethnic, and other minority groups (Amaro, 1988; Cochran & Mays, 1989; Guinan & Hardy, 1987a, 1987b; Mantell *et al.*, 1988; Mays & Cochran, 1988; Zuckerman & Gordon, 1988), creates a dual set of unique psychosocial problems attributable to their status both as women and as minority group members. Third, the pattern of transmission of HIV infection in women is changing, such that heterosexual transmission is expected to increase (Mays & Cochran, 1988). Fourth, as the number of HIV-infected women increases, the number of pediatric AIDS cases is also expected to increase, creating yet another set of problems for both women and children affected by HIV infection (Mays & Cochran, 1988). Finally, given the link between risk reduction and sexual and contraceptive behaviour in women, it is important to gain knowledge about women's contraceptive behaviours in relation to risk reduction in HIV infection (Mays & Cochran, 1988).

The challenge to caregivers working with heterosexuals with HIV infection is to understand and determine the specific psychological needs of different subgroups of heterosexuals, and to develop services which are tailored to meet these differing needs. Women with HIV infection, in particular, are an even more psychologically vulnerable group in need of services that reduce isolation and stigmatization through empowerment. As the voices at the beginning of this chapter suggest, HIV is being increasingly less viewed as a gay disease but one whose psychological impact is now reaching 'the person next door'. Innovative mental health services need to be developed to address the changing picture of HIV infection and its effects on psychological well-being and quality of life in persons with HIV-infection. The mental health agenda is particularly urgent for women with HIV infection.

ACKNOWLEDGEMENTS

We would like to acknowledge the invaluable contributions of several individuals involved in the national study including: M. Sewitch, E. Clark, B. Ryan, P. Di Meco, and M. Hamel who provided research assistance; Dr N. Gilmore, Dr S. Grover, Dr J. I. Williams, and C. Meister who formed the Steering Committee; and members of the Federal Centre for AIDS Working Group on HIV Infection and Mental Health (Chair: Dr S. Woo). We would also like to thank the HIV caregivers in several cities across Canada for their willing and generous cooperation in providing access to respondents and distributing questionnaires. We especially appreciate the participation of those with HIV infection, and the family members, significant others, and caregivers who responded to the national survey.

REFERENCES

Adams, M. L. (1986). Plagued by the new right: Politics, women and AIDS. *Horizons*, 4, 1–2; 27; 32.

Agle, D., Gluck, H., Pierce, G. F. (1987). The risk of AIDS: Psychologic impact on the haemophiliac population. *General Hospital Psychiatry*, 9, 11–17.

Amaro, H. (1988). Considerations for prevention of HIV infection among Hispanic women. *Psychology of Women Quarterly*, 12, 429–443.

Batki, S. L., Sorensen, J. L., Faltz, B., Madover, S. (1988). Psychiatric aspects of treatment of IV drug abusers with AIDS. *Hospital and Community Psychiatry, 39*, 439–441.

Battle, C. U. (1986). Women and AIDS. *Journal of the American Medical Women's Association, 41*, 37; 61.

Black, J. L., Dolan, M. P., DeFord, H. A. (1986). Sharing of needles among users of intravenous drugs. *New England Journal of Medicine, 314*, 446–447.

Buckingham, S. L., Rehm, S. J. (1987). AIDS and women at risk. *Health and Social Work, 12*, 5–11.

Caputo, L. (1985). Dual diagnosis: AIDS and addiction. *Social Work, 30*, 361–364.

Cochran, S. D., Mays, V. M. (1989). Women and AIDS-related concerns: Roles for psychologists in helping the worried well. *American Psychologist, 44*, 529–535.

Des Jarlais, D. C., Friedman, S. R., Strug D. (1986). AIDS and needle sharing within the IV-drug use subculture. *The social dimensions of AIDS*, (pp. 111–124). New York: Praeger.

Des Jarlais, D. C., Wish, E., Friedman, S. R., Stoneburner, R., Yancovitz, S. R., Mildvan, D., El-Sadr, W., Brady, E., Cuadrado, M. (1987). Intravenous drug use and the heterosexual transmission of the human immunodeficiency virus: Current trends in New York City. *New York State Journal of Medicine, 87*, 283–286.

Evans, K. M. (1987). The female AIDS patient. *Health Care for Women International, 8*, 1–7.

Federal Centre for AIDS. (May 28, 1990). *Surveillance update: AIDS in Canada*. Ottawa: Federal Centre for AIDS.

Flavin, D. K., Frances, R. J. (1987). Risk-taking behaviour, substance abuse disorders, and the acquired immune deficiency syndrome. *Advances in Alcohol and Substance Abuse, 6*, 23–32.

Friedman, S. R., Des Jarlais, D. C., Sotheran, J. L. (1986). AIDS health education for intravenous drug users. *Health Education Quarterly, 13*, 383–393.

Ginzburg, H. M. (1984). Intravenous drug users and the acquired immune deficiency syndrome. *Public Health Reports, 99*, 206–212.

Greif, G. L., Price, C. (1988). A community-based support group for HIV positive I.V. drug abusers: The HERO programme. *Journal of Substance Abuse Treatment, 5*, 263–266.

Guinan, M. E., Hardy, A. (1987a). Epidemiology of AIDS in women in the United States: 1981–1986. *Journal of the American Medical Association, 257*, 2039–2042.

Guinan, M. E., Hardy, A. (1987b). Women and AIDS: The future is grim. *Journal of the American Medical Women's Association, 42*, 157–158.

Hamel, M. (1992). *La fiabilité et la validité de deux nouvelles échelles pour évaluer la santé mentale des personnes affectées par le virus de l'immuno-déficience humaine*. Unpublished master's thesis, Université du Québec à Montréal, Montréal, QC.

Hays, L. R., Lyles, M. R. (1986). Psychological themes in patients with acquired immune deficiency syndrome [Letter to the editor]. *American Journal of Psychiatry, 143*, 551.

Health and Welfare Canada. (1992). *Ending the isolation: HIV disease and mental health in the second decade*. Ottawa: Ministry of Supply and Services.

Health and Welfare Canada and Statistics Canada. (1981). *The health of Canadians: Report of the Canada Health Survey*. Ottawa: Minister of Supply and Services.

Ickovics, J.R., Rodin, J. (1992). Women and AIDS in the United States: Epidemiology, natural history, and mediating mechanisms. *Health Psychology, 11*, 1–16.

James, M. E. (1988). HIV seropositivity diagnosed during pregnancy: Psychosocial characterization of patients and their adaptation. *General Hospital Psychiatry, 10*, 309–316.

Jordan, T. J., Grallo, R., Mashberg, D., Gordon, L., Kapila, R. (1987). Manifestations of AIDS in intravenous drug users: A psychological perspective. *Psychology and Health, 1*, 165–178.

Lamping, D.L., Hamel, M.A. (1991, September). *Development, reliability and validity of a scale to measure HIV-related mental health distress*. Paper presented at the First International Conference on Biopsychosocial Aspects of HIV Infection, Amsterdam.

Lamping, D.L., Hamel, M., Di Meco, P. (1990). *Addendum: HIV-related mental health needs and services in Canada: Needs assessment survey final report* (Federal Centre for AIDS Contract No. 2225; 164 pp.). Ottawa: Federal Centre for AIDS.

Lamping, D.L., Sewitch, M. (1990). *Review of the literature on HIV infection and mental health*. Ottawa: Health and Welfare Canada.

Lamping, D.L., Sewitch, M., Clark, E., Ryan, B. (1990a). *HIV-related mental health needs and services in Canada: Needs assessment survey final report* (Federal Centre for AIDS Contract No. 2225; 330 pp.). Ottawa: Federal Centre for AIDS.

Lamping, D.L., Sewitch, M., Clark, E., Ryan, B. (1990b). *Needs assessment study: Pretest study report*. (Available from Federal Centre for AIDS Working Group on HIV Infection and Mental Health).

Maire, M. (1988). Le SIDA et les femmes: Un entretien avec le Professeur Henrion. *Le Chirurgien-Dentiste De France, 428*, 38–45.

Mantell, J. E., Schinke, S. P. Akabas, S. H. (1988). Women and AIDS. *Journal of Primary Prevention, 9*, 18–40.

Mays, V. M., Cochran, S. D. (1988). Issues in the perception of AIDS risk and risk reduction activities by black and Hispanic/Latina women. *American Psychologist, 43*, 949–957.

Minkoff, H. L. (1987). Care of pregnant women infected with human immunodeficiency virus. *Journal of the American Medical Association, 258*, 2714–2717.

Mondanaro, J. (1987). Strategies for AIDS prevention: Motivating health behaviour in drug dependent women. *Journal of Psychoactive Drugs, 19*, 143–149.

Mulleady, G. (1987). A review of drug abuse and HIV infection. *Psychology and Health, 1*, 149–163.

Naji, S., Wilkie, P., Markova, I., Forbes, C., Watson, J. (1986). Coping strategies of patients with haemophilia as a risk group for AIDS (Acquired immune deficiency syndrome). *International Journal of Rehabilitation Research, 9*, 179–180.

Peterson, J. L., Marin, G. (1988). Issues in the prevention of AIDS among Black and Hispanic men. *American Psychologist, 43*, 871–877.

Rickert, E. J. (1989). Differing sexual practices of men and women screened for HIV (AIDS) antibody. *Psychological Reports, 64*, 323–326.

Sachs, B. P., Tuomala, R., Frigoletto, F. (1987). Acquired immunodeficiency syndrome: Suggested protocol for counseling and screening in pregnancy. *Obstetrics & Gynecology, 70*, 408–411.

Saint-Jarre, C. (1989). Une réalité qui dépasse la fiction. *Frontières, 2*, 52–53.

Selwyn, P. A., Feiner, C., Cox, C. P., Lipshutz, C., Cohen, R. L. (1987). Knowledge about AIDS and high-risk behaviour among intravenous drug users in New York City. *AIDS, 1*, 247–254.

Shaw, N., Paleo, L. (1986). Women and AIDS. In L. McKusick (Ed.), *What to do about AIDS: Physicians and mental health professionals discuss the issues* (pp. 142–154). Berkeley: University of California Press.

Silberstein, C. H., McKegney, F. P., O'Dowd, M. A., Selwyn, P. A., Schoenbaum, E., Drucker, E., Feiner, C., Cox, C. P., Friedland, G. (1987). A prospective longitudinal study of neuropsychological and psychosocial factors in asymptomatic individuals at risk for HTLV-III/LAV infection in a methadone programme: Preliminary findings. *International Journal of Neuroscience, 32*, 669–676.

Statistics Canada: Housing, Family, and Social Statistics Division. (1987). *Health and social support, 1985*. Ottawa: Ministry of Supplies and Services.

Velimirovic, B. (1987). AIDS as a social phenomenon. *Social Science and Medicine, 25*, 541–552.

Veroust, Ferragu. (1988). Conséquences psychologique de la contamination chez les enfants hémophiles. *Annales Mèdico-Psychologiques, 146*, 254–257.

Wofsy, C. B. (1987). Human immunodeficiency virus infection in women. *Journal of the American Medical Association, 257*, 2074–2076.

Zuckerman, C., Gordon, L. (1988). Meeting the psychosocial and legal needs of women with AIDS and their families. *New York State Journal of Medicine, 88*, 619–620.

14

Alcohol, AIDS and Sex

MARTIN A. PLANT

INTRODUCTION

The sharing of 'infected' injecting equipment by drug users has been an important factor in the heterosexual transmission of HIV infection in many areas (e.g. National Research Council, 1989; Plant, 1990; Strang and Stimson, 1990). As emphasized throughout this book, most HIV infection is attributable, not to intravenous drug use, but to unprotected sex (Mann, Tarantola and Netten 1992). It has long been believed that unprotected sexual encounters may be fostered by the use of alcohol or other psychoactive drugs, notably cannabis, cocaine and amphetamines. Much had been written about the possible drug-sex connection even before the recognition of AIDS (e.g. Cavan, 1966; Soloman and Andrews, 1973). Psychoactive drugs are widely used throughout the world primarily for recreational purposes, but also for reasons of ritual.

Alcohol is widely used in most countries, even though it is proscribed in some Islamic states. The consumption of alcohol is well established in industrial countries and has been increasing rapidly in many developing nations. Levels of per capita alcohol consumption vary considerably between different countries. For example in 1989 per capita consumption of pure alcohol ranged from 2.3 litres in Mexico to 13.2 litres in France (Brewers' Society, 1991). It must be noted that 'official' records fail to represent a considerable proportion of alcohol consumption in areas where alcoholic beverages are home produced, or illicit, or both. The consumption of alcohol is associated with leisure, enjoyment and sex in many areas of the world. This connection, supported very often by traditional mores, popular expectations and mythology, has for centuries fostered the view that alcohol may serve to increase sexual arousal, heighten sexual pleasure or increase the risk of unprotected sex. Concern about the possible impact of drinking on sexual behaviour has been heightened by the spread of HIV infection. This chapter examines available evidence on whether or not the consumption of alcohol might have an impact on sexual behaviour or be connected in other ways with the spread of HIV infection or the course of AIDS-related illnesses. The evidence considered is divided into three categories. These are firstly, the possible effects of alcohol on the immune system; secondly, the possible role of alcohol as a cofactor in AIDS-related illness and, thirdly, the possible association between alcohol and unprotected or risky sexual behaviour. This chapter highlights studies which relate to the possible impact of alcohol consumption on the sexual behaviour and HIV/AIDS-related risks amongst heterosexuals.

Two main issues are addressed in this chapter. The first is whether or not the use of alcohol makes people more likely to succumb to HIV infection if they are exposed to the virus, and whether or not HIV infection accelerates more rapidly to AIDS because of alcohol consumption levels. The second issue relates to the question of whether or not men and women are more likely to engage in unprotected or 'risky' sex after drinking than they would otherwise be.

ALCOHOL AND THE IMMUNE SYSTEM

The possibility that HIV infection may be fostered by psychoactive drug use has been acknowledged since the initial recognition of AIDS. As described by Schilts (1987) it was suspected that some of those who were first diagnosed with AIDS In the USA might have had their immune systems damaged through the use of 'poppers' (amyl nitrate). A fairly robust body of evidence indicates that heavy alcohol consumption may damage immune responses. This is significant because an individual whose immune defences are depressed may be more vulnerable to HIV infection if exposed to the virus.

It has been reported that high doses of alcohol produce harmful effects on the immunity of laboratory animals. Stimmel (1987) concluded that the numbers of lymphocytes were depressed by the administration of alcohol 'in doses sufficient to produce dependence within one week'. This conclusion needs to be considered in the light of the fact that although many humans are alcohol dependent, few if any, are likely to develop dependence in even remotely so short a time as a week. Animal research is often a valuable guide to drug effects and other factors in humans. Even so it is not always generalizable to humans.

Flavin & Frances (1987), reviewing the results of several studies, reached the following conclusions:

> "Various drugs of abuse, including alcohol, cocaine, cannabis, opiates and volatile solvents, have all been shown *in vitro* or *in vivo*, to demonstrate various properties of immune suppression. Chronic alcohol ingestion, for example, has been associated with an increased incidence of head and neck cancers, and infection, decreased numbers of circulating T lymphocytes and their reactivity to mitogenic stimulation and defects of humeral immune mechanisms". (p 24)

An Italian study by Stefani *et al.* (1989) compared 12 chronic alcohol dependent individuals with 15 non dependent controls. The authors concluded that alcohol did impede lymphocyte activation. Another study by Dunne (1989) described the following example:

> "Non-specific activation of B lymphocytes occurs in all patients who drink alcohol regularly in excess". (p 543)

Dunne who noted that the investigations by Tevari & Noble (1971) and Kay *et al.* (1984) also supported the conclusion that "Chronic alcohol abuse" reduced the B endorphines in the brain. These usually enhance immune responses. Studies by several other researchers have also indicated that chronic heavy drinking or alcohol-related liver disease are associated with weakened immune responses (Glukman, Dvorak and MacGregor, 1977; Palmer, 1978; Asch *et al.*, 1984).

Molgaard *et al.* (1988) have also concluded from reviewing earlier studies that individuals who abuse alcohol have an "enhanced susceptibility to infection".

Molgaard and his co-authors also cite a number of studies which indicate that individuals with alcoholic liver disease had reduced numbers of lymphocytes and circulating T-cells (Bernstein *et al.*, 1974; Berenyi, Straus and Avila, 1979). Molgaard *et al.*, further concluded that:

> ..."alcoholics display deficient primary immune reactions, exhibiting defects in the T-helper cell system, by depressed blastogenic transformation to mitogens such as concanavilin A (Con A) and phyto haemaglutinin (PHA), and by decreased delayed hypersensitivity reactions to new and recall antigens". (p 1148)

It has been noted that a high proportion of people with AIDS who are intravenous drug users have liver disorders, some of which may be attributable to heavy drinking (Novick *et al.*, 1986; Dworkin *et al.*, 1987). This view has, however, been challenged by Klimes *et al.* (1990). Beresford, Blow & Hall (1986) have reported that AIDS-related symptoms may be confused with symptoms associated with alcohol dependence. Worner (1989) has also noted that the rare Guillan-Barre's Syndrome in alcohol dependents may be "an early manifestation of AIDS".

A study by Bagasra, Kajdacsy-Balla & Lischner (1989) suggests that human immune responses are affected even by *moderate* alcohol consumption. This laboratory study related to a study group of three females and five males aged between 21 and 40. These individuals, all of whom were described as being 'healthy' and HIV seronegative, consumed from 0.7–3.1 litres of beer or its equivalent in the form of other beverages. Blood samples were drawn from the subjects and were subjected to a number of tests.

> "After moderate alcohol consumption there was increased human immunodeficiency virus (HIV) replication in peripheral blood mononuclear cells during 28 days of culture without mitogen stimulation indicated by overnight syncytium formation with SUP-T1 indicator cells and by increased levels of HIV p24 antigen in the culture supernates. There was also decreased ability of lymphocytes to produced interleukin 2 and soluble immune response suppressor activity after stimulation with concanavalin A, the former, possibly both, for over 4 days after alcohol ingestion. These preliminary data extend well-known immunosuppressive effects of chronic alcohol ingestion to acute ingestion and raise the question: Could even casual alcohol

consumption enhance HIV infectivity and/or enhance the progression of latent HIV infection?'' (p 636)

These authors noted that their results related only to low levels of alcohol consumption on a single occasion. They also concluded that their results did not appear to be beverage specific. They did emphasize, however, that it is not clear whether a weakened immune system is necessarily particularly susceptible to HIV infection. Bagasra and his colleagues also investigated the effects of consuming smaller quantities of beer and the duration of these effects. This work involved three subjects after consumption of an average of 1.1 litres of beer. This showed that blood samples exposed to HIV also had an increased susceptibility to infection and that immune responses were depressed. The increased susceptibility to infection "appeared to persist for at least 1.5 days after ingestion of beer and may not have peaked until that time". The authors also concluded that the depression of both helper and suppressor T-lymphocytes may last as long as 4.5 days after low levels of alcohol consumption. These results are noteworthy. They suggest that even mundane and unexceptional levels of alcohol consumption may depress immune responses. They also accelerate the progress of HIV replication after initial exposure to the virus.

A study of 4,462 male 'Vietnam era' US veterans has been reported. This lends strong support to the conclusion that there may be a dose-related effect of drinking on the immune system. The results of this investigation indicated that several measures of immune status varied at different levels of alcohol consumption (Mili *et al.*, 1992).

A major contribution of writings related to the possible connection between alcohol and the immune system was recently published (Seminara, Watson & Pawlowski, 1990). These authors noted that alcohol consumption has been associated with pronounced abnormalities of immune function, ranging from immune suppression to autoimmune phenomena.

This book presents an array of results from animal studies. Many of these support other evidence (e.g. Dehne *et al.*, 1989; Jerrells *et al.*, 1989; Aldo-Benson, 1989; Blank, Duncan & Meadows 1991; Jayasinghe, Gianutsos & Habhard, 1992) indicating that alcohol consumption may harm the immune system and otherwise increase susceptibility to infections. In addition further evidence is presented which supports the conclusion that chronic heavy drinking in humans is often associated with depressed immune responses. Additional evidence is provided by Bagasra *et al.* (1990) of the impact of moderate alcohol consumption of HIV-1 replication in human blood samples. In addition Prabhala & Watson (1990) described the results of a study of human subjects who were abstainers or 'moderate drinkers'. The latter consumed small quantities of alcohol, noted as ranging from 0.7–2.0 grammes per day. This indicated that alcohol consumption decreased the percentage of total T-lymphocytes. Even so the percentage of T-helper cells was increased by alcohol.

ALCOHOL AS A COFACTOR IN AIDS-RELATED ILLNESS

The fact that alcohol consumption depresses responses and may also increase susceptibility to HIV infection suggests that drinking may also be a cofactor in the development of AIDS. The implications of possible influences upon AIDS-related illness have been emphasized by Haverkos (1990).

Nair *et al.* (1990) have reported that available evidence suggests that alcohol might be a cofactor in HIV infection and the development of AIDS-related illnesses. This conclusion like those reported by Bagasra *et al.*, and Bagasra, Kaydacsy-Ball and Lischner (op cit) was based upon testing the effects of doses of alcohol an lymphocytes obtained from 'normal' human donors.

Kaslow *et al.* (1989) have described the results of a multicentre cohort study of homosexual men in the USA. This investigation examined the development of AIDS amongst HIV seropositive individuals in relation to psychoactive substance use. Analysis revealed that neither levels of the use of alcohol and illicit drugs were generally related to AIDS-related symptoms. In spite of this, amongst HIV infected subjects heavy drinking was found to be associated with "a lower prevalence of persistent generalized lymphadenopathy". The conclusions reached by Kaslow *et al.* have been criticized on several grounds. These include the possibly dubious value of self-reports of alcohol and drug use by alcohol dependents and the exclusion of people who seroconverted during the study (Drexler & Brown, 1990). These authors noted that "alcoholism may contribute to earlier central nervous system involvement by human immunodeficiency viruses in seropositive individuals". (Drexler & Brown, op. cit: 371).

Badgley (1990) also noted that Kaslow *et al.* did not present data related to any possible link between psychoactive drug use and seroconversion.

This book is concerned with heterosexual AIDS. Some evidence is available from studies of gay men. A selection of this is presented in this chapter because this helps to build up a fuller picture of the possible role of alcohol consumption in relation to sexual behaviour. As indicated below, such evidence also serves to emphasize the importance of examining the alcohol-sex connection with reference to different sub-groups of people. A study of sexually active gay men indicated that heavy drinking was associated with HIV seroconversion (Penkower *et al.*, 1991). This investigation also identified moderate to heavy illicit drug use, failure to use condoms and an increased number of sexual partners as being associated with seroconvertion. The connections between these types of variables are discussed further below. Another recent study by Williams *et al.* (1991) indicated no significant difference in lifetime alcohol or illicit drug abuse between homosexual men with and without HIV infection.

UNPROTECTED SEXUAL BEHAVIOUR

The suspicion that alcohol consumption may have an effect upon sexual behaviour is far from new. Ridlon (1988) has noted:

> "From the beginning of civilisation there has been a connection between drinking and involvement with sex". (p 27–28)

In many countries the consumption of alcoholic beverages is associated with dating, sexuality and often with prostitution. Many drinking locales, such as clubs and bars have explicit or implicit identities related to sex. Drinking and sex are frequently connected if only because both are commonplace facets of leisure time (Cavan, 1966; McKirnan & Peterson, 1989).

The concept of 'disinhibition' plays an important role in relation to the supposed link between alcohol and sexual behaviour. Disinhibition has been considered in detail elsewhere (Room & Collins, 1983). In relation to sexual behaviour 'disinhibition' is assumed to imply that drinking leads people to become less restrained, more sexually aroused or acquiescent. In other words individuals after drinking are more likely to engage in sexual acts which might not be seriously considered under other circumstances. As Room (1983) has noted the chemistry of alcohol "is often used to excuse or account for otherwise inexcusable behaviour" (pv).

Recent interest in the possible connection between alcohol consumption and unprotected sex has been greatly heightened by the spread of HIV infection and AIDS. Scientific impetus for the investigations of this topic as provided by Stall *et al.* (1986). These authors noted that 'high risk' sexual activity amongst homosexual men in the USA was associated with the use of alcohol and non-injected drugs such as cannabis (marihuana) and 'poppers' (amyl nitrate). These findings aroused considerable interest especially in the USA and the UK. This has been reflected by the publication of a series of study results related to this topic. These have related to both heterosexuals and to homosexuals. This book is *Heterosexual AIDS* but this chapter will refer to homosexual as well as to heterosexual studies since both provide important evidence in relation to the alcohol–sex connection. Some of this evidence is also cited elsewhere in this book by Strunin and Hingson.

For the purpose of this chapter the evidence considered is presented in the chronological order of year of publication to take into account overlapping or general coverage.

Arya *et al.* (1978) indicated that drinking was associated with failure to avoid unprotected sex amongst males treated for non-specific urethritis. Mott & Haurin (1988) conducted a study of young people in the USA and found no link between earlier sexual experience and first use of alcohol or illicit drugs. Even so the results did show that people who became sexually active later were more likely to have begun to drink or use illicit drugs at around the same age. A Scottish study by Robertson & Plant (1988) described a group of young people who had married while only teenagers. Those who had consumed alcohol immediately before their first experience of sexual intercourse were much less likely to have used any form of contraceptive than those who had not done so. The respective proportions were 13% and 57% (males) and 24% and 68% (females).

A US study of 69 sexually active women aged between 16 and 34 has been described by Harvey & Beckman (1986). This investigation collected information through daily log books and retrospective questionnaires. The results failed to show that alcohol produced significant effects on sexual arousal, sexual intercourse or orgasm. In addition women appeared to initiate *fewer* sexual activities after drinking. In spite of this respondents endorsed the view that alcohol enhanced sexual desire and activity. This study also indicated that drinking prior to sexual intercourse did not influence 'coitus–dependent' contraceptive use.

Additional support for the view that many women view alcohol as a disinhibitor has been provided by a study of sexual experience and drinking amongst women in a US national survey (Klassen & Wilsnack, 1986). This revealed that most women drinkers, especially heavier drinkers, reported that alcohol consumption reduces inhibition and "helps them feel close to others". Approximately a fifth reported becoming more sexually assertive after drinking, while 8% stated they were less particular in their choice of partners. Heavier drinkers also reported the highest levels of sexual dysfunction. The authors reported:

> "The study's findings may show the effects of a generalized moral value framework in which one large portion of the nation's population, especially females, is subject to pervasive proscriptions of behaviour, including their drinking and sexuality, while others vary in the freedom they find to drink and be sexual". (p 363).

A study of random samples of gay men in San Francisco indicated that those who continued to engage in unsafe sex were more likely than others to combine alcohol and/or illicit drugs with sex (Communication Technologies Inc., 1987).

A review by Crowe & George (1989) concluded that:

> "... alcohol disinhibits psychological sexual arousal and suppresses physiological responding, the former effect being stronger at lower doses and the latter effect at higher doses". (p374)

These authors also noted that disinhibition is both psychological and pharmacological. Its psychological aspects reflect "socially learned expectancies".

Ford (1989) conducted a survey of young people in the South West of England. This indicated that most respondents reported that alcohol consumption made them less sexually inhibited and also made sex more enjoyable. Most of the males and a large minority of females reported that alcohol consumption made them more likely to disregard the risks of HIV, AIDS and pregnancy. Half of the females and 64% of males reported that they were less likely to use condoms after drinking than they would otherwise have been. Ford reported that older individuals were particularly likely to regard alcohol as reducing sexual inhibitions. He also concluded that the heaviest drinkers were especially likely to view alcohol as influencing their sexual feelings.

Nakagawa *et al.* (1989) have described the results of a study of males in Japan. This study showed that heavier drinkers had experienced their first sexual intercourse significantly earlier than other men. Seigel *et al.* (1989) examined factors associated with risky sex amongst gay men in New York City. This revealed that illicit drug use in sexual contexts was a significant factor. Even so alcohol use was not. Windle (1989) concluded that a subset of heterosexual alcohol dependents (alcoholics) engaged in a variety of risky behaviours. These included high risk sex and frequent illicit drug use, including intravenous use.

The work of Hingson, Strunin and their colleagues has been elaborated in Chapter 8. Hingson *et al.* (1990) have reported that amongst teenagers in Massachusetts heavier drinkers were 2.8 times less likely than others to use condoms during sex. In addition 16% of drinkers reported that they were *less* likely to use condoms after imbibing alcohol than they would otherwise have been. A further survey by Hingson, Strunin & Berlin (1990) indicated that 13% of those who had combined sexual activity and drinking reported being less likely to use condoms under such circumstances. Another US study by Parker, Harford & Rosenstock (1990) reported that 'sexual risk-taking' amongst young people was associated with alcohol and illicit drug use. Cottler, Helzer & Tipp (1990) conducted a US general population survey of 3,000 people. This indicated that amongst females drinking habits were associated with having had multiple sexual partners.

A study of male and female prostitutes in Edinburgh, Scotland, has been described by Morgan Thomas (1990) and by Plant, Plant & Morgan Thomas (1990). These results indicated that many prostitutes were heavy drinkers and that most prostitute–client encounters involved drinking. Even so levels of condom use were *not* related to the self-reported levels of alcohol consumption of those providing sexual services. The same investigation also elicited data from a study group of sex industry clients. This revealed that amongst men who paid for sex with men, condom use was inversely related to alcohol consumption. Even so such an association was not evident amongst men who paid for sex with females (Morgan Thomas, Plant & Plant, 1990). These authors noted that although drinking and often heavy drinking were commonplace features of client–prostitute contacts, condom use appeared to be largely influenced by the negotiating power of male and female prostitutes. Such power depends upon many factors. These include the way in which prostitutes operate. For example those working in organized establishments such as brothels, saunas or massage parlours may be better able to enforce condom use than those working in isolation or those who enter clients' motor vehicles or homes.

Rolf *et al.* (1990) concluded from a study of US imprisoned male adolescents that having sex with 'high risk' individuals was associated with alcohol use. Flanigan *et al.* (1990) have cited several studies which suggest that females regard alcohol as being an aphrodisiac and that many consume alcohol before sexual intercourse. These authors have also concluded that alcohol or illicit drug use may be contributory factors in unplanned pregnancy.

A Scottish study examined a group of males and females aged between 25 and 27. This revealed that levels of alcohol consumption were not generally associated with levels of self-reported condom use. Even so males and females who reported a high frequency of combining drinking with sexual activity were *seven times* less likely to use condoms during vaginal sex than were other respondents. Females who had experienced higher levels of alcohol-related problems were more likely than other women to classify their own sexual activities as being 'risky'. Males who had experienced higher levels of alcohol problems reported having had more sexual partners in the past year than had other men (Bagnall, Plant & Warwick, 1990).

Temple & Leigh (1990) have described a general population study conducted in California. This indicated that sexual encounters with new partners were most likely to involve drinking. Even so this also indicated that alcohol consumption in itself was not associated with unprotected sex. Leigh (1990a,b) has described two other US studies. These related to 844 respondents to a mail survey, 117 volunteers who kept diaries, as well as respondents to the household survey. Alcohol consumption was not associated with unprotected sex amongst gay men. This finding contrasts with the influential results reported by Stall *et al.* (1986). Amongst heterosexuals alcohol consumption was only associated with risky sex amongst women in the mail survey who had consumed five or more drinks prior to sex. In contrast the diary study revealed that drinking was weakly associated with *safe* sex amongst both males and females. Individuals who kept diaries were not a representative group of people. They may also have been influenced in their behaviours by involvement in the research. Leigh concluded that the main predictor of risky sex amongst heterosexuals was the total frequency of sex. Alcohol or illicit drug use by a partner appeared to explain only a small proportion of total variance (Leigh, 1990c). The mail survey noted above indicated that males and females, both homosexual and heterosexual, differed in relation to their sex-related expectancies of alcohol. Homosexual men and women reported stronger expectancies of reduced nervousness and increased riskiness than did heterosexuals. Heavier drinkers appeared to be particularly willing to support the view that alcohol consumption would affect their sexual behaviour (Leigh, 1990d).

A US survey of over 5,000 college students indicated that alcohol use was positively associated with having had a larger number of sexual partners. Even so alcohol use was not related to levels of condom use (MacDonald *et al.*, 1990). A study of gay men in Boston, Massachusetts, indicated that those who reduced the frequency of their drinking were more likely to refrain from risky sexual practices (McCusker *et al.*, 1990). Clearly the frequency of drinking could have been a facet of visiting bars, or other social and/or sexual contacts. Gold *et al.* (1991) reported the results of another study of alcohol use by gay men in Melbourne, Australia. This did not indicate that drinking was associated with risky sex. Orr, Beiter and Ingersoll (1991) have examined factors associated with sexual experience amongst a study group of US boys and girls aged 12–16. This investigation indicated that such early sexual experience was associated with a number of behaviourial factors. These included the use of alcohol and illicit drugs and a variety of problem behaviours. A study of US high school students revealed that:

"The best predictor of sexual risk behaviour was alcohol and drug use" (Shafer and Bayer, 1991) (p 827)

These authors further concluded that:

"... several factors related to adolescent risks for STDs: the connection between peer influence and adolescent risk behaviors, the link between alcohol and drug use and sexual behavior, and the role of knowledge in determining non use of condoms". (p 826)

The existence of differences in alcohol-related sexual expectancies of homosexual and heterosexual people has been noted above. Trocki & Leigh (1991), reviewing available data together with the mail survey described by Leigh (op cit), concluded that it is necessary to elicit information about specific sexual encounters in order to produce "a better understanding of the dynamics of sexual encounters and the predictors of risky sex in the encounters" (p 981).

The mythology, or at least popular views, of the effects of alcohol and other drugs on sexual behaviour were examined by Bills & Duncan (1991) in relation to students in a university in the midwest of the USA. This revealed that 43.5% of 'experienced alcohol users' indicated that they believed that alcohol reduced sexual inhibitions. In addition some drinkers and non-drinkers endorsed incorrect views. These included the belief that alcohol increased sexual arousal and sexual drive so that it enhanced sexual performance. Another study of US students concluded that 47% of males and 57% of females reported that they and engaged in sexual intercourse "primarily because they were intoxicated" (Butcher, Manning & O'Neal, 1991). This finding lends further support to the view that many people *believe* that alcohol is an aphrodisiac or disinhibitor, but does not, in itself provide evidence to support the view that drinking necessarily affects sexual behaviour. Chopper & Lipsitt (1991) concluded from a study of 332 US male undergraduates that "older adolescent/young males may engage in riskier sexual behaviour when using alcohol" (p 91). This view was based upon an analysis of separate drinking occasions. The researchers concluded that the most powerful predictor of unprotected sexual intercourse was risk-taking. They noted that 10% of their respondents claimed to have had alcohol-influenced unprotected sex.

As noted above studies of alcohol use and sexual behaviour amongst homosexual men have produced conflicting results. A US study by Kelly, St. Lawrence & Brasfield (1991) examined the predictors of the resumption of high risk sexual activities. This indicated that intoxication preceding sex, together with several other behaviourial and psychological variables, were associated with such relapse. A survey of US adolescents indicated that sexual risk-taking was associated with alcohol use (Keller *et al.*, 1991). A Norwegian study of 3,000 adolescents indicated that age at first intercourse was associated with drinking and smoking behaviour as well as with educational qualifications, peer affiliation and the frequency of visiting a discotheque (Kraft, 1991). Casual sex amongst young Norwegians has been further examined by Traeen & Lewin (1992). Data were elicited from a representative sample of 2,997 people aged 17–19. The results of this investigation indicated that the amount of sexual experience was associated with "lifestyle factors such as smoking and drinking". The authors noted that drinking and smoking, together with sexual behaviour, mark the transition from childhood to adult status.

A postal and interview survey of 2,174 students in North East England examined the role of alcohol in relation to sexual behaviour. The postal survey revealed that heavier drinkers were more likely to engage in risky sex than were others. Similar results were obtained by the interview survey. The authors concluded:

> "There are three possible explanations of the association between drinking habits and unsafe sex: alcohol might disinhibit safe sex; young risk-takers may also drink more, or, drinking might be associated with unsafe sex by coincidence because sexual encounters often begin in licensed premises". (p 577)

An analysis of survey data from a representative group of households in the San Francisco area has been described by Ericksen & Trocki (1992). This showed that problem drinking was a risk factor for sexually transmitted diseases independent of the pattern of alcohol or illicit drug use. Both men and women who had histories of alcohol problems were more likely than other respondents to have had sexually transmitted diseases and to have had multiple sexual partners.

A notable theme emerging from the literature under review is the association of both alcohol use and risky sexual behaviour with other forms of risk-taking. A study of 602 young people in the USA indicated that several high-risk behaviours clustered together. These included alcohol or drug misuse symptoms, anxiety, intravenous drug use and engaging in prostitution. (Stiffian, Dore, Earls & Cunningham, 1992). A study of 42 Nature American adolescents showed that heavy drinkers were most likely to report that drinking makes sexual activity more enjoyable. This investigation also showed that a substantial proportion of this small study group agreed that alcohol increased sexual arousal and led to sexual disinhibition (Conner & Conner, 1992).

A Scottish study examined the sexual behaviours and psychoactive drug use of 1,378 people aged 16–30 in two deprived urban areas. This indicated that 22% of males and 15% of females reported being less likely to use condoms during sex after drinking (Bagnall & Plant, 1991). The same study also indicated that sexual risk-taking was associated with heavier use of alcohol, tobacco and illicit drugs. Even so the precise pattern of such associations differed between the two sexes and the two areas surveyed (Plant *et al.*, 1993) alcohol consumption was *not* associated with individual condom use on specific occasions (Miller, 1993). Weatherburn (1992) has analysed diary records of over 4,000 sexual encounters kept by a study group of gay men in Britain. This revealed no significant differences between levels of sexual risk taking in relation to the use or non-use of alcohol.

CONCLUSIONS AND DISCUSSION

The preceding evidence indicates that chronic heavy drinking or dependent drinking associated with reduced immune functioning. Perhaps more disturbing is the fact that even 'moderate' or 'social' alcohol consumption also appears to reduce the effectiveness of the human immune system and may increase HIV progression. It is, however, not clear whether this fact in itself increases vulnerability to HIV infection although *in vitro* studies suggest that alcohol may increase such susceptibility. Limited current evidence suggests that alcohol consumption may not be a cofactor in the development of HIV-related illnesses, but this conclusion can only be provisional at this stage.

Abundant survey data support the conclusion that alcohol consumption is often, though not always, associated with various measures of unprotected or 'risky' sexual activity. Findings in this respect are not uniform, especially in relation to gay men. Even so a persuasive body of evidence supports the conclusion that sexual risk-taking is associated, in some study groups of both heterosexual and homosexuals, with a number of other risky behaviours, including heavy drinking as well as the use of other psychoactive drugs.

At present it has not been demonstrated whether alcohol consumption makes an individual, or a pair of partners, more likely to engage in unprotected sex than they would otherwise be. Very few studies have examined specific sexual encounters. Those which have (e.g. Robertson & Plant, 1988; Harvey & Beckman, 1987; Leigh, 1990c; Gold *et al.*, 1991; Trocki & Leigh, 1991; Weatherburn, 1992; Miller, 1993) have produced varied results. So too have studies which have examined *general* patterns of alcohol consumption and general patterns of sexual behaviour.

The relationship between drinking and sex is complex. Available evidence supports the view expounded by Jessor & Jessor (1977) that some people are especially likely to engage in a variety of problem behaviours. As noted by Plant & Plant (1992) alcohol consumption may be a proxy variable or a marker for a constellation of risk-taking behaviours. Moreover risk-taking in different forms is commonplace, and even normal, amongst young adults.

Alcohol is linked with sexual activity for many reasons. It is clear that in some cultures there is a widespread belief that alcohol disinhibits, fosters and enhances sexual activity. In spite of this the inter-relationship between drinking and sex remains scientifically problematic. As noted by Gillies (1991) and by Plant & Plant (op cit) no clear causal relationship has been delineated, even if there is abundant evidence of an *association* between drinking and risky sex. It should be noted that much of this evidence does not relate to specific events. Moreover the main conclusion indicated by available findings is that some people take more risks than others.

At present research has failed to support the popular belief that alcohol consumption does in fact foster risky sex. This still remains an unresolved issue (World Health Organization, 1993). The roles of intoxication and disinhibition should not be dismissed. Drinking *may* impair judgement and certainly does influence sexual responses (Robertson 1990). Inexperienced adolescents and other young adults commonly regard drinking as having a confidence boosting, relaxing or other instrumental role in sexual contexts. There is evidence that blood alcohol levels associated with specific quantities of alcohol vary markedly at different points in the female's menstrual cycle (nb. Sutker, Goist & King, 1987). This variation may make it harder for females to cope with, or to predict the effects of alcohol consumption, than it is for males. More generally young women in many cultures face great difficulties, even if they are motivated, to negotiate or insist upon condom use with their male partners, whether the latter are drunk or sober.

Further research is needed to investigate the multitude of factor which may mediate the alcohol–sex connection. These include the details of specific sexual encounters, the nature of relationships, the self-efficacy and negotiating power of the actors and the role of alcohol-related expectancies in different situations amongst specific sub-groups. In the meantime care should be taken not to promulgate messages suggesting that drinking per se is an excuse for unprotected sex. Conversely in many contexts AIDS prevention activities could also be usefully targeted at drinking locales such as clubs and bars since these are often linked with casual or unprotected sex for social reasons (nb. Honnen & Kleinke, 1990).

ACKNOWLEDGEMENTS

The compilation of this review was assisted by Dr Jan Gill of the Alcohol Research Group, University of Edinburgh and Mr Peter Weatherburn of the South Bank University, London. Mrs Janis Nichol is thanked for her fast and efficient word processing from a nearly illegible manuscript.

REFERENCES

Aldo-Benson, M. (1989) Mechanisms of alcohol-induced suppression of B-cell response. *Alcoholism: Clinical and Experimental Research*, 13, 469–475.

Arya, O.P., Abergant, C.D., Annels, E.H., Chovey, P., Gosh, A.K., Goddard, A.D. (1978) Management of non-specific urethritis in men. *British Journal of Venereal Diseases*, 54, 414–421.

Aschah, K.J., Hyland, R.H., Hutcheson, M.A., Urbanski, S.J., Pruzanski, W., St. Louis, E., Jones, D.P., Keystone, E.C. (1984) Invasive aspergillois in a 'healthy' patient. *Canadian Medical Association Journal*, 131, 332–335.

Badgley, L.E. (1990) Psychoactive drug use and AIDS (letter), *Journal of the American Medical Association*, 263, 371.

Bagasra, O., Kajdacsy-Balla, A., Lischmer, H.W. (1989) Effects of alcohol ingestion on in vitro susceptability of peripheral blood mononuclear cells to infection with HIV and of selected T-cell functions, *Alcoholism: Clinical and Experimental Research*, 13, 636–643.

Bagasra, O., Whittle, P., Kajdacsy-Balla, A., Lischner, H.W. (1990) Effects of alcohol ingestion on in vitro susceptibility of peripheral blood mononuclear cells to infection with HIV-1 and on CD4 and CD8 lymphocytes, In: Seminara, D., Watson, R.R. and Pawlowski, A. (eds) *Alcohol, Immunomodulation with AIDS*, New York, Alan R. Liss Inc., 351–358.

Bagnall, G.M., Plant, M.A. (1991) AIDS risk, alcohol and illicit drug use amongst young adults in areas of high and low rates of HIV infection, *AIDS Care*, 3, 355–361.

Bagnall, G., Plant, M.A. and Warwick, W. (1990) Alcohol, drugs and AIDS-related risks: results from a prospective study. *AIDS Care*, 2, 309–317.

Berenyi, M.R., Straus, B., Avila, T. (1975) T-Rosettes in alcoholic cirrhosis of the liver. *Journal of the American Medical Association*, 232, 44–46.

Beresford, T.P., Blow, E.C., Hall, R.C.W. (1986) AIDS encephalitis mimicking alcohol dementia and depression. *Biological Psychiatry*, 21, 394–397.

Bernstein, I.M., Webster, K.H., Williams, R.C. Jnr., Strickland, R.G. (1974) Reduction in circulating T-lymphocytes in alcoholic liver disease. *Lancet*, 2, 488–490.

Bills, S.A., Duncan, D.F. (1991) Drugs and sex: A survey of college students beliefs, *Perceptual and Motor Skills*, 72, 1293–1294.

Blank, G.E., Duncan, D.A., Meadows, G.G. (1991) Suppression of natural killer cell activity by ethanol consumption and food restriction. *Alcoholism: Clinical and Experimental Research*, 15, 16–22.

Brewers' Society (1991) *Statistical Handbook*, London, Brewers' Society.

Butcher, A.H., Manning, D.T., O'Neal, E.C. (1991) HIV-related sexual behaviour of college students. *Journal of Americal College of Health*, 491, 115–118.

Cavan, S. (1966) Liquor License: An Ethnography of Bar Behavior, Chicago, Aldine.

Clapper, R.L., Lipsitt, L.P. (1991) A retrospective study of risk-taking and alcohol-mediated unprotected intercourse. *Journal of Substance Abuse*, 3, 91–96.

Communication Technologies Inc (1987) *Report on Designing and Effective AIDS Prevention Campaign Strategy for San Francisco: Results from the Fourth Probability Sample of an Urban Gay Male Community*, Communication Technologies.

Conn, H.O., Fessel, J.M. (1976) Spontaneous bacterial peritonitis in cirrhosis: variations on a theme. *Medicine*, 50, 160–197.

Conner, J.L., Conner, C.N. (1992) Expected benefits of alcohol use on sexual behaviour: Native American adolescents. *Psychological Reports*, 70, 91–98.

Cottler, L.B., Helzer, J.E., Tipp, J. (1990) Lifetime patterns of substance abuse among general population subjects engaging in high risk sexual behaviours. *American Journal of Drug and Alcohol Abuse*, 16, 207–222.

Crowe, L.C., George, W.H. (1989) Alcohol and human sexuality: Review and integration. *Psychological Bulletin*, 105, 374–386.

Dehne, N.E., Mendenhall, C.L., Roselle, G.A., Grossman, C.J. (1989) Cell-mediated immune responses associated with short-term alcohol intake: time course and dose dependency. *Alcoholism: Clinical and Experimental Research*, 13, 201–205.

Draper, L.R., Gyure, L.A., Hall, J.G., Robertson, D. (1983) Effect of alcohol on the integrity of the intestinal epithelium. *Gut*, 24, 399–404.

Drew, D.A., Clifton, P.M., La Brooy, J.T., Sherman, D.J.C. (1984) Polyclonal B cell activation in alcoholic patients with no evidence of liver dysfunction. *Clinical and Experimental Immunology*, 57, 479–486.

Drexler, K.P.G., Brown, G.R. (1990) Psychoactive drug use and AIDS (letter). *Journal of the American Medical Association*, 263, 371.

Dunne, F.J. (1989) Alcohol and the immune system, *British Medical Journal*, 298, 543–544.

Erickson, K.P., Trocki, K. (1992) Behavioural risk factors for sexually transmitted diseases in American households. *Social Science and Medicine*, 34, 843–853.

Flanigan, B., McLean, A., Hall, C., Propp, V. (1990) Alcohol use as a situational influence on young women's pregnancy risk-taking behaviours. *Adolescence*, XXV, 97, 205–14.

Flavin, D.K., Francis, R.J. (1987) Risk-taking behavior, substance abuse disorders and the Acquired Immune Deficiency Syndrome. *Advances in Alcohol and Substance Abuse*, 6, 23–32.

Gillies, P. (1991) HIV Infection, alcohol and illicit drugs. *Current Opinion in Psychiatry*, 4, 448–453.

Glassman, A.B., Bennett, C.E., Randall, C.L. (1985) Effects of ethyl alcohol on human peripheral lymphotytes, *Archives of Pathology and Laboratory Medicine*, 109, 540–542.

Glukman, S.J., Dvorak, V.C., MacGregor, R.R. (1977) Host defences during prolonged alcohol consumption in a controlled environment. *Archives of International Medicine*, 137, 1539–1543.

Gold, R.S., Skinner, M.J., Grant, P.J., Plummer, D.C. (1991) Situational factors and thought processes associated with unprotected intercourse in gay men. *Psychology and Health*, 5, 259–278.

Harvey, S.M., Beckman, L.J. (1986) Alcohol consumption, female sexual behaviour and contraceptive use. *Journal of Studies on Alcohol*, 47, 327–332.

Haverkos, H.W. (1990) The search for cofactors in AIDS, including an analysis of the association of nitrate inhalent abuse and Kaposi's Sarcoma, In: Seminara, D., Watson, R.R., and Pawlowski, A. (eds) *Alcohol, Immunomodulation on AIDS*, New York, Alan R. Liss Inc. 93–102.

Hingson, R., Strunin, L., Berlin, B. (1990) Changes in knowledge and behaviours amongst adolescents, Massachusetts Statewide Surveys, 1986–1988. *Pediatrics*, 89, 24–29.

Hingson, R., Strunin, L., Berlin, B., Heeren, T. (1990) Beliefs about AIDS, use of alcohol, drugs and unprotected sex amongst Massachusetts adolescents, *American Journal of Public Health*, 80, 295–299.

Honnen, T.J. and Kleinki, C.L. (1990) Prompting bar patrons with signs to take free condoms. *Journal of Applied Behavior Analysis*, 23, 215–217.

Jayasinghe, R., Gianutsos, G., Hubbard, A.K. (1992) Ethanol-induced suppression of cell-mediated immunity in the mouse. *Alcoholism: Clinical and Experimental Research*, 16, 331–335.

Jerrells, T.R., Marietta, C., Bone, G., Weight, F.F., Eckhart, M.J. (1988) Ethanol-associated immune suppression. *Advances in Biochemistry and Psychopharmacology*, 44, 173–185.

Jerrells, T.R., Peritt, D., Marietta, C., Eckardt, M.J. (1989) Mechanisms of suppression of cellular immunity induced by ethanol, *Alcoholism: Clinical and Experimental Research*, 13, 490–493.

Jessor, R., Jessor, S.L. (1977) Problem Behavior and Psychosocial Development: A Longitudinal Study of Youth, New York, Academic Press.

Kaslow, R. A., Blackwelder, W.C., Ostrow, D.G., Yerg, D., Palenicek, J., Clulsen, A.H., Valdiserri, R.O. (1987) No evidence for a role of alcohol or other psychoactive drugs in accelerating immunodeficiency in HIV-1 positive individuals. *Journal of the American Medical Association*, **261**, 3424–3429.

Kay, N., Allan, J., Morley, J.E. (1984) Endorphines stimulate normal human peripherals blood lymphocyte natural killer activity, *Life Science*, **35**, 53–59.

Keller, S.E., Bartlett, J., Schlerfer, S.J., Johnson, R., Pinner, E., Delaney, B. (1991) HIV-related sexual behaviour among a healthy inner city heterosexual adolescent population in an endemic area of HIV. *Journal of Adolescent Health*, **12**, 44–48.

Kelly, J.A., St. Lawrence, J.S., Brasfield, T.L. (1991) Predictors of vulnerability to AIDS risk behaviour relapse. *Journal of Consulting and Clinical Psychology*, **59**, 163–166.

Klassen, A.B., Wilsnack, S.C. (1986) Sexual experience and drinking among women in a US national survey. *Archives of Sexual Behavior*, **15**, 363–392.

Klimas, N.G., Morgan, R., Blaney, N.T., Chitwood, D., Page, J.B., Milles, K., Fletcher, NM.A. (1990) Alcohol and immune function in HIV-1 seronegative and HTLV-I/II seronegative and positive men on methadone, In: Seminara, D., Watson, R.R., and Pawlowaki, A. (eds) *Alcohol, Immunomodulation and AIDS*, New York Alan R. Liss Inc. 103–111.

Kraft, P. (1991) Age at first experience of intercourse among Norwegian adolescents: A lifestyle perspective. *Social Science and Medicine*, **33**, 207–213.

Leigh, B.C. (1990a) Venus gets in my thinking: drinking and female sexuality in the age of AIDS. *Journal of Substance Abuse*, **2**, 129–145.

Leigh, B.C. (1990b) Alcohol use and sexual behaviour in descrete events: II. Comparison of three samples, Paper presented at the Alcohol Epidemiology Symnposium, ICAA. Kettil Bruun Society, Budapest, Hungary.

Leigh, B.C. (1990c) The relationship of substance use during sex to high risk sexual behaviour, *Journal of Sex Research*, **27**, 199–213.

Leigh, R.C. (1990d) The relationship of sex-related alcohol expectancies to alcohol consumption and sexual behaviour, *British Journal of Addiction*, **85**, 919–928.

Liu, Y.K. (1980) Effects of alcohol on granulocytes and lymphocytes, *Seminars on Hematology*, **17**, 130–136.

Lundy, J., Raaf, J.H., Deaken, S. (1975) The acute and chronic effects on alcohol on the human immune system. *Surgical Gynaecology and Obstetrics*, **141**, 212–218.

McKirnan, D.J., Peterson, P.L. (1989) Alcohol and drug use amongst homosexual men and women: epidemiology and population characteristics. *Addictive Behaviors*, **14**, 545–553.

MacGregor, R.R., Gluckman, S.J., Senior, J.R. (1978) Granulocyte function and levels of immunoglubulins and complement in patients admitted for withdrawal from alcohol, *Journal of Infectious Diseases*, **138**, 747–753.

McCusker, J., Westenhouse, J., Stoddard, A.M., Zapka, J.G., Zorn, M.W., Majer, K.H. (1990) Use of drugs and alcohol by homosexually active men in relation to sexual practices, *Journal of Acquired Immune Deficiency Syndromes*, **3**, 729–736.

MacDonald, N., Wells, G., Fisher, W., Warren, W., King, M., Doherty, J., Bowie, W. (1990) High-risk STD/HIV behaviour among college students. *Journal of the American Medical Association*, **263**, 3155–3159.

McEwan, R., McCallum, A., Bhopal, R., Madnok, R. (1992) Sex and a risk of HIV infection: the role of alcohol, *British Journal of Addiction*, **87**, 577–584.

Mann, J., Tarantola, D.J.M., and Netten, T.W. (eds) (1992) *AIDS in the World*, Cambridge, Harvard University Press.

Mili, F., Flanders, D., Baring, J.R., Annest, J.L., DeStefano, F. (1992) The associations of alcohol drinking and drinking cessation to measures of the immune system in middle aged men, *Alcohol: Clinical and Experimental Research*, **16**, 688–694.

Miller, P. (1993) *Alcohol, Illicit Drugs as Rising Sex*, London, Mental Health Foundation (in press).

Molgaard, C.A., Nakamura, C., Howell, M., Elder, J.P. (1988) Assessing alcoholism on a risk factor for acquired immunodeficiency syndrome (AIDS), *Social Science and Medicine*, **27**, 1147–1152.

Morgan Thomas, R. (1990) AIDS risks, alcohol, drugs and the sex industry: A Scottish study, In: Plant, M.A. (ed) AIDS, Drugs and Prostitution, London, Tavistock/Routledge, 88–108.

Morgan Thomas, R., Plant, M.A., Plant, M.L. (1990) Alcohol, AIDS risks and sex industry clients: results from a Scottish study, *Drug and Alcohol Dependence*, **26**, 265–269.

Mott, F.L. and Haurin, R.J. (1988) Linkages between sexual activity and alcohol and drug use amongst American adolescents, *Family Planning Perspective*, **20**, 128–136.

Nair, M.P.N., Schwartz, S.A., Kronfol, Z.A, Heiner, E.P., Pottathil, R. and Greden, J.F. (1990) Immunoregulatory effects of alcohol on lymphocyte responses to human immunodeciciency virus proteins, In: Seminara, D., Watson, R.R. and Pawlowski, A. (eds) *Alcohol, Immunomodulation and AIDS*, New York, Alan R. Liss Inc, 221–230.

Nakagawa, S., Watanabe, H., Obe, H. and Nako, M. (1989) Sexual behaviour in Japanese males relating to area, occupation, smoking drinking and eating habits, *Andrologia*, **22**, 21–28.

National Research Council (1989) AIDS: Sexual Behavior and Intravenous Drugs Use, Washington, D.C, National Acadamy Press.

Orr, D.P., Beiter, M. and Ingersoll (1991) Preventive sexual activity as a indicator of psychosocial risks, *Pediatrics*, **87**, 141–147.

Palmer, D.L. (1978) Alcohol consumption and cellular immunoacceptence, *Immunology*, (Supple 8) 13–17.

Parker, D.A., Harford, T.C. and Rosenstock, G.M. (1990) Alcohol and other drugs and sexual risk-taking among young adults in the United States. Paper presented at the Alcohol Epidemiology Section ICAA/Kettil Bruun Society, Budapest, Hungary.

Penkower, L., Dew, H.A., Kingsley, L., Becker, J.T., Satz, P., Shaerf, F.W. and Sheridan, K. (1991) Behavioural, health and psychological factors and risk for HIV infection amongst sexually active homosexual men: The Multicenter AIDS cohort study, *American Journal of Public Health*, **81**, 194–196.

Plant, M.A. (ed) (1990) AIDS, Drugs and Prostitution, London, Tavistock/Routledge.

Plant, M.A., Duffy, J., Mason, W.W., Miller, P. (1993) Dangerous liaisons: sex, alcohol, tobacco and illicit drugs use amongst young adults in two urban areas, *AIDS Care* (Submitted).

Plant, M.A. and Plant, M.L. (1992) Risk-Takers: Alcohol, Drugs, Sex and Youth, London, Tavistock/Routledge.

Plant, M.L., Plant, M.A. and Morgan Thomas, R. (1990) Alcohol, AIDS risks and commercial sex: some preliminary results from a Scottish study, *Drug and Alcohol Dependence*, **25**, 51–55.

Prabhala, R.H. and Watson, R.R. (1990) Effects of various alcohols applied in vitro on human lymphocyte subtypes and mito genesis, In: Seminara, D., Watson R.R. and Pawlowski, A (eds) *Alcohol, Immunomodulation and AIDS*, New York, Alan R. Liss Inc., 155–164.

Ridlon, F.V.C. (1988) A Fallen Angel: The Status Insularity of the Female Alcoholic, London, Bricknell University Press.

Rimland, D. (1983) Mechanisms of ethanol induced defects of olvestar macrephage function, *Alcoholism*, **8**, 73–76.

Ristov, S.S., Starkey, J.R. and Hass, G.M. (1982) Inhibition of natural killer cell activity *in vitro* by alcoholics, *Biochemical and Biophysical Research Communications*, **105**, 1315–1321.

Robertson, J.A. (1990) *The Role of Alcohol and other Psychoactive Substance Use in the Marital Adjustment of Young People*, Edinburgh, M.Phil Thesis.

Robertson, J.A. and Plant, M.A. (1988) Alcohol, sex and risk of HIV infection, *Drug and Alcohol Dependence*, **22**, 75–78.

Rolf, J., Nanda, J., Baldwin, J., Chandra, A. and Thompson, L. (1990) Substance misuse and HIV/AIDS risks among delinquents: a preventive challenge, *International Journal of the Addictions*, **25**, 533–558.

Room, R. (1983) Introduction. In: Room, R. and Collins, G. (eds) *Alcohol and Disinhibition: Nature and Meaning of the Link*, Research Monograph 12, Department of Health and Human Services, Washington, D.C., NIAAA, v–viii.

Room, R. and Collins, G. (eds) (1983) *Alcohol and Disinhibition: the Nature and Meaning of the Link*, Research Monograph 12, US Department of Health and Human Services, Washington, D.C., NIAAA.

Roselle, G.A. and Mendenhall, C.L. (1982) Alteration of *in vitro* human lymphocyte function by ethanol, acetaldehyde and acetate, *Journal of Clinical and Laboratory Immunology*, **9**, 33–37.

Schilts, R. (1987) *And The Band Played On*, Harmondsworth, Penguin.

Seminara, D. and Pawlowski, A. Preface, In: Seminara, D., Watson, D.D. and Pawlosksi, A. (eds) (1990) *Alcohol, Immunomodualtion and AIDS*, New York, Alan R. Liss, Inc.

Seminara, D., Watson, R.R. and Pawlowski, A. (eds) (1990), *Alcohol, Immunomodulation and AIDS*, New York, Alan R. Liss, Inc.

Siegel, K., Mesagno, F.P., Chen, J-Y and Christ, G. (1989) Factors distinguishing homosexual males practising risky and safer sex, *Social Science and Medicine*, **28**, 561–569.

Smith, F.E. and Palmer, D.L. (1976) Alcoholism, infection and altered host defences: a review of clinical and experimental observations, *Journal of Chronic Disorders*, **29**, 35–49.

Soloman, D. and Andrews, G. (2973) *Drugs and Sexuality*, Herts, Panther.

Stacey, N.H. (1984) Inhibition of antibody dependent cell-mediated cytotoxicity by ethanol, *Immunopharmacology*, **8**, 155–161.

Stall, F., McKusick, L., Wiley, J. *et al.* (1986) Alcohol and Drug use during sexual activity and compliance with safe sex guidelines for AIDS: the AIDS Behaviourial Research Project, *health Education Quarterly*, **13**, 359–371.

Stefani, G., Mazzetti, M., Zunarelli, P., Piccini, G., Amorati, S., Capelli, G.C., and Gasbarrine, G. (1989) In vivo effect of chronic ethanol abuse on membrande I- Glycoprotein of lymphocytes and immune responses to various stimulatory agents, *Alcoholism: Clinical and Experimental Research*, **13**, 444–448.

Stiffman, A.R., Dare, P., Earls, F. and Cunningham, R. (1992) The influence of mental health problems on AIDS-related risk behaviours in young adults, *Journal of Nervous and Mental Disease*, **180**, 314–320.

Stimmel (1987) AIDS, alcohol and heroin: a particularly deadly combination (editorial), *Advances in Alcohol and Substance Abuse*, **6**, 1–5.

Strang, J. and Stimson, G.V. (eds) (1990) *AIDS and Drug Misuse*, London, Tavistock/Routledge.

Sutker, P.B., Goist, K. and King, A.R. (1987) Acute alcohol intoxication in women: Relationships to dose and menstrual cycle phase, *Alcoholism: Clinical and Experimental Research*, **11**, 74–79.

Temple, M. and Leigh, B.C. (1990) Alcohol and sexual behaviour in discrete events. I. Characteristics of sexual encounters involving and not involving alcohol, Paper presented at Alcohol Epidemiology Symposium, ICAA/Kettil Bruun Society, Budapest, Hungary.

Tewari, S. and Noble, E.P. (1971) Ethanol and brain protein synthetics, *Brain Research*, **20**, 469–479.

Traeen, B. and Lewin, B. (1992) Casual sex among Norwegian adolescents, *Archives of Sexual Behavior*, **21**, 253–269.

Trocki, K. and Leigh B.C. (1991) Alcohol consumption and unsafe sex: A comparison of heterosexual and homosexual men, *Journal of Acquired Immune Deficiency Syndromes*, **4**, 981–986.

Watson, R.R., Jackson, J.C., Hartman, B., Samplimer, R., Nobley, D. and Gokebon, C. (1985) Cellular immune functions, endorphines and alcohol consumption in males, *Alcoholism: Clinical and Experimental Research*, **9**, 248–254.

Watson, R.R. and McMurray, D.N. (1979) The effects of malnutrition on the secretory and cellular immune processes, *CRC Review of Food Service and Nutrition*, **12**, 113–159.

Weatherburn, P., (1992) Personal Communication. Project Sigma, University of South Bank, London.

Williams, J.R.W., Rubkin, J.G., Remien, R.H., Gorman, J.M. and Ehrhardt, A.A. (1991) Multidisciplinary baseline assessment of homosexual men with and without human immunodeficiency virus infection, *Archives of General Psychiatry*, **48**, 124–130.

World Health Organization (1993) *Alcohol and HIV/AIDS*, Copenhagen, World Health Organization (in press).

Worner, T.M. (1989) Guillian-Barre's Syndrome in alcoholics, (letter) *Drug and Alcohol Dependence*, **23**, 93.

15

Is There An Ethics Of Heterosexual AIDS?[1]

CHARLES A. ERIN AND JOHN HARRIS

THE THREAT OF AIDS IS GENDER NEUTRAL

It seems that in the West the once widely accepted view that AIDS is predominantly a disease affecting homosexuals may be returning reinforced with the conviction that AIDS is a syndrome affecting only those heterosexuals who indulge in 'deviant practices' — promiscuity, intravenous drug use, or association with prostitutes. Various scientific reports lend support to this view, and this in turn makes it a point of discussion for ethicists and jurists. Consider, for example, the following passage from Orr (1990):

> It is often claimed that prostitutes and intravenous drug-users are the means through which AIDS will be heterosexually transmitted to the general public. Recent studies suggest that it is, in fact, intravenous drug use which poses the vastly greater risk.[95]

And Orr's note 95 (Orr (1990)):

> According to the Centers for Disease Control, heterosexual transmission of the virus in the United States is mostly from intravenous drug-users (75 per cent) — A.R. Moss, 'AIDS and intravenous drug use: the real heterosexual epidemic' BMJ 294 (1987) 389.

The complacency of the general population appears to be sustained by any reports which tend to marginalize those believed to be at risk of infection, and the perceived insulation that results from the view that HIV/AIDS is a problem for *others* is, manifestly, dangerous. Such an attitude can lead heterosexuals who do not believe themselves to be promiscuous, do not use intravenous drugs or associate with prostitutes to feel a false sense of security, perhaps even to believe that they are immune to the threat of infection by HIV. Whilst it may be true that certain groups within society — homosexuals, intravenous drug users — are *more* at risk of infection, the fact remains that the entire world population *is* at risk to this pandemic, irrespective of sexual orientation. Whilst lifestyle may affect the *level* of risk, the *absolute* risk of HIV infection is independent of such considerations.

Two issues have, however, emerged as special problems for AIDS as it affects the heterosexual population although, as indicated, they are by no means confined to that population. The first is consequent upon the probability that it is a widely, though quietly, accepted (but not scientifically confirmed), rule of thumb that the risk to a woman of becoming infected with HIV through unprotected sexual intercourse ('unsafe sex') with an infected man is greater than that to a man of contracting HIV through unprotected sexual intercourse with an infected woman. This may be thought of as an important feminist dimension of heterosexual AIDS.

The second problem is one that has been highlighted in a number of press reports and scare stories (e.g. Graves, 1992; Hunt, 1992; Mullin, 1992; Seaton, 1992). It is the problem of apparently (or, in any event, allegedly) deliberate attempts to infect others via sexual intercourse or, possibly, by other reckless or deliberate means. Both these issues will be examined in turn.

FEMINISM AND HETEROSEXUAL AIDS

Almond (1990) points out:

> ... following the phase in which AIDS has been seen as a discrimination issue and, in particular, a homosexual or gay rights issue, it should now be regarded as a feminist issue. For the next stage of the virus is one in which the pattern is increasingly one of men infecting women.

Even if the 'rule of thumb' was accepted as an established scientific fact, considering AIDS as a feminist issue in this way is still to ignore the fact that AIDS affects us all. Relative infectivity may vary according to such features as gender or sexual orientation, but the vulnerability to transmission does not, and it is this fact which is of overriding importance.

The moral principles germane to a discussion of the ethics of AIDS are universal principles of justice and individual responsibility which are not altered by application to one particular group within society.

Almond continues in the same passage:

> This will be a transitory phase, however, for in the end AIDS is *everyone's* issue. Even complacent mature heterosexuals looking back on twenty or more years of settled marriage will find that the virus affects *their* lives too, in the threat that it poses to their sons and daughters.

This is true, but 'complacent mature heterosexuals' in 'settled' relationships are themselves exposed to the *threat* posed by HIV/AIDS even if they do not 'stray'. They may, perhaps, require a blood transfusion at some time and the recent French experience (e.g. Webster 1992; Witcher & Petre 1992) is evidence that it is not just their children who are at *risk* to AIDS. But this is not our point: those who do not consider themselves to be at risk — those who may choose to abstain from sexual intercourse, intravenous drug use, are not haemophiliacs, and never need a blood transfusion — remain under *threat* from HIV/AIDS. Indeed those who understand the transmission of HIV, will regard this threat as a reason for not 'straying'.

The *ethics* of AIDS are then the same for heterosexuals and homosexuals alike. The mode of transmission — heterosexual relations, homosexual relations, transfusion of infected blood, intravenous drug use — do not alter the ethics. Justice is of its very nature universal and morality cannot be simply relative to particular groups. It is worth digressing for a moment to say why this must be so.

THE IMPOSSIBILITY OF MORAL RELATIVITY

While it is true that there are many different moral outlooks and perspectives, and perhaps equally many and various moral theories, all presuppose the possibility of moral argument. This is because if something is right or wrong, good or bad, there must be some reason why this is so. And once reasons enter into the discussion, moral argument has begun. Reasons can always be scrutinised for their adequacy. There are better or worse reasons, reasons supported by better or worse arguments, reasons underpinned by more or less established or plausible evidence. Of course, arguments may not always be resolved. Sometimes the evidence relevant to a solution is unclear or unevenly balanced or the particular arguments deployed on either side are inconclusive. But moral arguments, if they are genuine, are always in principle resolvable. It is not coherent, for example, to believe that murder is wrong, but think that it is only wrong here and now, but not in another time or place, or for another culture or group; wrong only for people of this society and time, or for people with those beliefs (Harris, 1985).

Neither can citing God as a source of moral conviction or of particular moral imperatives help us to avoid the inevitability of moral argument. As Russell (1957) borrowing an argument originally used by Socrates[2], so eloquently demonstrated:

> The point I am concerned with is that, if you are quite sure there is a difference between right and wrong, you are then in this situation: is that difference due to God's fiat or is it not? If it is due to God's fiat, then for God Himself there is no difference between right and wrong, and it is no longer a significant statement to say that God is good. If you are going to say, as theologians do, that God is good, you must then say that right or wrong have some meaning that is independent of God's fiat, because God's fiats are good and not bad independently of the mere fact that he made them.

This leaves the inevitable task of trying to formulate the ethical principles that should guide society's response to heterosexual HIV/AIDS.

JUSTICE AND INDIVIDUAL RESPONSIBILITY

The two most apposite moral considerations seem to be, on the one hand, the moral responsibilities of the individual towards others and, secondly, justice, which is here relevant to the way a community treats its individual members (Erin & Harris, in press). To summarize, they are as follows:

i. Central to any conception of justice is the ethical principle of equality which demands that each person within a community should be shown the same respect, concern, and protection as is accorded to any other;
ii. Consequently, no individual or group within the community should be unfairly discriminated against;
iii. Irrespective of premeditation or intent, the individual is responsible for what he/she *knowingly or recklessly* causes, either through his/her action or inaction.

Justice, Individual Responsibility And Deliberate Or Reckless HIV Transmission

So what are the implications of the principle of justice and the moral imperative of individual responsibility for HIV/AIDS? One can consider here the case of deliberate or reckless transmission of HIV. It should be emphasized that what is said here bears application to both heterosexually and homosexually transmitted HIV.

Responsibility And The Individual

Individual responsibility has two aspects in this context. There are the responsibilities both of potential transmitters of HIV and of potential receivers to be accounted for. Consider potential transmitters first. This group may be sub-divided into those who *know* they are HIV seropositive and those who do not. However, among the members of this latter sub-group are those who *have reason to believe* that they may be HIV seropositive. There is no morally relevant difference between the obligations of this group and of those who have had their HIV seropositive status confirmed. Members of both groups know that they may constitute a mortal danger to others in certain circumstances.

It is this feature of AIDS that makes it almost unique among diseases and which imposes strict obligations on the individual.

Quite simply, the individual who knows that he[3] is HIV seropositive or who has reason to believe that he may be, has a moral duty to forewarn prospective partners of his HIV status and is responsible for their fate if he does not. It is important to be clear about just why this is so.

ANALOGIES WITH LAW AND HEALTH CARE PRACTICE

It is tempting to draw analogies with law and with health care practice here, although it will be argued that ultimately such analogies fail.

In common law, any 'laying on of hands' or for that matter of other bodily parts is battery (and the threat of it is assault) unless the recipient has freely and full-heartedly consented. In current health care practice it is now almost universally accepted that for such consent to be valid it must be fully informed. At the very least this must mean that the subject of the touching must know all relevant facts including the likely consequences of such touching (Harris, 1985). Clearly, the fact that illness and almost certain death are a significant risk of the touching in question must be a relevant fact upon which any valid consent would have to be based. Whether the common law regarding assault and battery coincides with what would be regarded as acceptable current health care practice is a moot point. The law relating to consent to sexual intercourse where there is a danger of sexually transmitted disease, for example, is based on a number of Victorian cases and on the sexually transmitted diseases envisaged in those cases which were not fatal. These cases are a poor guide to what the courts would decide today although, in one, a man called Bennet was convicted of indecent assault for having sex with a thirteen year old girl while infected with a sexually transmitted disease. The court held that although the girl was below the 'age of consent', such consent as there was had been obtained by fraud and was therefore invalid (Arnheim, 1992). Arguably, no consent to intercourse could be valid if it was made in ignorance of the HIV seropositive status of one of the partners or in ignorance of the known probability of such status, whether or not the law would today regard lack of information or the withholding of information about HIV seropositive status as vitiating consent to intercourse. However, there is perhaps a better legal precedent for thinking about the responsibilities of the potential transmitter of HIV.

Another approach might be to regard the law and ethics of battery and its relationship to consent as irrelevant because of the specially serious risks associated with AIDS. It may be that a better guide would be the law regarding either grievous bodily harm or the administration of a 'noxious' thing. Both of these perspectives are covered in English law by the *Offences Against The Person Act 1861*. Under this act, the most serious of the assault genus of offences is that where the intent is to cause grievous bodily harm. Hence the consent of the 'victim' is probably irrelevant to the commission of the offence. The 1861 Act also deals with the administration of "any Poison or other destructive or noxious Thing" (*Offences Against The Person Act 1861*, s. 23). Clearly, if a person poisons another's coffee, he needs neither to assault nor batter her. Moreover, his act is not the less culpable because she consents to drink the coffee in ignorance of its possibly lethal contents.[4] This seems a better analogy for the knowing or reckless exposure by one person of another to HIV/AIDS. However, again, it is perhaps not quite close enough.

It might well be claimed that the HIV seropositive individual or the person who has reason to believe that she might be such an individual, lacks or may lack, the intent to harm that is requisite for the commission of the offences against the person under consideration. The moral, as opposed to the legal question is as to whether lack of the requisite intent is relevant.

THE MORAL CULPABILITY OF HIV TRANSMISSION

People are responsible for what they knowingly bring about (Harris, 1980). The individual who knows he is HIV seropositive and has sexual intercourse with another person without forewarning that person of his status has disregarded his moral obligation to disclose HIV status, and has thus undermined the autonomy of his sexual partner and put that partner at risk of HIV infection. Such an individual is responsible for the wrong done to the person he or she places at risk. He is responsible for the death of that person if, as a result of contracting HIV through sexual contact with him, she dies of AIDS. Even if they do not consequently contract HIV there is still responsibility for knowingly exposing another person to considerable risk.

That this is a separate and considerable wrong whether or not the risk materialises can be seen by considering the case of other hazards. Suppose someone were to allow a possibly lethal chemical effluent to run off into a public street. They would be culpable whether or not anyone actually succumbed to its effects.

The potential transmitter has neglected her moral obligation to forewarn and is to blame for any detriment to her sexual partner directly consequent upon her lack of disclosure. The individual who has reason to believe she may be HIV seropositive and neglects to forewarn her sexual partner of her at-risk status is equally at fault and equally culpable for any detrimental consequences to her sexual partner resulting directly from her lack of disclosure.

It might be thought that the current less than complete understanding of infectivity, particularly the apparent variation in infectivity during the various stages after infection with HIV, undermines this claim; that the fact that it is not certain that sexual intercourse with an HIV seropositive person *will* result in transmission of HIV nullifies the obligation to forewarn and thus provides extenuation of the infector's responsibility and culpability. But this is analogous to saying that an individual who, without warning, fires a machine gun indiscriminately into a crowd mortally wounding someone is not responsible for that person's injury and not guilty of murder (or at the very least manslaughter) when she dies of her wounds because he could not know for sure when firing that anyone would actually be hit.[5]

RESPONSIBILITY AND THE POTENTIAL RECEIVER

What of the responsibilities of the potential receiver? To begin, it is perhaps worth noting that not all those who might be considered potential receivers of deliberate HIV infection are 'victims' of deliberate infection[6]. There will be, it seems fair to assume, those who will have been infected previously by whatever transmission mode, but who have not previously had their HIV status confirmed one way or the other. All those who have suffered a lack of forewarning are, however, victims to an assault on their autonomy, but, to simplify matters, consider the case of a person whose HIV seronegative status has been confirmed.

CONTRIBUTORY NEGLIGENCE: A DUTY OF SELF-PROTECTION?

In the United Kingdom, as elsewhere, government AIDS education campaigns have focused on convincing the individual citizen of the wisdom of practising 'safe sex'. There is no such thing as *safe* sex, of course, merely *safer* sex, and while one cannot provide oneself with total protection against HIV transmission through sexual intercourse, one can considerably reduce the chances of transmission by that mode by, for example, the use of condoms. Practising protected intercouse may be thought of as the 'common sense' approach. It is far from clear, however, that the individual has a *duty* to do so. If this was the case, it might be claimed that the individual's duty of self-protection relieves the potential transmitter of the duty to forewarn. Such a claim is fundamentally flawed, as has been discussed elsewhere (Erin & Harris, in press):

> It is sometimes claimed that every individual has the obligation to protect herself and that there is consequently no duty to warn. This principle has two major flaws. The first is that it assumes that people will actually protect themselves in obedience to the principle. The second is that it assumes that the protective steps that they might take will be adequate.

> We will just look a little more closely at both these flaws. It may be the case, for example, that all workers at a nuclear plant should wear protective clothing at all times. It does not follow from the soundness of such a rule that worker A, seeing that worker B is without her protective clothing on this particular occasion, has no obligation not to turn on a machine that emits dangerous radiation or to warn worker B before turning on the machinery. Or, even if all *are* wearing protective clothing, that there is no obligation not to increase the dangerous radiation above the levels to which the workers have consented to be exposed and are expecting to receive.

> The second flaw is equally important. Since there is no such thing as '*safe* sex', merely less hazardous sex, it is important that each individual makes his/her own informed judgement about the level of risk they are prepared to run in each particular case. One might, for example, think that the risk that one's partner has AIDS is low and that this combined with the further lowering of the risk by practising protected intercourse was an aggregate risk worth running. One's assessment might be different if one knew that the first of the two risks was not small but, rather, 100%. This is why health care professionals often want to know (and rightly) the HIV status of patients for particular procedures even though they take routine precautions against infection during those procedures. Equally, and for the same reasons, patients have a legitimate interest in knowing the HIV status of health care professionals.

If this were not true, it would follow that, for example, a woman who walks alone at night has no cause for complaint if she is assaulted. It was, so it might analogously be claimed, her duty to protect herself by avoiding such conduct and she has only herself to blame.

DISCHARGING ONE'S RESPONSIBILITIES

Whilst individuals clearly have an interest in self-protection, it should not be afforded the same moral stature as the duty to forewarn others of the risks they are, or may be taking on by agreeing to sexual relations. Such disclosure is necessary for an individual to make an informed, autonomous judgement as to whether she is prepared to run those risks in the particular instance. Uninfected individuals are justified in being interested. That is, they have a right to demand that their sexual partners are open and honest with them regarding HIV status and risk category. It is only on this basis that their autonomy is safeguarded. And it is only on this basis that 'common sense' comes into play: whilst it is sensible, and advisable, that all persons educate themselves in the epidemiology of HIV/AIDS, particularly in the known HIV transmission modes, the decision of whether or not to indulge in sexual intercourse with a partner, and whether or not to practise 'saf*er* sex', depends on frank disclosure from one's partner.[7]

VOLENTI NON FIT INJURIA

If an HIV seropositive individual *does* inform any sexual partner of his HIV status, and the partner nevertheless indulges in sexual intercourse, whether protected or unprotected, he is a volunteer to the respective risks. This latter individual has made an informed consent and must bear responsibility for any consequences detrimental to himself. The HIV seropositive person who discloses his HIV status has discharged his responsibilities to his partner.

DELIBERATE TRANSMISSION AND THE CRIMINAL LAW

Should the deliberate or reckless transmission of HIV be considered a criminal offence in law; if so, what type of criminal offence? It is necessary to be explicit as to what is meant by *deliberate* transmission: it refers to the case of a person who knows she is HIV seropositive and, despite this knowledge, knowingly or recklessly does something where there is a possibility of passing on the virus, by whatever transmission mode, to another person (whom she does not know to be HIV seropositive) and does not shoulder her moral responsibility to disclose her HIV status to that person *prior* to that act. It is clear that where ignoring a moral responsibility can jeopardize the very lives of others and can lead to their deaths, this is a sufficiently serious matter, other things being equal, to justify criminalization. But are other things equal?

Firstly, assuming the moral symmetry of acts and omissions (Harris, 1980 *passim*), we are forced to accept that it does not make a moral difference whether non-disclosure was a result of misrepresentation (denying HIV seropositive status when asked) or as a result of non-representation (not offering the information in the absence of solicitation). Non-disclosure thus most nearly constitutes fraud in law.

There are three potential ways of considering the criminalization of deliberate HIV transmission. The first hinges on the issue of fraudulent representation. There is precedent (although by no means a conclusive precedent) for considering fraudulent representation as the basis of the charge of rape where sexual intercourse is the mode of transmission. Thus, if a woman consents to sexual intercourse with a man who has represented himself as single when he is actually married, and she would not have consented if she had been made aware of his married status, there is a case for saying she has been raped. Equally, if a person consents to sexual intercourse with an HIV seropositive individual who has not disclosed his HIV status, and that person would not have consented if she had been apprised of this information, there is a case for charging rape. Note that this approach encompasses the rape of both females and males. And note also that this approach would deem a crime to have been committed whether or not the victim of that crime contracted HIV as a result of intercourse with the perpetrator and whether or not the victim eventually died of AIDS.

The second alternative is to consider deliberate transmission as either attempted manslaughter or murder, or actual manslaughter or murder. If ('attempted') transmission is done recklessly, then the appropriate charge would likely be (attempted) manslaughter; if ('attempted') transmission is done knowingly, the appropriate charge would likely be (attempted) murder. It should be noted here that the *attempted* charge can, in principle, be brought where transmission has not occurred. Where sexual intercourse does result in transmission of HIV from a non-disclosing HIV seropositive individual to a seronegative individual, it is a moot point whether the crime committed could be considered in law as manslaughter (if done recklessly) or murder (if done knowingly), the point being that the manslaughter/murder victim is likely to be a living person for some considerable time after the putative crime is committed. However, taking into consideration the current state of the art of HIV/AIDS epidemiology which indicates strongly that the person who contracts HIV *will* eventually die of AIDS leads us to believe that, if the manslaughter/murder option is to be taken up, this is how the crime in this scenario should be viewed. The victim of the crime has, after all, been given a 'death sentence'.

The third option is to borrow a concept from American law, and create a new offence specifically to fit the circumstances of this new disease and perhaps call it 'reckless endangerment'.

THE POINT OF CRIMINALIZATION

It is likely that, whichever of the above approaches was to be chosen, the chances of a successful conviction would be slim. Firstly, it would need to be shown that the alleged victim of the crime was not HIV seropositive prior to the crime being committed. Secondly, it would probably need to be shown that the crime's perpetrator knew that he was HIV seropositive. Finally, there are various problems thrown up by the fact that transmission usually occurs during acts which are private and usually intimate. However, just as the charge of rape within marriage may be a difficult charge to prove one way or the other, the point of criminalizing such an act is to send out the emphatic message that rape within marriage is *morally wrong*, that it is a crime, whether or not it is likely to be successfully prosecuted in any particular case.

The key question is not "whether what has occurred is a criminal offence but whether it should be made a crime" (Brazier, 1992). In this paper it has been argued that the deliberate or reckless transmission of HIV, or 'attempts' at such transmission are not only a most serious moral wrong but also, in all probability, a crime.

Whether it should be made, or where it already is, remain a criminal offence in law is a further and separate question and one it seems on balance should be answered in the negative.[8]

Knowing HIV Transmission Should Not Be A Criminal Offence

There would be immense practical, social and even moral difficulties in the way of making the knowing transmission of HIV into a criminal offence. In the first place it is probably undesirable and dysfunctional to take any steps which would have the effect of further stigmatizing those with HIV/AIDS by treating them all as potential rapists or murderers.[9] Just as part of the point of criminalizing an activity is to send out clear and emphatic messages about what is tolerable behaviour in a society, so part of the point of not criminalizing an activity is to secure an analogous outcome: in this case, to try to minimize such wrongful and unjustified stigmatization as already exists. This is particularly appropriate where criminalization, while understandable and perhaps even defensible, is in fact unlikely to do any good in the sense of reducing the prevalence of such 'crimes' or in compensating victims (e.g. Orr, 1990).

There are a number of reasons to suppose criminalization would be ineffective. If intent were made the essence of the crime it would be difficult to prove. If recklessness were sufficient there would be so many mitigating circumstances alleged in every case as to render any deterrent effect problematic.

It would be difficult to improve upon Brazier's account of the scenario for any alleged victim in such a trial (Brazier, 1992): "The defence would say it was not *their* client who infected Ms X but one of several other men who they would show she slept with".

This said, two firm and inescapable conclusions follow, and these are the conclusions of this paper also. The first is that, while knowing transmission of HIV is a crime both in morality and probably also in law, it should not become, or, where it already is, remain a criminal offence. It should be recognised on all sides that those who are HIV seropositive or who believe that they may be should accept their responsibility not to endanger the lives of others. It may seem harsh to emphasize this point where those on whom the burden of disclosure falls are already themselves sufferers of a terrible disease and likely also to be victims of unfair and indefensible discrimination insofar as their HIV status is known. It is essential that society recognises that it has special and powerful obligations to those who are HIV seropositive. Such people should receive substantial protections against discrimination in employment, housing, health care and in all other respects be treated as equals in any society. These protections have been outlined in detail elsewhere (Erin & Harris, in press; Harris, 1992) and for this reason will not be rehearsed here.

The second is that *anyone* and *everyone* has the most powerful of motives to protect innocent third parties from becoming the objects of knowing or reckless transmission. This will include those such as doctors and other health care workers who come by their knowledge of someone's HIV seropositive status in a confidential or quasi-confidential role. The duty of confidentiality is not absolute and where it conflicts with the obligation to protect people at risk of their very lives it surely must give way to such an overwhelming moral priority (Harris, 1985).

As Brazier (1992) has suggested in the context of the Birmingham case in which a man who, contrary to medical and other advice, allegedly continued to have unprotected sex with several women without warning them of his condition:

> To protect such women, doctors might have to publish his name in the press and perhaps include a photograph.

However, it should be reaffirmed that the most effective means of preventing the spread of HIV and of protecting people from contracting it is to encourage those who are HIV seropositive "to come forward and seek diagnosis of their condition and advice on how to care for themselves and others"(Brazier, 1992). And, more importantly, we must ensure that, when they do, they are protected against discrimination and ensure also that they are able to provide for themselves and their families, and this we must do at public expense if necessary (Erin & Harris, in press, *passim*).

NOTES

1. This paper was written as part of the development of the project for the Commission of the European Communities entitled "AIDS: Ethics, Justice and European Policy". The authors gratefully acknowledge the stimulus and support provided by the Commission.

2. Plato (1954) *The Euthyphro*, in *The Last Days Of Socrates*, transl. H. Tredennick (Harmondsworth: Penguin) 10B–11B.

3. We have switched the gender of the personal pronouns throughout for the sake of equality and elegance.

4. Here, as elsewhere, we are grateful to our colleague Margaret Brazier for her stimulating legal advice.

5. Steinbock comes to similar conclusions for slightly different reasons (Steinbock (1989) pp 27ff.). Steinbock locates the obligation to disclose in a duty of concern for welfare rather than, as do we, in an obligation not to harm.

6. Or of infection on the occasion in question.

7.The assumption here is that it is autonomous individuals which are under consideration, that is, individuals capable of authentic action. Insofar as they are not, it is, of course, pointless to make any recommendations as to what they should do. However, it is often too readily assumed that those under various sorts of pressure lose their autonomy.

8. Despite the fact that in the United States, for example, there is precedent for the (attempted) knowing transmission of HIV being considered in law as attempted manslaughter and attempted murder (Hermann, 1991, pp 296–297) and 20 states have already passed laws making knowing transmission of HIV a criminal offence (Bayer, 1991, p 46).

9. In the hysterical way that some feminists have sought to stigmatize all men as potential rapists.

REFERENCES

Almond, B. (1990) 'Introduction: War of the world' in Brenda Almond (ed.) *AIDS: A Moral Issue — The Ethical, Legal And Social Aspects* (London: MacMillan) p 1–21.

Arnheim, M. (1992) *The Guardian*, 24 June.

Bayer, R. (1991) 'AIDS, public health, and civil liberties' in F.G. Reamer (Ed.) *AIDS & Ethics* (New York: Columbia University Press) p 26–49.

Brazier, M. (1992) *The Guardian*, 24 June.

Erin, C.A., Harris, J. (in press) 'AIDS: Ethics, Justice, and Social Policy', *Journal of Applied Philosophy*.

Graves, D. (1992) 'Dilemma over Aids man who infected four women', *The Daily Telegraph*, 23 June, p. 1, cols. 1–7.

Harris, J. (1980) *Violence & Responsibility* (London: Routledge & Kegan Paul).

Harris, J. (1985) *The Value of Life: An Introduction to Medical Ethics* (London: Routledge).

Harris, J. (1992) *Wonderwoman & Superman: The Ethics of Human Biotechnology* (Oxford: Oxford University Press).

Hermann, D.H.J. (1991) 'AIDS and the law' in F.G. Reamer (Ed.) *AIDS & Ethics* (New York: Columbia University Press) p 277–309.

Hunt, L. (1992) 'HIV victim on "revenge" sex spree may be detained', *The Independent*, 23 June, p. 1, cols. 2–4.

Mullin, J. (1992) 'Man "set out to spread HIV"', *The Guardian*, 23 June, p. 1, cols. 4–6.

Orr, A. (1990) 'The legal implications of AIDS and HIV infection in Britain and the United States' in Almond (1990) p 112–139.

Russell, B. (1957) "Why I am not a Christian" in Paul Edwards (Ed.), *Why I am not a Christian* (London: George Allen and Unwin).

Seaton, C. (1992) 'Woman dies as HIV man ignores advice and spreads Aids', *The Times* [London], 23 June, p. 3, cols. 1–3.

Steinbock, B. (1989) 'Harming, wronging and AIDS', in James M. Humber & Robert F. Almeder (Eds.) *AIDS And Ethics, Biomedical Ethics Reviews 1988*, (Clifton, New Jersey: Humana Press).

Webster, P. (1992) 'French doctors go on trial in case of Aids-infected blood', *The Independent*, 23 June, p. 7, cols. 5–7.

Witcher, T., Petre, J. (1992) 'Doctors on trial over HIV-infected transfusions', *The Daily Telegraph*, 23 June, p. 10, col. 8.

16

Knowledge, Attitudes and Behaviour in Heterosexual Men and Women: The Research Evidence

MICHAEL W. ROSS AND MARGARET KELAHER

The linking of knowledge, attitudes and beliefs, and behaviour together as a unit implies a degree of interconnection between them. However, as the research evidence will illustrate, in the case of heterosexual men and women and in many other situations, the linkage may imply more about popular beliefs about health-related behaviours than the empirical research. The link between knowledge and behaviour is not necessarily a strong one. It may be important to bear in mind the barriers and the enabling characteristics which may be more important determinants of behaviour (Green *et al.*, 1980).

This chapter will review a number of research studies on the knowledge, attitudes and beliefs, and behaviours of heterosexual people and seek to identify the central issues involved. The focus will be on knowledge attitude and behaviour studies in pattern 1[1] countries. The effects of gender, ethnicity, and socio-economic status on knowledge, attitudes, and beliefs about HIV/AIDS risk behaviour will not be discussed in detail although these variables also have a strong impact on these latter variables. The first section will discuss the extent to which heterosexuals are at risk of contracting AIDS. The second section will address the effects of HIV/AIDS knowledge and personal engagement in these issues on ameliorating this risk. The third section will discuss the limitations of studies of knowledge. A fourth section will examine studies of attitude.

---

[1] countries where the epidemic was first manifest in men who have sex with men and users of blood products, then injecting drug users.

HETEROSEXUALS RISK OF CONTRACTING HIV/AIDS

The major problem in assessing behaviour change in heterosexuals is that it is often difficult to judge the extent to which heterosexual people are at risk. In most western societies, the effects of the HIV pandemic have been greatest for homosexually active men and on injecting drug users. These groups (which are traditionally but inaccurately referred to as "risk groups", although it is the *risk behaviour* and not the "risk group" which confers the risk) have been seen as the source and focus of HIV infection. There has been a tendency for heterosexual people to oscillate between complacency and panic according to media trends (Lupton, 1992).

The risk posed to heterosexuals by HIV/AIDS remain relatively low in pattern 1 countries although it is not as remote as many heterosexuals believe. For example, estimates of the probability of transmission per sexual act in the European community are 0.002(0.001–0.004) for male to female and 0.001(0.003–0.003) for female to male transmission (De Vincenzi, Ancelle-Park and Brunet, 1992). HIV/AIDS is a considerable public health issue for heterosexuals. For example, in a Danish study of 115 women who had become infected with HIV, 31% had been infected through heterosexual intercourse. Of these, 71% had become infected by contact with a male who himself had behaviour which put him at risk for HIV (Smith *et al.*, 1990).

Fanning, Cosler, Gallagher, Chiarella & Howell (1991) reported grave concerns about increases in the incidence rates of heterosexual infection especially in urban minorities in the US. This is supported by Cochran, Mays and Leung (1991) study of Asian-Americans which found that 15% of this group reported engaging in anal intercourse. This figure which is supported by data from studies in the U.K. However, a longitudinal study carried out by Samuel *et al.* (1991) in 209 single heterosexual men San Francisco indicates positive changes in sexual behaviours. There was a significant decrease in men who had two or more partners from 53% to 41%, and condom use for the previous six months increased from 48% to 61%. Anal intercourse declined from 25% to 9%. This study was carried out over a 60 month period, which may have provided more time for significant changes to occur, and while it occurred in a city with high HIV seroprevalence and a highly politically and socially visible AIDS epidemic, it does suggest that risk behaviour is decreasing in this heterosexual population.

Mathematical models of heterosexual transmission of AIDS taking into account implicit sexual behaviour change have been developed by Lepont & Blower (1991). These models suggest that if HIV transmission is slow (due to inefficient transmission or low numbers of partner changes) then seroprevalence would rise very slowly. However if HIV transmission was high then seroprevalence would rise rapidly with a high incidence of early mortalities. This suggests that effective interventions may be critical to altering the course of the epidemic in heterosexuals. Although, a study by Johnson *et al.* (1989) suggested the modal number of partners for heterosexuals was one and that the mean number of partners decreased as age and socioeconomic status increased. This suggests that high rates of transmission might be restricted to a small number of multi-partnered heterosexuals who are also likely to be young.

Overall, these findings suggest that heterosexual transmission of HIV/AIDS is likely to be a considerable problem without changes in sexual behaviour. This has lead to an interest in applying public health models which emphasise the role of knowledge and attitudes in changing health risk behaviours to issues concerning heterosexuals and HIV.

THE EFFECTS OF KNOWLEDGE OF AND ENGAGEMENT WITH HIV/AIDS RISKS ON BEHAVIOUR

Initially, there was a strong belief on the part of health educators that adequate knowledge about HIV/AIDS would lead to a reduction in risk behaviours. This assumption was true in the sense that for an individual to change their behaviour, it is necessary to know that behaviour is risky. However the potency of knowledge to change behaviour was limited. This is demonstrated in a number of studies.

A telephone-based study of 9,416 people in Scotland between 1987 and 1990 by Uitenbroek & McQueen (1992) used education as a proxy variable for measuring the effects of HIV knowledge on HIV risk behaviours. The sample consisted of participants aged between 18 and 44. Over this time period, they report an increase in condom use for both genders among respondents with greater education. There was also an increase in condom use by multi-partnered respondents who were less educated, although this increase was considerably higher among women than men. Less educated respondents showed a decrease in their numbers of sexual partners, suggesting that HIV risk reduction strategies may differ across education levels.

A major study of 1,127 young adults at 12 geographically diverse universities across the US by DiClemente *et al.* (1990) provided data on 1,059 who were heterosexual (one third of whom were male, two thirds female). Their median age was 21, four-fifths were Caucasian, and they were well informed about the risks of HIV transmission and the principal modes of transmission. However, their knowledge was poor about casual contact and risk of HIV transmission, particularly about the likelihood of transmission through casual or social contact. While most believed that HIV would spread to the general population, there was a relatively high level of risk, with 93% of non-virgins reporting sex in the past year and of these, 43% reporting multiple partners (with one in ten reporting over five). Condom use was not common, with 37% reporting never using them and only 8% reporting using them all the time. On the other hand, over a third reported behaviour change, specifically a reduction in sex without condoms, and a reduction in the number of partners. The predictor of change was perceived personal susceptibility to HIV infection. There was no relationship between knowledge and reported behaviour change, and in fact those with the *lowest* knowledge reported the greatest changes! This result may indicate that the extent to which a person is engaged by HIV/AIDS information, as indicated by perceived personal susceptibility, may be a more important predictor of behaviour change than knowledge *per se*.

A second major United States study of HIV/AIDS knowledge and behaviour changes among adults was carried out by Hingson *et al.* (1989). They surveyed 1,323 northeastern residents using random telephone sampling. The results were consistent with previous studies in that almost all respondents were aware of the routes of transmission of HIV. Those who continued risky behaviour were just as aware of the transmission routes and about HIV/AIDS as others, but were as might be expected less worried about contracting HIV infection. This again indicates the importance of being personally engaged by information about risk. Six percent of respondents reported unprotected sex with multiple partners in the past six months. Hingson *et al.* also noted that Hispanics were less knowledgeable than other respondents. When knowledge deficits occurred, as in the sample of DiClemente *et al.*, they were usually limited to inaccurate anticipation of casual or social transmission. Of the heterosexuals in Hingson *et al.*s' sample, only 21% indicated that they had adopted safer sexual practices (monogamy, condom use or abstinence). These findings are commonly reported. In a major review of knowledge and attitudes towards AIDS in university students in the United States, Edgar, Freimuth and Hammond (1988) concluded that while the majority of people are knowledgeable about the transmission of HIV and preventive measures, only a small minority translated their knowledge into behavioural change.

As in the studies already described, perceived susceptibility was also a major belief which was associated with change in HIV-related risk behaviour in a study of 574 sexually transmissible disease clinic attenders in the United Kingdom. James, Gilles & Bignell (1991) carried out a study on this population in 1989. The majority of the sample by virtue of being exposed to STD were at risk of HIV infection. However, only 19% perceived themselves as susceptible. Knowledge of the modes and risks of HIV infection was described as adequate, with knowledge highest among the better educated, and lowest among the unemployed. Older individuals had better HIV knowledge. Despite adequate knowledge, of those with multiple partners, 79% did not see themselves at risk of HIV infection, and 64% infrequently used condoms with casual partners. Compounding this risk, those with more partners had a significantly higher rate of both vaginal and oral sex without condoms. Multiple partner use was more common among men (67%) than women (44%).

Hookyas *et al.* (1991) conducted a longitudinal study of 340 multiple partnered heterosexuals who attended a sexually transmitted disease clinic in the Netherlands. Over the mean 4.2 months of follow-up period, they found that while private (non-commercial) partner numbers decreased, there was no change in condom use and no change in sexual practices, although there was a disproportionate loss of subjects from ethnic minorities. Disturbingly, less than 10% always used condoms, and 40% used them irregularly (with significantly less women than men using them). The HIV seroprevalence in this population was low (less than 1%), which is likely to provide a false sense of security to heterosexuals who believe that the risk of infection is too low to require a change in behaviours. During the course of the study there was a major public health campaign and those at higher risk were given more intensive preliminary counselling regarding sexual risk behaviours. Hookyas *et al.* attribute the lack of change to the failure of public health campaigns to provide information that was regarded as personally relevant by those at risk. Although it should be noted that the time of follow-up was relatively short which may have restricted that size of any behavioural effects.

The data on heterosexual men and women mirror those on homosexual men with regards to the relative importance of knowledge and variables indicating engagement with an issue such as perceived personal susceptibility. Ross and Rosser (1989) concluded a major review of HIV/AIDS health education and behaviour change by arguing that the critical variable in promoting behaviour change was not provision of information but providing motivation through personalisation of information to activate the information and translate it into behaviour change. This assertion also accurately reflects the outcomes of the studies presented here. However, it is important from a public health perspective and for the design of interventions to understand why knowledge may have had limited impact on heterosexuals HIV/AIDS risk behaviour.

LIMITS ON THE ABILITY OF KNOWLEDGE TO AFFECT BEHAVIOUR

There are a number of reasons why knowledge may have had a limited effect on behaviour change. First, the time it was established that AIDS was caused by HIV in 1983–4, there had already been wide media coverage of the disease. Consequently, in studies which date from later than the mid-1980s accurate knowledge of HIV/AIDS was generally reported. Where knowledge is universally high there may be insufficient variance to produce statistically significant relationships with other variables, such as changes in HIV/AIDS related risk behaviour. This statistical attenuation may explain the disappointing results attributed to the provision of information. However a number of recent studies (e.g. Hingson *et al*. 1989) have found variation between levels of knowledge suggesting that this explanation is not applicable.

An alternative theoretical explanation is that knowledge only predicts stages in the process of behaviour change but not behaviour change itself. For example Weinstein's (1988) precaution adoption model consists of five stages: (1) unaware of the issue; (2) aware of the issue and personally engaged; (3) engaged and deciding what to do; (4) planning to act and not yet having acted; and (5) acting. The provision of information affects decision making only in the first two stages. Thus the lack of consistent effects due to knowledge may be due to the selection of the wrong outcome variables, that is actual behaviour change rather then transitions between preliminary stages in the choices processes.

Finally, the failure of increased HIV/AIDS knowledge to facilitate appropriate changes in behaviour maybe due to the type of information provided or the characteristics of the person who perceives it. Clift & Stears (1988) reported that following accurate information on HIV/AIDS to university students, concern about casual or social transmission decreased, but attitudes remained unchanged. On the other hand, Rigby *et al*. (1989) compared people on level of AIDS knowledge both before and after a major nationwide Australian AIDS campaign based on a fear-providing message. They found that levels of knowledge about HIV/AIDS, in general, remained unchanged, although there was an increase in the acceptance of the safety of blood transfusions. Ross *et al.* using the same sample a year later found some evidence of change in beliefs about how much was known about HIV transmission by the medico-scientific community, as well as lower concern about casual transmission (as also found by Clift and Stears, 1988). The data suggested that fear campaigns have little impact.

Very similar findings were reported in a previous study in the United Kingdom by Sherr (1987), who reported that the government's health education campaign on AIDS had no measurable impact in improving the public's knowledge of HIV/AIDS, although in Switzerland, Lehmann *et al.* (1987) did find a public health education campaign significantly increased public knowledge of the disease. Sherr's study questioned groups of respondents at higher and lower risk before and after the campaign and found that significantly more of those at higher risk (50% compared with 31%) noticed and read the campaign, suggesting that those at higher risk are more likely to be vigilant for relevant information.

It is possible that the differences in studies on the effects of HIV-related knowledge on attitudes, beliefs and behaviour are dependent on cultural factors and differences in the presentation of HIV and the stage of the pandemic. In a three city comparison of knowledge and attitudes about HIV/AIDS (London, New York and San Francisco), Temoshok, Sweet & Zich (1987) found that both fear of AIDS and anti-homosexual attitudes were associated with knowledge about AIDS, and that in London, these were associated with both sexual and general health behaviour change. In New York, sexual behaviour change was also associated with fear of AIDS, while there was no such association in San Francisco. Temoshok, Sweet & Zich suggest that these data may be explained by differences in the time elapsed since becoming concerned about AIDS. In the first stage, they postulate, fear is associated with *less* knowledge. In the second stage, people seek and obtain more information but are still fearful; and in the third stage, there is a sufficiently long period with AIDS as a salient health risk in the community for fear to have dissipated and for a more informed stance to have occurred. It is important to emphasise that cultural, temporal and situational variables will all influence the relationships between knowledge, attitudes and beliefs, and behaviours.

There is a common link between all of the explanations given of the ways knowledge may interact with HIV risk behaviour. They all suggest further interventions which focus solely on the provision of knowledge are unlikely to facilitate behaviour change unless the target audience perceives that information as personally relevant. This assertion is reflected in changing trends in research and interventions.

THE EFFECTS OF ATTITUDE ON HIV/AIDS RISK BEHAVIOURS

The fact that variables like perceived personal susceptibility appeared to be better predictors of behaviour change than knowledge alone has led to a greater focus on the role of attitudes in motivating behaviour change. These studies usually focussed on the relationship between attitudes and adherence to particular safer sex practices. Earlier attitudinal studies were criticised because they were individualistic and over-emphasized the role of rationality and intentionality in adherence to preventive measures. Such studies failed to account for the fact that sexual encounters are highly emotionally charged, often occur in suboptimal conditions with regard to safer sex (e.g. when participants are intoxicated or when the availability of condoms is low) and involve the interaction between at least two people (Salt, Boyle & Ives, 1990). Consequently, decisions not to adhere to the safer sex advice maybe unintentional, the result of social and situational constraints. However these criticisms have been addressed by more recent studies which are intervention orientated.

The importance attitudes and beliefs relating to altering risks of HIV transmission were illustrated in a study by Basen-Engquist (1992) in the United States. Basen-Engquist's study maintained an indivudalistic and intentional focus using the Health Belief model of Janz & Becker (1984), the social learning theory of Bandura (1977) and the Theory of Reasoned Action of Ajzen & Fishbein (1973). However, she also incorporated cognitive theories of coping strategies into the study, allowing aspects of individuals' responses to their environment to be taken into account. Basen-Engquist studied the HIV-protective behaviours (condom use and discussion of AIDS and sexual history with sexual partners) in 275 university students with a mean age of 22 years. She found that significant predictors of intention to use a condom were an information avoiding coping style and perceived barriers which were inversely related, and perceived susceptibility which was positively related. Significant predictors of intention to discuss AIDS and sexual history with partners were perceived self-efficacy and social support which were both positively related. Basen-Engquist's study indicates that condom use and discussions with partners are independent HIV preventive actions. HIV preventive behaviours are thus multidimensional and are associated with different predictors as indicated by her study. Consequently, interventions should target specific behaviours and the associated group of predictors.

Attitudes and beliefs about condoms as HIV prophylaxis are important determinants of protective behaviour. In a study of 408 young adults in Australia, Chapman *et al.* (1990) used an anonymous sealed envelope interviewing technique. This study addressed variables concerned with the communicative subtext of condom use (e.g. that condoms were unerotic or associated with juvenile sexuality). They found that there were three dominant attitudes which differentiated regular and irregular or non- condom users. These were seeing condom use as a positive action (a reinforcing factor); seeing condom use as a cue to embarrassment; and seeing condom use as antithetical to good sex (both barriers). They also found that perceived personal susceptibility to AIDS but not other STDs was a predisposing factor in condom use. Chapman *et al.* suggest that these specific dimensions of attitudes toward condoms may be useful predictors of their use. Although it should be noted that another Australian study found that there were still large discrepancies between having a positive attitude towards condom use and actually using condoms most of the time (Lupton *et al.*, 1992).

Gold *et al.*(1992) studied the beliefs and thought processes immediately associated with the decision to have unprotected sexual intercourse and the types of occasion when they were likely to occur. This enabled attitudes about HIV/AIDS to be examined in their situational and social context. Gold *et al.* asked 340 university students in the United Kingdom to recall a safe and an unsafe sexual encounter, and recorded the type of situation and justifications for unprotected intercourse in the unsafe encounter. The most common self-justification was that contraceptive measures had already been taken and that heterosexuals are a low risk group, suggesting that young heterosexual adults still see condoms as contraceptives rather than prophylactics. The first factor extracted from analysis of responses related to using perceptible characteristics (such as apparent intelligence, education and appearance) to infer that the partner was not the sort of person who would be infected. The type of partner also distinguished between safe and unsafe encounters. This is a similar finding to that of Chapman & Hodgson (1988), who found that appearance of partner was used as an important index to determine the probability of the partner being infected with HIV or an STD, with the more respectable the appearance, the lower chance of infection. Gold *et al.*s' study also indicated that when type of partner was controlled for there was greater intimacy with partners in the unsafe encounter and increased level of intoxication. The most common justifications for the unsafe encounter related to the low probability of heterosexuals will contract HIV. Gold *et al.* argue that the results of the study indicate the importance of attending to the thoughts and processes involved during sexual encounters in HIV interventions.

It is important to note that explanation of safer sexual behaviours must also take into account attitudes and their associated social skills. In a study of the relationship between attitude, assertiveness and condom use, Treffke, Tiggemann & Ross (1992) looked at both homosexual and heterosexual men. They found that for the homosexual men, intention to use condoms was associated with favourable attitudes toward condoms and condom-related assertiveness. In contrast, the heterosexual men general social assertiveness was *negatively* related to attitudes toward condoms. Condom use was common among the homosexual, but not among the heterosexual, men. These data provide a caution against extrapolating data from homosexual to heterosexual populations. This may suggest that the relationships between attitudes, assertiveness and condom use may either differ between heterosexuals and homosexuals or, more probably, differ in regard to the stage of the pandemic in different populations.

It seems that studies of the relationship between attitudes and HIV/AIDS risk behaviour in heterosexuals can provide an important basis for the development of intervention initiatives. These studies indicate that attitudes and beliefs do not exist in a vacuum but arise as result of strategic, social and situational circumstances and individuals' ability to cope with these. The results of attitudinal studies also suggest that health promoters need to project messages which specifically relate to particular protective behaviours. This may mean being selective about which behaviours are promoted given differences in adherence to and the effectiveness of different strategies.

CONCLUSION

It is apparent that while there are a wide range of findings on attitudes, beliefs and behaviours of heterosexual women and men with regard to HIV/AIDS, there are a number of common elements. First, the relationship between knowledge and behaviour change is poor, with knowledge having only a threshold effect. Further, while there has been some behaviour change in the direction of safer sex, it is generally low and inconsistent. Attitudes and beliefs about HIV/AIDS appear to be among the major mediating variables between knowledge and behaviour, and of particular importance are the perception that one is at risk (personal susceptibility) and the belief that one can carry out behavioural changes successfully (self-efficacy). There is also some evidence to suggest that social skills in negotiating safer sex are important, and that future research might most profitably look at the interactions between attitudes and beliefs and situational and social variables in determining their impact on safer sexual behaviours.

REFERENCES

Ajzen, I., Fishbein, M. (1973). Attitudinal and normative variables as predictors of specific behaviours. *Journal of Personality and Social Psychology* 27, 41–57.

Bandura, A. (1977). Self-efficacy: toward a unifying theory of behavioural change. *Psychological Review* 84, 191–215.

Basen-Engquist, K. (1992). Psychosocial predictors of "safer sex" behaviours in young adults. *AIDS Education and Prevention* 4, 120–134.

Chapman, S., Hodgson, J. (1988). Showers in raincoats: attitudinal barriers to condom use in high-risk heterosexuals. *Community Health Studies* 12, 97–105.

Chapman, S., Stoker, L., Ward, M., Porritt, D., Fahey, P. (1990). Discriminant attitudes and beliefs about condoms in young, multi-partner heterosexuals. *International Journal of STD & AIDS* 1, 422–428.

Clift, S.M., Stears, D.F. (1988). Beliefs and attitudes regarding AIDS among British college students: a preliminary study of change between November 1986 and May 1987. *Health Education Research* 3, 75–88.

Cochran, S.D., Mays, V.M., Leung, L. (1991). Sexual practices of heterosexual Asian-American young adults: implications for risk of HIV infection. *Archives of Sexual Behaviour* 20, 381–391.

De Vincenzia, I., Ancelle-Park, R.A., Brunet, J.B. (1992). Concerted action on heterosexual transmission in *Commission of the European Communities: AIDS research within the biomedical and health research programme*.

DiClemente, R.J., Forrest, K.A., Mickler, S., Principal site investigators. College students' knowledge and attitudes about AIDS and changes in HIV-preventive behaviours. *AIDS Education and Prevention* 2, 201–212.

Edgar, T., Freimuth, V.S., Hammond, S.L. (1988). Communicating the AIDS risk to college students: the problem of motivating change. *Health Education Research* 3, 59–66.

Fanning, T.R., Cosler, L.E., Gallagher, P., Chiarella, J., Howell, E.M. (1991). The epidemiology of AIDS in the New York and California Medicaid programmes. *Journal of Acquired Immune Deficiency Syndromes* 4, 987–999.

Gold, R.S., Karmiloff-smith, A., Skinner, M.J., Morton, J. (1992). Situational factors and thought processes associated with unprotected intercourse in heterosexual students. *AIDS Care* 4, 305–323.

Green, L.W., Kreuter, M.W., Deeds, S.G., Partridge, K.B. (1980). *Health education planning: a diagnostic approach. Palo Alto: Mayfield.*

Hingson, R., Strunin, L., Craven, D.E., Mofenson, L., Mangione, T., Berlin, B., Amaro, H., Lamb, G.A. (1989). Survey of AIDS knowledge and behaviour changes among Massachusetts adults. *Preventive Medicine* 18, 806–816.

Hookyas, C., van der Linden, M.M.D., van Doornum, G.J.J., van der Velde, F.W., van der Pligt, J., Couthino, R.A. (1991). Limited changes in sexual behaviour of heterosexual men and women with multiple partners in the Netherlands. *AIDS Care* 3, 21–30.

James, N.J., Gilles, P.A., Bignell, C.J. (1991). AIDS-related risk perception and sexual behaviour among sexually transmitted disease clinic attenders. *International Journal of STD & AIDS* 2, 264–271.

Janz, N.K., Becker, M.H. (1984). The Health Belief Model: a decade later. *Health Education Quarterly* 11, 1–47.

Johnson, A.M., Wadsworth, J., Elliott, P., Prior, L., Wallace, P., Blower, S., Webb, N.L., Heald, G.I., Miller, D.L., Adler, M.W., Anderson, R.M. (1989). A pilot study of sexual lifestyle in a random sample of the population of Great Britain. *AIDS* 3, 135–141.

Kaslow, R.A., Francis, D.P. (eds) (1989). *The epidemiology of AIDS: expression, occurrence, and control of Human Immunodeficiency Virus Type 1 infection.* New York: Oxford University Press.

Lehmann, P., Hauser, D., Somaini, B., Gutzwiller, F. (1987). Campaign against AIDS in Switzerland: an evaluation of a nationwide educational programme. *Btitish Medical Journal* 295, 1118–1120.

Lepont, F., Blower, S. (1991). The supply and demand dynamics of sexual behaviour: Implications for heterosexual HIV epidemics. *Journal of Acquired Immune Deficiency Syndromes* 4, 987–999.

Lupton, D. (1992). From Complacency to Panic: AIDS and heterosexuals in the Australian Press, July 1986 to June 1988. *Health Education Research* 7(1): 9–20.

Lupton, D., Chapman, S., Donavon, B., Mulhall, B. (1992). Attitudes to and use of condoms in multi-partnered heterosexuals in Sydney Australia. *Venereology* 5(2): 41–45.

Rigby, K., Brown, M., Anagnostou, P., Ross, M.W., Rosser, B.R.S. (1989). Shock tactics to counter AIDS: The Australian Experience. *Psychology and Health* 3, 145–159.

Ross, M.W., Rosser, B.R.S. (1989). Education and AIDS risks: a review. *Health Education Research* 4, 273–284.

Ross, M.W., Rigby, K., Rosser, B.R.S., Brown, M., Anagnostou, P. (1990). The effect of a national campaign on attitudes toward AIDS. *AIDS Care* 2, 339–346.

Salt, H., Boyle, M. Ives, J. (1990). HIV prevention: Current health promoting behaviour models for understanding the psychosocial determinants of condom use. *AIDS Care* 2(1): 69–76.

Samuel, M.C., Guydish, J., Ekstrand, M., Coates, T.J. and Winkelstein, W. (1991). Changes in sexual practices over 5 years of follow-up among heterosexual men in San Francisco. *Journal of Acquired Immune Deficiency Syndromes* 4, 896–900.

Sherr, L. (1987). An evaluation of the UK government health education programme on AIDS. *Psychology and Health* 1, 61–72.

Smith, E., Kroom, S., Gerstoft, M.J., Kvinesdal, B. and Mathiesen, L.R. (1990). Heterosexually acquired human immunodeficiency virus infection in women in Copenhagen: sexual behaviour and other risk factors. *International Journal of STD & AIDS* 1, 416–421.

Temoshok, L., Sweet, D.M., Zich, J. (1987). A three city comparison of the public's knowledge and attitudes about AIDS. *Psychology and Health* 1, 43–60.

Treffke, H., Tiggemann, M. Ross, M.W. (1992). The relationship between attitude, assertiveness and condom use. *Psychology and Health* 6, 45–52.

Uitenbroek, D.V., McQueen, D.V. (1992). Changing patterns in reported sexual practices in the population: multiple partners and condom use. *AIDS* 6, 587–592.

Weinstein N. (1988). The precaution adoption process *Psychology & Health* 7, 355–386.

17

Partner Management

KRISTINA RAMSTEDT AND JOHAN GIESECKE

INTRODUCTION

Any health care environment must aim to meet everyone who attends with empathy and understanding for his/her special situation. Partners of HIV patients are often, unlike many other patients, very lonely in their knowledge about their exposure to a potentially lethal virus. Health care providers who meet these partners must be more than usually alert: it is far from certain that they disclose the reason why they e.g. attend for HIV testing. The preparedness for HIV infection in a partner is often lower among heterosexuals than among gay men, and if such partners are met with nonchalance this will only serve to increase their anxiety. Since an HIV test may not become positive until several months after a transmission, and since the last contact with the HIV patient may have been quite recent, the partner often has to wait for a long time to find out about his/her serostatus. Anxiety often culminates during this period and the risk of suicide should not be neglected.

The HIV-negative partner who has been able to talk and work through all his/her anxieties and questions while waiting for the test result has the best opportunity also to be able to refrain from exposure to HIV in the future. Special support must be offered to the partner who has a continuing relation with an HIV patient, with opportunities to discuss issues relating both to him-/herself and the partner. An existing programme for partner notification adds to the responsibility to take care of those partners who never asked to be told that they have had sex with an HIV positive partner.

There are thus a number of specific points to observe when caring for partners of HIV patients. However, we believe that health care providers who have met critically ill patients and their relatives before, and who are not without empathy, should be able to handle most of the situations that arise. The rather more special points about partners of HIV patients concern the risk of transmission of the virus and the possible advantages of early detection of the infection. The rest of this chapter will thus mainly cover partner notification for HIV infection.

One strategy in the management of sexual partners or needle-sharing contacts of an HIV-positive patient consists of identifying them and offering them counselling and medical examination. *Contact tracing* or *partner notification* are the terms generally used to describe this strategy for dealing with partners of a patient with any sexually transmitted disease (STD), and its aims are to halt spread and prevent complications. The basic strategy has been discussed both in the United States and in the United Kingdom (Burgess, 1963; Wigfield, 1972; Satin, 1977; 1978; Mills, 1978). In the UK it was first put forward in January 1948, when the Ministry of Health sent a letter to the local authorities, medical officers of health, and physicians-in-charge of special treatment centres entitled "Expiry of defence regulation 33 B. Suggested method of continuing to trace sources of venereal infection" (Burgess, 1963).

Partners to Patients with other STDs

Contact tracing has been used for STD control activities in Europe (Wigfield, 1972; Coutinho, 1987) as well as in developing countries (Winfield, 1985). The method has been shown effective in the control of outbreaks of infection due to antibiotic-resistant gonococcal strains and for the identification of 'core-groups' (Handsfield, 1982; Rothenberg, 1983; Ramstedt, 1985; Zenilman, 1988; Handsfield, 1989). Re-interviewing patients with gonorrhoea or syphilis has been found to increase the number of reported partners (Muspratt, 1967; Capinski, 1970, Hammar, 1972). The study by Capinski tremendously well documents the importance of letting an experienced interviewer qualified in psychology interview the patient: 160 patients with syphilis who had failed to name any contacts while talking to the physician were re-interviewed by this skilled person. This led to the naming of 208 contacts, 189 of whom were brought for examination, and among whom 88 cases of syphilis were detected. Efficacy depends as much on who is doing the interview and a commitment to success, as it does on methods.

Katz (1988) compared three strategies of contact tracing for chlamydia trachomatis infection. When calculating the total cost of each strategy, the field follow-up (i.e. a strategy where the clinic assumed responsibility to assure that all partners attended for examination) was the cheapest and most effective. Another study compared three alternative approaches to tracing the partners. The follow-up strategy was again the most effective and also cheapest, especially if nurses did the work (Montesinos, 1990).

When the STD act 1988 in Sweden was expanded to include Chlamydia trachomatis infections the average number of reported partners per woman who came for information and examination increased substantially (Ramstedt, 1991).

Partners to HIV Patients

Contact tracing for HIV infection has been controversial, especially in the USA (Osborne, 1988; Brandt, 1990). Two editorials in major medical journals have, however, stressed the need for research on the method's applicability to HIV infection (Adler, 1988; Rutherford, 1988). A concise account of the arguments has been published by Potterat (1989). Several studies have shown that HIV patients are able to identify their partners and some authors have also stressed the educational value to the HIV negative partners (Wykoff, 1988; CDC, 1988; Toomey, 1989; Jones, 1990; Judson, 1990) especially in heterosexual populations (Clumeck, 1989). In patient groups where it is common to have a large number of anonymous sexual partners, contact tracing can fail as an isolated control measure (Andrus, 1990).

In January 1989 the WHO held a consultation session on partner notification for patients with HIV infection, which stated that: "Partner notification programmes, a form of contact tracing, should be considered, but within the context of comprehensive AIDS prevention and control programmes" (WHO, 1989). Already in the previous year, Adler had written a thoughtful editorial which discussed the efficacy of contact tracing for STDs, and contrasted this with issues surrounding HIV infection (Adler, 1988).

The statement on contact tracing from the National Venereology Council of Australia has been discussed by Bradford. He supports contact tracing as a valuable tool in the control of all STDs including HIV, provided that the traditional high standards of venereological practice are preserved. These standards must include the maintenance of confidentiality, tactful sympathetic management of index cases and their contacts, and opposition to legislative and punitive measures (Bradford, 1990).

Bayer and Toomey have described the complex problems provoked by attempts in the past decade to implement contact tracing for HIV. By examining vicissitudes of two distinct approaches which excist to notifying partners of possible risk they come to the conclusions that:

> "Early identification of HIV infection in asymptomatic individuals will become increasingly beneficial in the changed clinical climate produced by the availability of antiviral therapy, prophylactic antimicrobials, and other therapeutic interventions. The case for partner notification becomes especially important as the incidence of HIV infection shifts from gay middle-class men to other populations, in which the level of awareness is lower and the capacity to act on whatever awareness exists may be limited" (Bayer 1992).

DEFINITIONS

Contact tracing has been the term commonly used in connection with gonorrhoea or syphilis, but WHO has recommended *partner notification* for HIV infection.

Index patient: This is the patient who is first diagnosed with HIV infection, and who becomes the starting point of the partner notification.

Partner: In the context of HIV infection, we use the term partner to include not only sexual partners of the index patient, but also persons with whom he/she has been sharing needles or injection equipment. If a partner is found seropositive on testing, he/she becomes a new index patient.

Note that in some epidemiological literature 'index patient' is taken to mean the first person in a chain of infections, but this need not be the case here.He/she is simply the first one to be diagnosed with HIV infection.

Many authors make a difference between 'steady' and 'casual' relationships, but they are notoriously difficult to define. More useful terms are:

On-going relationship: A partner with whom the index patient thinks he/she is going to have sex again, and

Previous partner: A partner with whom the index patient thinks he/she is not going to have sex in the future.

There are also two different types of referral possible:

Patient referral: The index patient contacts the possibly infected partners, and encourages them to have a medical appointment.

Provider referral: The health care worker (physician, nurse, counsellor) contacts the partner for the index patient.

PARTNER NOTIFICATION

Partner notification can never be seen as an isolated activity; it must always be a part of a meeting between two persons, encompassed within a wider frame of psycho-social care for the patient. It is an extraordinary task to ask a person about some of their best-guarded secrets: with whom they have had sex , when, how often, and in what ways.

It is a time-consuming activity and its feasibility is often limited by resource constraints. The main purpose is epidemiological and preventive: to attempt to stop further spread of the virus, but this purpose must not take precedence over the patient's well-being. However, if the interview and subsequent notifications are well performed, this could become an important part of the future relation between patient and counsellor. At best it can help the patient to cope better with his/her crisis reaction.

In this chapter we will give our views on the prerequisites for success in this sometimes very difficult task.

A FUNDAMENTAL ASSUMPTION

The epidemiological merits of contact tracing for gonorrhoea, syphilis, or chlamydia are obvious: by finding persons who are infected – often unwittingly since infection with these bacteria may well be asymptomatic – and offering them treatment, the number of potential sources of infection in the population decreases. Also, in on-going relationships it is futile to treat only the patient not the partner for an STD, since he or she will immediately become re-infected.

For HIV infection (as for genital warts or herpes), matters are different. The infective persons cannot be treated to take away their infection. The epidemiological rationale for partner notification in HIV infection rests on one fundamental assumption: That people who become aware of their seropositivity will take precautions not to infect others in the future. If this is true, then partner notification for HIV infection should carry the same public health benefits as contact tracing for treatable STDs.

Although some studies have been made of how knowledge of HIV status affects behaviour change, they are not very conclusive and the fundamental assumption above will have to rest on belief. In the end it comes down to your general view on human nature.

In the past there has been much debate about the balance between public benefits of partner notification versus the negative consequences for the individual, who might not want to know that he/she is HIV positive. This balance is now shifting more and more in favour of notification, since advances in treatment of early HIV infection now seem to confer an advantage in early diagnosis also to the patient him/herself.

The rest of this chapter builds on the belief that early diagnosis of asymptomatic HIV infection *is* beneficial to the seropositive person and to society.

TWO EPIDEMIOLOGICAL APPROACHES

The basic fact is that partners of HIV patients constitute a high-risk group for being HIV positive, which makes it worth while to put in resources to find them. This has been repeatedly documented: In one study from USA an investigation starting with one HIV-positive patient and his 19 male contacts ended in the identification of 62 partners, 8 of whom were HIV positive (Wykoff, 1988). In our own study every third partner was found HIV positive, and half of them were unaware of their infection before they were notified (Giesecke, 1991).

There are two – conceptually somewhat different – approaches to partner notification:

1. The aim of 'classical' contact tracing for an STD is to establish the chain of infection, following the pathogen from patient to patient backwards and forwards in time. In Figure 17.1 (where filled circles denote infected people) this approach would mean that one must identify and test all partners of the index patient to make sure who is the source of the infection and to whom the disease has been transmitted. This also includes going on with the same accuracy for each positive partner backwards and forwards in time.
2. The second strategy is better regarded as one of offering counselling and testing to a high-prevalence group, namely those who have been partners of a verified HIV patient. With this approach (Figure 17.2) it becomes less important to know who has transmitted the virus to whom. The main goal is not even to test all partners, but to offer counselling and testing to as many partners as possible.

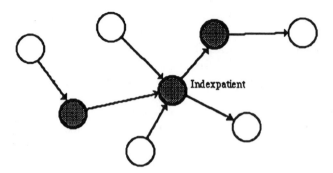

Fig. 1   Classical contact tracing

Since it is often impossible to ascertain when an HIV patient was infected, and thus to know which partners could have been exposed (even if the patient remembers them), this approach is often more appropriate. In real life one often uses a mixture of the two approaches.

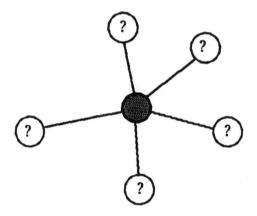

Fig. 2   Counselling and testing approach

ETHICAL PROBLEMS

The ethical dilemma in partner notification for HIV infection is that the unwittingly HIV-positive partner is often feeling quite healthy and may remain so for several years. He/she may have no wish to be notified about an exposure to a potentially lethal virus, and even less to be diagnosed as being HIV positive. 'The right not to know' has been one of the important objections to partner notification.

However, the opposite view is just as possible – and maybe just as common: "If some doctor (or nurse, or counsellor) knows that I have been a partner of an HIV-positive patient, I should have the right to know also". The problem is that you can never know which opinion the partner will have. It is not feasible simply to call him/her and ask "If you had had sex with an HIV-positive patient, would you want to know that?"

Another objection against the strategy is that one should not rely on testing programmes or partner notification as epidemiological tools: In a country which has been hit by the HIV epidemic, everyone has a responsibility to live as if they themselves, or their partners, were seropositive. It then becomes immaterial to know who is seropositive and who is not, and resources should better be spent on health education campaigns about condom usage, restricting number of partners, and other aspects of the concept 'safer sex'.

DESCRIPTION OF THE METHOD

What is so special about the partner notification sessions? Are they not just ordinary talks between two people?

Yes, at least initially they are just like any other counselling sessions, and the issue of partners may not be touched upon at all. The difference is that you must bear in mind that partners will have to be discussed at some point during your sessions with the patient. You cannot leave that to somebody else. You will also have to take care of all administrative work yourself, such as keeping records (which are always to be kept under heavy lock, separate from all other medical records), writing letters to partners, talking to all partners yourself, and so on.

Some of the patients are so preoccupied thinking about who could have infected them – or who they themselves might have infected – that it can be a relief to be able to discuss this already during the first appointment. For these patients the thought that they might have infected their partner even overshadows the graveness of their own situation. The burden of guilt can be hard to bear, and some of the patient's anguish can be alleviated if these feelings can be talked about openly. However, in our experience it is almost always better to wait a while after the patient has received his/her diagnosis before beginning to talk about partners, and it might actually be a good idea to ask those patients who want to notify all their partners immediately to reconsider for a couple of days. The right moment to start the partner notification interview may vary considerably from patient to patient. However, it is extremely important always to mention at some point during the initial stages of contact with the patient that eventually – when he/she is feeling somewhat more in balance – the issue of sexual partners will be returned to. Otherwise it may well be that after the first sessions of supportive character, when confidence has been established, the patient feels betrayed to get questions which he/she did not expect.

In order to make partner notification at all possible, you must first have established a good relationship with the patient so that he/she wants to cooperate, i.e. being prepared either to contact partners or to supply information about them so that you can contact them. It is crucial that the patient feels safe in his/her relationship with the person to whom he/she is divulging the very sensitive information about partners, especially for reasons of confidentiality.

The patients must also feel that he/she is participating in a campaign to try to stop the spread of the virus — this is the viewpoint of general prevention. Another aspect is to make the patient realise that it is essential for his partners to know if they are infected, thus giving them the opportunity to receive early medical care, making it possible for them to refrain from becoming infected with other diseases, and giving them a chance to change their lifestyle.

A great deal of time, energy and factual knowledge about the disease may have to be put into informing the patient about this latter aspect. Accurate information about the risks of infection, and why it is important to know whether one is infected or not, is the best way to motivate the patient to cooperate in the partner notification. This puts demands on you to be well read up on the medical literature on HIV infection and AIDS.

PATIENT REFERRAL

When the question of partner notification is first raised, some patients are very apprehensive about revealing the name of their partner: they often wish to make this contact themselves, and this applies to practically everyone with a steady partner. Discuss with the patient how he/she is going to inform his/her partner. A good idea is to perform a small role-play where you act the role of the partner.

If the index patient has a steady partner, then this person will almost always accompany the patient to one of the first visits after diagnosis. This is the ideal opportunity to suggest that the partner should also be tested.

Some pros and cons of patient referral are:

Advantages	The patient is active in the process. He/she does not have to worry about the partner's reaction, since he/she will be there. Low cost for the health care system.
Disadvantages	There is a risk that the patient's crisis will worsen. No confidentiality (the index patient's HIV status is revealed to the partner).

PROVIDER REFERRAL

Complete information must be acquired about those partners that the index patient does not want to inform personally. If the patient has only been able to supply fragmentary information, such as a first name or a telephone number, it is important to go on trying to establish that the right person is being sought by asking the patient for a description of the partner, or by other means of identification.

The choice of procedure to approach a named contact is important. You should always discuss with the index patient how each partner should best be contacted, trying to get as much information as possible about their social life. Married? Living single? Work environment? The best way is usually to send a letter asking the partner to telephone or write to set up a time for a meeting. This is better than giving an appointment directly, since we feel that the partner should be the one to choose a suitable time.

Do not reveal the reason for the appointment in the letter. The wrong person may open it and even if it is opened by the addressee, a letter is never adequate for informing someone that he/she has been a contact of an HIV patient. This should be done in a conversation, where one is able to calm the person down, to explain further and to give direct support. The letter should be sent in a plain, hand-written envelope (not an official one) without the sender's name. It is important that the contacted partner can get an appointment with you straight away – do not mail it so that he/she receives it on a Friday.

The identity of the index patient must never be revealed to the partner (even if there are situations where this must be obvious). Likewise, an index patient who has chosen provider referral must never be told the result of this partner's HIV test.

Some pros and cons of provider referral:

Advantages ,   Confidentiality is preserved.
            The index patient is spared the strain of having to talk to partners.

Disadvantages   Higher cost, since it can involve a lot of work for the health care provider.

PARTNER'S REACTIONS AFTER BEING NOTIFIED

Very different reactions can be expected from the contacted partners. Many partners are anxious to find out who gave you their names, but this information can never be disclosed. As the intercourse with an HIV-infected person could have occurred a long time ago, there may be several partners to choose among. If provider referral is used, the contacted person often wants to know the approximate time when intercourse with the infected person took place, but this information must also be withheld for reasons of confidentiality.

It may be tempting for the partner to brush aside the suggestion to be tested with the excuse: "Even if I am infected, there is nothing to be done anyway". Studies also show that many individuals at increased risk for HIV infection have already changed to safer sex habits, especially homosexual men (Martin, 1987). It may sometimes take a great deal of effort to convince a partner to be tested, and also to explain the importance of knowing whether or not he/she is infected, both for his/her own sake and for the sake of future partners.

The contacted partner may show different reactions such as anxiety, fear, or even aggression, or may complain that the matter is being dealt with in the wrong way, etc. Most people tell no one that they have been notified, and they become very isolated and frightened individuals. These partners need a lot of support. You should ask the partner if he/she has told anyone about the notification, and if this person could be there when he/she is getting the test result and be supportive during the waiting time.

Finally, a consultation as a result of partner notification with a negative test result could possibly be a turning point towards more careful sexual relationships in the future. The notion of a 'near miss' tends to give a very personal dimension to otherwise abstract information.

DEALING WITH PARTNERS IN THE FUTURE

If a steady partner turns out to be seronegative we usually let him/her return 1–3 times per year for a new examination, possibly including testing, and counselling. If the sexual relationship ceases, the partner should be tested some 3 to 6 months after the last sexual contact with the index patient.

CONCLUSIONS

If the interviews with the patient about his sexual contact/s are performed by a committed and well educated health care worker with an ambition also to be a counsellor, partner notification for HIV may well be as good an epidemiological tool as it has been for treatable STDs. No legislation can force a patient to tell with whom he/she has had sex! The bedrock of the method is confidentiality and trust between the patient and the health care worker performing the interviews. The success of the partner-locating efforts is based only on the patient's willingness to cooperate. To have this cooperation the programme has to ensure that the identity of the index patient would under no circumstances be disclosed, and it also has to offer different models for referral. One study has shown that if the index patient's identity is revealed to a partner, then this partner will not continue to have risky sex with the known HIV-positive index patient, but might instead assume that all other partners are not infected and thus have risky sex with them. Also, this partner may be less likely to practise safe behaviour with future partners (Cates, 1990). In the same study of 25 HIV-positive women, 68% said that they would give the names of their partners if their own identity were not revealed. If their names were given to the partners, only 20% said they would cooperate in the partner notification process. Landis (1992) compared two methods of notifying sexual contacts of individuals with HIV: In a group using patient referral only 7% of contacts were notified, despite legal requirements to notify. In contrast, provider referral resulted in 50% of contacts being notifed.

Our view is that the index patient must maintain ultimate control over the process, including referral methods.

The early identification of those with HIV infection has become important in a rapidly changing clinical context, and in the context of the changing epidemiology of the epidemic efforts at partner notification will play an important public health role.

REFERENCES:

Adler, M., Johnson, A. (1988) Contact tracing for HIV infection. *BMJ* 296, 1420–1421.

Andrus, J.K., Fleming, D.W., Harger, D.R. *et al.* (1990) Partner notification: can it control epidemic syphilis? *Ann Intern Med* 112,539–543.

Bayer, R., Toomey K. (1992) HIV prevention and the two faces of partner notification. *Am J Public Health* 82,1158–1164.

Bradford, D. (1990) Contact tracing in HIV infection (Editorial) *Venereology* 3, 3.

Brandt. Editorial (1990) Sexually transmitted disease: Shadow on the land, revisited. *Ann Intern Med* 112, 481–483.

Burgess, J.A. (1963) A contact tracing procedure. *Br J Vener Dis* 39, 113–117.

Capinski, T.Z., Urbanczyk, J. (1970) Value of re-interviewing in contact tracing. *Br J Vener Dis* 46, 138–140.

Cates, W., Toomey, K., Havlak, R.G., Bowen, G.S., Hinman, A.R. (1990) Partner notification and confidentiality of the index patient: Its role in preventing HIV. *Sex Transm Dis* 17, 113–114.

Centers for Disease Control. (1988) Partner notification for preventing human immunodeficiency virus (HIV) infection — Colorado, Idaho, South Carolina, Virginia. *MMWR* 37, 393–396 and 401–402.

Clumeck, N., Taelman, H., Hermans, P., Piot, P., Schoumacher, M., DeWit, S. (1989) A cluster of HIV infection among heterosexual people without apparent risk factors. *N Engl J Med* 32, 1460–1462.

Coutinho, R.A., Schoonhoven, F.J., Hoek, J.A.R., Emsbroek, J.A. (1987) Influence of special surveillance programmes and AIDS on declining incidence of syfilis in Amsterdam. *Genitourin Med* 63, 210–213.

Giesecke, J., Ramstedt, K., Granath, F., Ripa, T., Rådö, G., Westrell, M. (1991) Efficacy of partner notification for HIV infection. *Lancet* 338, 1096–1100.

Hammar, H., Ljungberg, L. (1972) Factors affecting contact tracing of gonorrhoea. *Acta Derm Venereol* (Stockh) 52, 233–240.

Handsfield, H.H., Sandström, E., Knapp, J.S., Perine, P.L., Whittington, W.L., Sayer, D.E. Holmes, K.K. (1982) Epidemiology of penicillinase-producing *Neisseria gonorrhoeae* infections. *N Engl J Med* 306, 950–954.

Handsfield, H.H., Rice, R.J., Roberts, M.C., Holmes, K.K. (1989) Localized outbreak of Penicillinase-producing *Neisseria gonorrhoeae*. *JAMA* 261, 2357–2361.

Jones, J.L., Wykoff, R.F., Hollis, S.L., Longshore, S.T., Gamble, W.B., Gunn, R.A. (1990) Partner acceptance of health department notification of HIV exposure, South Carolina. *JAMA* 264, 1284–1286.

Judson, F.N. (1990) Partner notification for HIV control. *Hosp Pract* 12, 63–70,73.

Katz, B.P., Danos, C.S., Quinn, T.S., Caine, V., Jones R.B. (1988) Efficiency and cost-effectiveness of field follow-up for patients with *Chlamydia trachomatis* infection in a sexually transmitted diseases clinic. *Sex Transm Dis* 15, 11–16.

Landis, S., Schoenbach, V.J., Weber, D. *et al.* (1992) Results of a randomized trial of partner notification in cases of HIV infection in North Carolina. *N Engl J Med* 326, 101–106.

Martin, J.L. (1987) The impact of AIDS on gay male sexual behaviour patterns in New York City. *Am J Public Health* 77, 578–581.

Mills, A., Satin, A. (1978) Measuring the outcome of contact tracing. 2: The responsibilities of the health worker and the outcome of contact investigations. *Br J Vener Dis* **54**, 192–198.

Montesinos, L., Frisch, L.E., Greene, B.F., Hamilton, M. (1990) An analysis of and intervention in the sexual transmission of disease. *J Appl Behav Anal* **3**, 275–284.

Muspratt, B., Ponting, L. (1967) Improved methods of contact tracing. *Br J Vener Dis* **43**, 204–208.

Osborne J. (1988) Sounding Board. AIDS: Politics and science. *N Engl J Med* **318**, 444–447.

Potterat, J.J., Spencer, N.E., Woodhouse, D.E., Muth, J.B. (1989) Partner notification in the control of human Immunodeficiency virus infection. *Am J Public Health* **79**, 874–876.

Ramstedt, K., Hallhagen, G., Bygdeman, S. *et al.* (1985) Serologic classification and contact tracing in the control of microepidemics of Betalactamase-producing N.gonorrhoeae. *Sex Transm Dis* **12**, 209–214.

Ramstedt, K., Forssman, L., Johannisson, G. (1991) Contact tracing in the control of genital Chlamydia trachomatis infeciton. *Int J STD Aids* **2**, 116–118.

Rothenberg, R.B. (1983) The geography of gonorrhoea. Empirical demonstration of core group transmission. *Am J Epidemiol* **117**, 688–694.

Rutherford, G.W., Woo, J.M. (1988) Contact tracing and the control of human immunodeficiency virus infection. *JAMA* **259**, 3609–3610.

Satin, A. (1977) A record system for contact tracing. *Br J Vener Dis* **53**, 84–87.

Satin, A., Mills, A. (1978) Measuring the outcome of contact tracing. 1: A description of the patient and contact populations studied. *Br J Vener Dis* **54**, 187–191.

Toomey, K.E., Cates, W. (1989) Partner notification for the prevention of HIV infection. *AIDS* **3** (suppl 1), S57–S62.

Wigfield, A.S. (1972) 27 years of uninterrupted contact tracing: The "Tyneside Scheme". *Br J Vener Dis* **48**, 37–50.

Winfield, J., Latif, A.S. (1985) Tracing contacts of persons with sexually transmitted diseases in a developing country. *Sex Transm Dis* **12**, 5–7.

World Health Organization. Report of the consultation on partner notification for preventing HIV transmission. Geneva 11–13 January 1989. WHO/GPA/ESR/89.2.

Wykoff, R., Heath, C., Hollis, S., Leonard, S., Quiller, C., Jones, J., Artzrouni, M., Parker, R. (1988) Contact tracing to identify human immunodeficiency virus infection in a rural community. *JAMA* **259**, 3563–3566.

Zenilman, J.M., Bonner, M., Sharp, K.L., Rabb, J.A., Alexander, E.R. (1988) Penicillinase-producing *Neisseria gonorrhoeae* in Dade county, Florida: Evidence of core-group transmitters and the impact of illicit antibiotics. *Sex Transm Dis* **15**, 45–50.

Index